HAUSER, P.   0010962.

This book is to be returned on or before
the last date stamped below.

10. SEP. 1999

Thyroid Diseases of Infancy and Childhood

Effects on Behavior and Intellectual Development

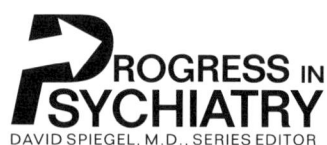

PROGRESS IN PSYCHIATRY
DAVID SPIEGEL, M.D., SERIES EDITOR

Thyroid Diseases of Infancy and Childhood

Effects on Behavior and Intellectual Development

Edited by
Peter Hauser, M.D., and
Joanne Rovet, Ph.D.

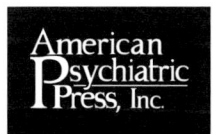

Washington, DC
London, England

Note: The authors have worked to ensure that all information in this book concerning drug dosages, schedules, and routes of administration is accurate as of the time of publication and consistent with standards set by the U.S. Food and Drug Administration and the general medical community. As medical research and practice advance, however, therapeutic standards may change. For this reason and because human and mechanical errors sometimes occur, we recommend that readers follow the advice of a physician who is directly involved in their care or in the care of a member of their family.

Books published by the American Psychiatric Press, Inc., represent the views and opinions of the individual authors and do not necessarily represent the policies and opinions of the Press or the American Psychiatric Association.

Copyright © 1999 American Psychiatric Press, Inc.
ALL RIGHTS RESERVED
Manufactured in the United States of America on acid-free paper
First Edition
01 00 99 98   4 3 2 1

American Psychiatric Press, Inc.
1400 K Street, N.W.
Washington, DC 20005
www.appi.org

Library of Congress Cataloging-in-Publication Data
Thyroid diseases of infancy and childhood: effects on behavior and intellectual development / edited by Peter Hauser and Joanne Rovet. — 1st ed.
     p.   cm.
  (Progress in psychiatry series; no. 57)
  Includes bibliographical references and index.
  ISBN 0-88048-767-4 (alk. paper)
  1. Behavior disorders in children—Etiology. 2. Cognition disorders in children—Etiology. 3. Thyroid gland—Diseases—Psychological aspects.   I. Hauser, Peter, 1955- . II. Series.
  [DNLM: 1. Thyroid Diseases—in infancy & childhood. 2. Thyroid Diseases—complications. 3. Thyroid Hormones—physiology. 4. Child Behavior Disorders. 5. Cognition.   W1PR6781L no.57 1998]
  RJ506.B44T48 1998
  618.92—44—dc21
  DNLM/DLC   98-26778
  for Library of Congress   CIP

British Library Cataloguing in Publication Data
A CIP record is available from the British Library.

P.H.—To Jirina and Susi Hauser, Susi Hauser-Devrient,
David Korn, Cathy Ostroski, and my friends
J.R.—To Ernest, Benjamin, Heather, and Jennifer,
and to Janie Rigler
Both—To Audrey McMahon and her family

Contents

Contributors ix

Introduction to the Progress in Psychiatry Series xi
David Spiegel, M.D.

Introduction xiii
Peter Hauser, M.D., and Joanne Rovet, Ph.D.

Part I
Thyroid Hormone Physiology and Function

1   Overview of Thyroid Disease in
    Pregnancy and Childhood 3
    Robert W. Lash, M.D.

2   Thyroid Hormone and Development:
    Brain and Peripheral Tissues 29
    Christoph A. Meier, M.D.

Part II
Clinical Studies of Thyroid Diseases in Infancy and Childhood

3   Overview of Newborn Screening for
    Congenital Hypothyroidism 59
    Kenneth Pass, Ph.D.

4   Behavioral and Cognitive Abnormalities
    Associated With Congenital Hypothyroidism 85
    Joanne Rovet, Ph.D.

5	Resistance to Thyroid Hormone: Implications for Child Psychiatric Research 127
	Peter Hauser, M.D.
6	Behavioral and Cognitive Abnormalities Associated With Juvenile Acquired Hypothyroidism 163
	Joanne Rovet, Ph.D., and Denis Daneman, M.D.
7	Behavioral and Cognitive Abnormalities Associated With Pediatric Thyrotoxicosis 187
	Vinod S. Bhatara, M.D., M.S., and J. Michael McMillin, M.D., F.A.C.P.
8	Neurodevelopmental Changes Associated With Thyroid-Disrupting Contaminants 221
	Vinod S. Bhatara, M.D., M.S., J. Michael McMillin, M.D., F.A.C.P., and Peter Hauser, M.D.
	Conclusions 285
	Peter Hauser, M.D., and Joanne Rovet, Ph.D.
	Index 295

Contributors

Vinod S. Bhatara, M.D., M.S.
Co-Director of Child Psychiatry Division, Director of Research (Child Psychiatry), and Associate Professor of Psychiatry (Child Psychiatry), Department of Psychiatry, University of South Dakota School of Medicine, Sioux Falls, South Dakota

Denis Daneman, M.D.
Department of Psychiatry, Hospital for Sick Children, University of Toronto, Toronto, Ontario, Canada

Peter Hauser, M.D.
Professor of Psychiatry and Internal Medicine (Endocrinology), University of Maryland School of Medicine; Chief of Psychiatry, Psychiatry Service, Veterans Administration Medical Center, Baltimore, Maryland

Robert W. Lash, M.D.
Assistant Professor of Medicine, University of Michigan Medical Center, Ann Arbor, Michigan

J. Michael McMillin, M.D., F.A.C.P.
Professor of Internal Medicine (Endocrinology), University of South Dakota School of Medicine, Sioux Falls, South Dakota

Christoph A. Meier, M.D.
Endocrine Division, Massachusetts General Hospital, Boston, Massachusetts

Kenneth Pass, Ph.D.
Director, Laboratory of Newborn Screening and Genetic Services, Wadsworth Center for Laboratories and Research, New York State Department of Health, Albany, New York

Joanne Rovet, Ph.D.
Departments of Pediatrics (Endocrinology) and Psychiatry,
University of Toronto, Toronto, Ontario, Canada

Introduction to the Progress in Psychiatry Series

The Progress in Psychiatry Series is designed to capture in print the excitement that comes from assembling a diverse group of experts from various locations to examine in detail the newest information about a developing aspect of psychiatry. This series emerged as a collaboration between the American Psychiatric Association's (APA) Scientific Program Committee and the American Psychiatric Press, Inc. Great interest is generated by a number of the symposia presented each year at the APA annual meeting, and we realized that much of the information presented there, carefully assembled by people who are deeply immersed in a given area, would unfortunately not appear together in print. The symposia sessions at the annual meetings provide an unusual opportunity for experts who otherwise might not meet on the same platform to share their diverse viewpoints for a period of 3 hours. Some new themes are repeatedly reinforced and gain credence, whereas in other instances disagreements emerge, enabling the audience and now the reader to reach informed decisions about new directions in the field. The Progress in Psychiatry Series allows us to publish and capture some of the best of the symposia and thus provide an in-depth treatment of specific areas that might not otherwise be presented in broader review formats.

Psychiatry is, by nature, an interface discipline, combining the study of mind and brain, of individual and social environments, of the humane and the scientific. Therefore, progress in the field is rarely linear—it often comes from unexpected sources. Furthermore, new developments emerge from an array of viewpoints that do not necessarily provide immediate agreement but rather expert examination of the issues. We intend to present innovative ideas and data that will enable you, the reader, to participate in this process.

We believe the Progress in Psychiatry Series will provide you with an opportunity to review timely, new information in specific fields of interest as they are developing. We hope you find that the excitement of the presentations is captured in the written word and that this book proves to be informative and enjoyable reading.

David Spiegel, M.D.
Series Editor
Progress in Psychiatry Series

Introduction

The study of neuroendocrinology has long been at the forefront of psychiatric research and has served to bridge the gap between brain and behavior. Abnormalities of various hormones have been implicated in the pathophysiological processes underlying the symptom picture of certain psychiatric disorders. The focus of this research has been on the immediate hormonal changes associated with the onset of adult psychiatric disorders in order to establish specific diagnostic indicators or to improve treatment. The role of hormones in the etiology of childhood psychiatric disorders has been far less actively studied. In thyroid diseases, behavioral and cognitive symptomatology have been recognized as cardinal manifestations as early as the late 1700s. Although it was originally believed that certain thyroid diseases were precipitated by extreme stress or psychic trauma, a syndrome of specific endocrine origin was not distinguished from the psychiatric group of illnesses until the late 19th century. With the obvious exception of untreated congenital hypothyroidism, the role of thyroid hormone in the etiology of childhood psychiatric disorders has received far less attention until recently.

The effects of thyroid hormone on early brain growth and development and later cognitive functioning are well characterized and suggest that thyroid hormone and the thyroid hormone receptor are essential to normal behavioral and intellectual development. There is a growing body of literature that suggests that, in humans, disturbances of the thyroid system adversely affect neurodevelopment. Although outcome in children with congenital hypothyroidism is markedly improved by newborn screening and prompt treatment, the long-term effects of thyroid deficiency and replacement therapy have only recently been studied. Despite early replacement therapy, children with congenital hypothyroidism have lower IQs, nonverbal learning disabilities, and attentional and school problems. Like congenital hypothyroidism, resistance to thyroid hormone—an autosomal dominant disease caused by mutations in the thyroid hormone receptor gene on chromosome 3—is also associated with lowered IQs (but not mental retardation) and school problems, as well as attention-deficit/hyperactivity disorder and language disorders. Similar abnormalities have been described in hypothyroidism and hyperthyroidism acquired during childhood or adolescence. These findings suggest that perturbations of thyroid homeostasis during critical periods of neurodevelopment may be of etiologic significance for certain childhood behavioral disorders. Therefore, elucidating the role of thyroid hormone in these disorders holds the promise of contributing greatly to our understanding of the underlying pathophysiologic mechanisms.

This book consolidates the research studies of the behavioral consequences associated with congenital and acquired thyroid diseases and also introduces more recent studies relating to the neurodevelopmental toxicity caused by exposure to synthetic chemicals that disrupt the thyroid hormone system. This book does not review the thyroid state of children with psychiatric disorders (although it does include suggestions for areas of study of these disorders based on the behavioral findings associated with thyroid diseases). It has been written to give the reader a basic understanding of congenital and childhood thyroid diseases and their behavioral manifestations. It is primarily a compilation of the contributors' most recent findings in this field and, as such, is not meant as a comprehensive survey.

The book is divided into two parts. Part I, Thyroid Hormone Physiology and Function, reviews the mechanisms of thyroid hormone action at molecular genetic and physiologic levels, with a particular focus on selected aspects related to the developing brain and central nervous system. In Part II, Clinical Studies of Thyroid Diseases in Infancy and Childhood, research studies pertaining to the relationship between thyroid diseases and abnormalities of behavioral, brain, and intellectual development are reviewed with an emphasis on the original research conducted by the particular chapter authors.

Part I, which consists of two chapters, provides the reader with a foundation for the subsequent clinical chapters. In Chapter 1, Dr. Lash reviews the thyroid axis and thyroid hormone physiology and discusses the clinical and laboratory tests used to diagnose fetal, neonatal, and childhood thyroid diseases. Chapter 2, by Dr. Meier, concisely summarizes the research studies that have elucidated the molecular mechanisms of thyroid hormone action with an emphasis on the regulation, by thyroid hormone, of genes necessary for neurodevelopment.

Part II reviews clinical aspects of thyroid diseases of infancy and childhood. In Chapter 3, the first of the clinical chapters in Part II, Dr. Pass reviews the history and rationale for newborn screening, with a focus on newborn screening for congenital hypothyroidism. He then presents preliminary data on a newborn screening study of subjects with resistance to thyroid hormone, who are at high risk for developing attention-deficit/hyperactivity disorder (ADHD). This study suggests that it is feasible to identify individuals at birth who have gene mutations associated with behavioral disorders, particularly if these mutations are associated with obvious hormonal or biochemical abnormalities. This is important for the study of childhood psychiatric disorders, because the lack of clear biological or genetic markers has prevented the performance of prospective studies of infants at risk for these disorders. Identification of newborns at risk for particular psychiatric disorders permits prospective assessment and evaluation and also provides a description of the early manifestations and consequences of these disorders. Predictors of these disorders in infancy and childhood can then be determined.

Chapter 4, by Dr. Rovet, and Chapter 5, by Dr. Hauser, present the most recent behavioral studies found in two congenital thyroid diseases, congenital hypothyroidism and resistance to thyroid hormone. These two diseases represent complementary models to study the effects of in utero thyroid abnormalities on neurodevelopment. In congenital hypothyroidism, the thyroid receptor is intact but there is an absence of the ligand, thyroid hormone, that activates the receptor. In resistance to thyroid hormone, there is an excess of thyroid hormone, but it cannot be optimally utilized because the mutant thyroid receptor protein has a decreased affinity for thyroid hormone. The congenital hypothyroidism model allows us to study the effects of fetal and early postnatal absence of thyroid hormone on behavioral, brain, and cognitive development, whereas the resistance to thyroid hormone model allows us to study the effects on neurodevelopment of a defective thyroid receptor and resultant inability to utilize circulating thyroid hormone adequately.

Chapters 6 and 7 describe acquired thyroid diseases of childhood. Chapter 6, by Drs. Rovet and Daneman, is a concise review of juvenile acquired hypothyroidism; Chapter 7, by Drs. Bhatara and McMillin, examines the cognitive and behavioral manifestations of hyperthyroidism. Both chapters are based on case studies in the literature and the experiences of the authors. They are of interest to mental health clinicians because they describe disorders that must be ruled out before the diagnosis of a childhood psychiatric disorder is confirmed.

Chapter 8, the final chapter, by Drs. Bhatara, McMillin, and Hauser, discusses an issue of increasing concern and controversy for clinicians and parents: the role of environmental toxicants—in particular, dioxin-like compounds—on the behavior and welfare of our children. There is increasing evidence that exposure during the perinatal period to certain synthetic compounds, including dioxins and polychlorinated biphenyls (PCBs), can lead to impaired learning, memory, and attentional processes in the offspring. Recent animal and human studies suggest that exposure to these environmental toxicants impairs normal thyroid function. Although the precise mechanism of action of these toxicants on neurodevelopment has not yet been elucidated, it is possible that they are partially or predominantly mediated by alterations of the thyroid axis. This chapter describes the convergence of studies that examine the neurodevelopmental consequences of moderate impairment of thyroid function with studies that demonstrate the adverse behavioral and cognitive effects of perinatal exposure to dioxins and PCBs. It provides new insights into the basic pathogenesis of developmental neurotoxicity following exposure to thyroid-disrupting synthetic compounds.

In conclusion, by examining the behavioral and intellectual consequences of thyroid diseases, it is possible to gain new insights into the underlying pathophysiologic mechanisms of various psychiatric disorders, including ADHD and learning disabilities. This ultimately promises to improve the quality of life for children with these disorders. It is the intent of this book to present a thorough review of fetal, neonatal, and childhood thyroid diseases and their behavioral, intellectual, and neurodevelopmental manifestations, which will serve as a reference for clinicians and researchers in the fields of endocrinology, mental health, neurology, neuroscience, and pediatrics. The authors also hope that this book will serve to generate new hypotheses about the role of thyroid hormone in neurodevelopment and childhood psychiatric illnesses that can be tested in a research setting. Further research ultimately promises to improve the quality of life for our children.

Acknowledgments: This book could not have been written without the contributions of Drs. Bhatara, Daneman, Lash, McMillin, Meier, and Pass. Their expertise and studies have contributed greatly to our understanding of thyroid hormone and neurodevelopment. We wish to thank the American Thyroid Association for their continuing support of our research. Dr. Hauser wishes to thank the University of Maryland School of Medicine and the Baltimore VA Medical Center for their generous support of his research efforts. Dr. Rovet wishes to thank the Research Institute of the Hospital for Sick Children, the Ontario Mental Health Foundation, the Medical Research Council of Canada, the Ontario Ministries of Health and of Community and Social Services, and Health and Welfare Canada. We also would like to thank Ms. Mary Beth Schultheis for her editorial assistance and the staff of the American Psychiatric Press.

Peter Hauser, M.D., and
Joanne Rovet, M.D.

Part I

Thyroid Hormone Physiology and Function

Chapter 1

Overview of Thyroid Disease in Pregnancy and Childhood

Robert W. Lash, M.D.

The Hypothalamic-Pituitary-Thyroid Axis

Thyroid hormone homeostasis is maintained by the interaction of hormones secreted by the hypothalamus, pituitary gland, and thyroid gland (Figure 1–1). At the "top" of this hypothalamic-pituitary-thyroid axis is the hypothalamus, which releases thyrotropin-releasing hormone (TRH) into a portal system connecting the hypothalamus and pituitary. TRH binds to specific receptors on thyrotropin-secreting cells (thyrotrophes) in the pituitary gland, stimulating the synthesis and secretion of thyrotropin, also called thyroid-stimulating hormone (TSH). TSH, in turn, is released into the systemic circulation, where it stimulates growth of the thyroid and the synthesis and release of thyroid hormone. The euthyroid state is maintained by the feedback effects of thyroid hormone on the hypothalamus and pituitary, where it reduces synthesis of TRH (Koller et al. 1987; Segerson et al. 1987) and TSH (Shupnik et al. 1985).

TRH is a modified peptide consisting of three amino acids: a pyroglutamyl residue, histidine, and a proline amide (Figure 1–2) (Boler et al. 1969; Burgus et al. 1969). It is initially synthesized as a prohormone that contains six copies of the TRH tripeptide (Yamada et al. 1990). Enzymatic processing of this prohormone releases the TRH tripeptides and modifies their glutamine and proline residues yielding active TRH molecules.

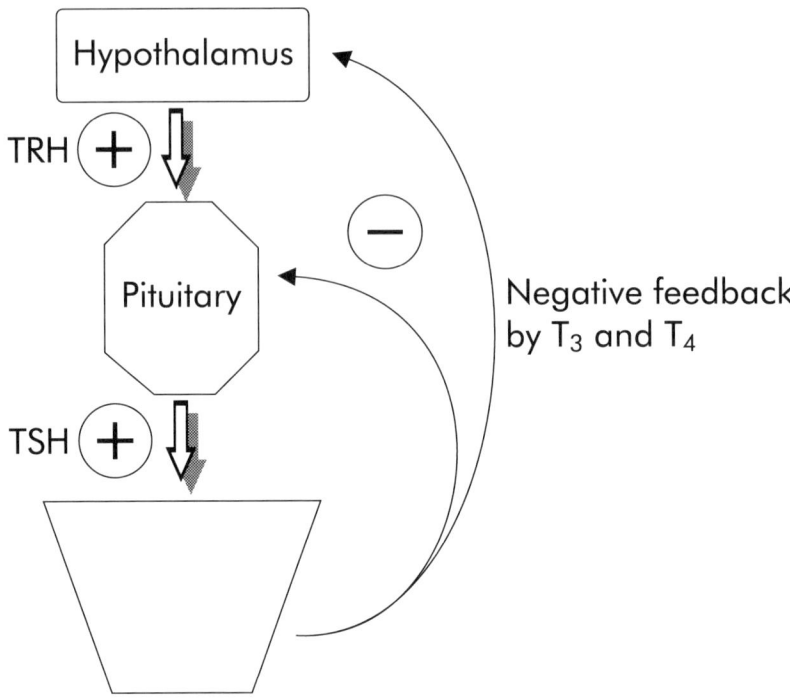

Figure 1–1. The hypothalamic-pituitary-thyroid axis. Thyrotropin-releasing hormone (TRH) is released by the hypothalamus, stimulating the synthesis and secretion of thyroid-stimulating hormone (TSH) by the pituitary. TSH, in turn, stimulates thyroid gland growth and the production of the thyroid hormones thyroxine (T_4) and triiodothyronine (T_3). Thyroid homeostasis is maintained through negative feedback on the hypothalamus and the pituitary by thyroid hormones, particularly T_3 (see text for details).

TSH, in contrast, is a much larger protein composed of non-covalently linked α and β subunits. The α subunit is 92 amino acids in length and is also present in each of the other glycoprotein hormones: luteinizing hormone (LH), follicle-stimulating hormone (FSH), and chorionic gonadotropin (CG). The β subunit of each of these hormones is unique and confers biological and immunological specificity (Pierce and Parsons 1981). The TSH-β subunit is composed of 112 amino acids.

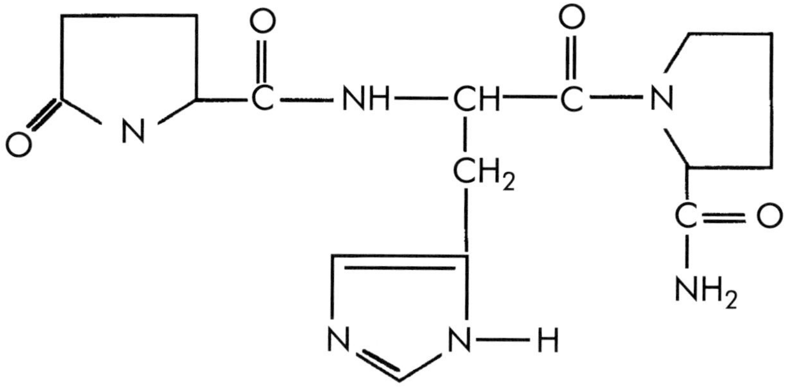

Figure 1–2. Chemical structure of the thyrotropin-releasing hormone (TRH) tripeptide.

The genes for the α and β subunits of TSH are present on chromosomes 6 and 1, respectively (Dracopoli et al. 1986; Fiddes and Goodman 1979) and are regulated by a variety of intracellular messengers. Thyroid hormone reduces the transcription of both genes but has a much greater effect on the β subunit gene (Shupnik et al. 1985). The mechanisms by which thyroid hormone negatively regulates the expression of the TSH-α and β subunit genes remain poorly understood. It was originally proposed that a complex of triiodothyronine and its receptor "got in the way" of the protein complex that starts gene transcription. However, more recent studies suggest that this process may have additional levels of complexity (Carr et al. 1992).

The TSH molecule is the major regulator of thyroid gland function, activating both the cyclic adenosine monophosphate (cAMP) and phosphoinositol signal transduction pathways in thyroid cells (Laurent et al. 1987). Other molecules, such as adenosine triphosphate (ATP) and catecholamines, also play a role in modulating thyroid physiology (Raspé and Dumont 1992). However, TSH is necessary for normal thyroid function, including the synthesis of thyroid hormone.

TSH stimulates each of the major steps in thyroid hormone synthesis as outlined in Figure 1–3. Thyroid hormone synthesis begins with the active transport of iodide molecules against a large concentration gradient into thyroid follicular cells (thyrocytes). These iodide molecules are rapidly oxidized by the enzyme thyroid peroxidase and are covalently linked to tyrosine residues present on the protein thyroglobulin on the apical side of the thyrocyte. Thyroglobulin is a large protein (660 kd) with multiple tyrosine residues, many (but not all) of which can be iodinated (reviewed in Dunn 1996). Tyrosine residues can bind either one iodide, yielding monoiodotyrosine (MIT), or two iodides to give diiodotyrosine (DIT). These MITs and DITs, in turn, are oxidatively coupled to one another, yielding triiodothyronine (T_3) or thyroxine (T_4) bound to thyroglobulin.

Iodinated thyroglobulin is stored as colloid within the lumen of the follicular cells. This colloid serves as a large reservoir of thyroid hormone. Thus, the inhibition of thyroid hormone synthesis by drugs such as the thionamides has little immediate effect on thyroid hormone levels, unless thyroid hormone release is also blocked. The final step in thyroid hormone synthesis is the reuptake of iodinated thyroglobulin into thyrocytes, where it is hydrolyzed, releasing T_4 and T_3. These thyroid hormones are then transported across the basal membrane of the thyrocyte and into the systemic circulation.

T_4 is the predominant form of thyroid hormone synthesized and released by the thyroid gland. Although the thyroid gland also synthesizes small amounts of T_3, most is derived from the deiodination of T_4. There are two major 5'-deiodinases: Type I 5'-deiodinase is present in a variety of tissues but is most abundant in liver and kidney. Type II 5'-deiodinase is present in the brain (including the pituitary gland), where it produces T_3 from T_4 for use within the central nervous system. T_4 can also undergo deiodination to become reverse T_3 (rT_3). Reverse T_3 does not bind to the thyroid hormone receptor, and its function is unknown. However, it is found in elevated concentrations during fetal development.

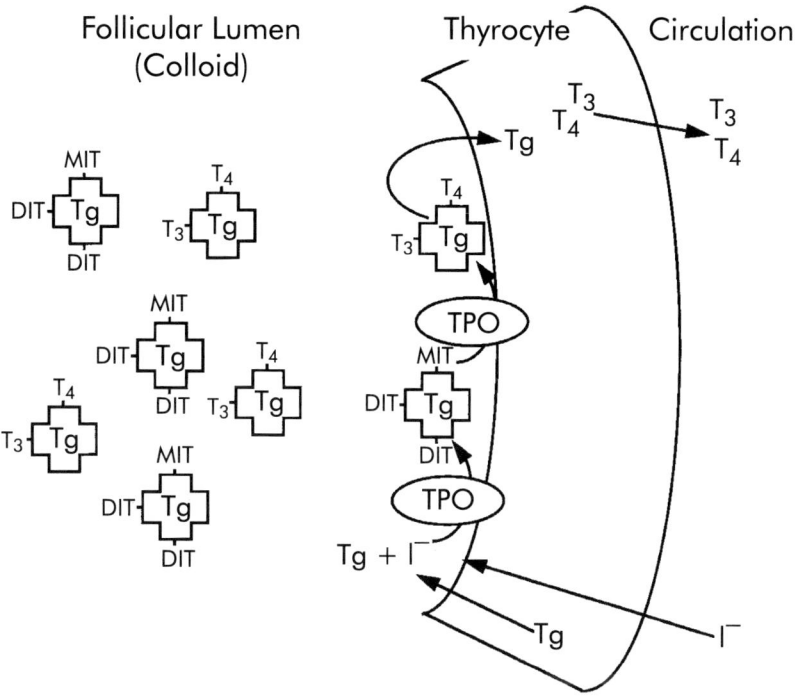

Figure 1–3. Schematic diagram showing the major steps in thyroid hormone synthesis. Iodine (I) is pumped against a concentration gradient into the thyroid cell (thyrocyte). It then undergoes oxidation by thyroid peroxidase (TPO) and becomes covalently bound to one of multiple thyroid residues on the thyroglobulin (Tg) molecule. These monoiodotyrosine (MIT) and diiodotyrosine (DIT) residues on the Tg molecule then couple to each other to form thyroxine (T_4) and triiodothyronine (T_3). This reservoir of thyroid hormone is stored in the follicular lumen until it is taken up by the thyrocyte, cleaved from Tg, and released into the circulation (see text for details).

T_4 circulates in higher concentrations (10,000 ng/dL) than T_3 (150 ng/dL) and has a longer half-life (7 days versus 18 hours). More than 99.5% of both T_4 and T_3 circulates as protein-bound molecules. About 70% of circulating thyroid hormones are bound to thyroxine-binding globulin (TBG), with thyroxine-binding pre-

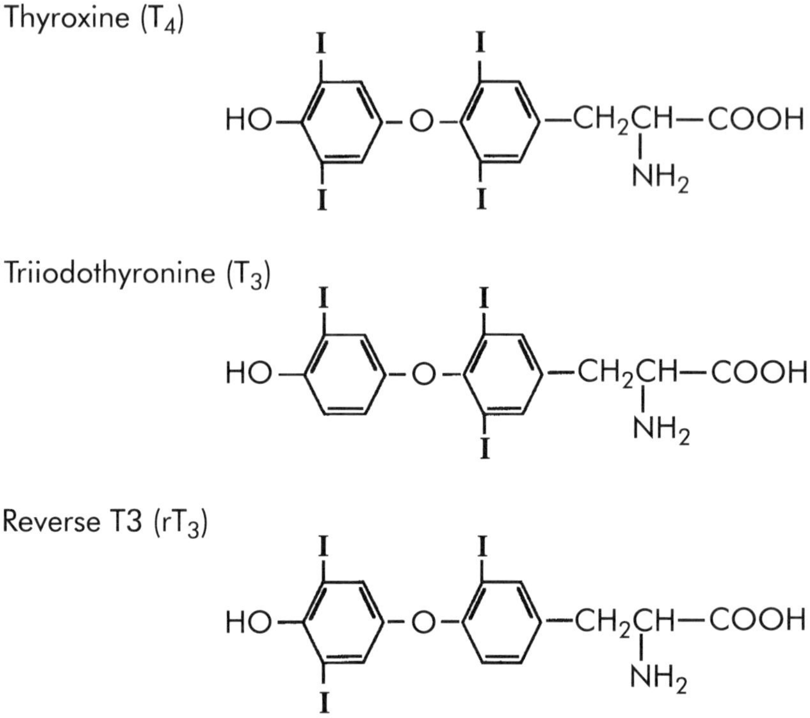

Thyroxine (T$_4$)

Triiodothyronine (T$_3$)

Reverse T3 (rT$_3$)

Figure 1–4. Chemical structures of thyroxine (T$_4$), triiodothyronine (T$_3$), and reverse T$_3$ (rT$_3$).

albumin (TBPA or transthyretin) and albumin each carrying about 15%. Because only the free forms of T$_4$ and T$_3$ are biologically available, the protein-bound portion can be considered a reservoir of thyroid hormone that can be released as needed to maintain thyroid hormone homeostasis.

The biologically active form of thyroid hormone is T$_3$, which binds to the thyroid hormone receptor with far greater affinity than does T$_4$. As opposed to the receptors for TRH and TSH, which lie on cell surfaces, the thyroid hormone receptor is intracellular, exerting its effects directly on gene transcription (Sap et al. 1986; Weinberger et al. 1986). To reach its receptor, the T$_3$ molecule must therefore cross the cell membrane. Although some T$_4$ may enter cells and subsequently be converted to T$_3$, it appears that circulating T_3 is the predominant source of intracellular T_3 outside the central nervous system. As discussed above, within the brain and pituitary gland, T_3 is derived from the intracellular conversion of T_4 to T_3 by type II 5'-deiodinase.

Fetal Thyroid Function in Utero

The embryological precursor of the fetal thyroid is present by 4 weeks of embryonic development. The fetal thyroid is a central structure that starts as an outpouching from the base of the pharynx and moves caudally along what will become the thyroglossal duct. After the fetal thyroid tissue completes its migration from the pharynx to the base of the neck, the thyroglossal duct dissolves. This primitive thyroid is capable of thyroglobulin synthesis, but its ability to organify iodine and synthesize iodotyrosines does not develop until about 10–12 weeks' gestation (Shepard 1967). TSH is also first detected at about 10 weeks (Fisher and Klein 1981). The absence of TSH during early thyroid development indicates that TSH is not necessary for organogenesis. However, the temporal relationship between the presence of TSH and the onset of iodine organification and thyroid hormone synthesis strongly suggests that thyroid *function* is dependent on the action of TSH. Fetal TSH levels rise steadily through at least the second trimester, reaching a peak of about 15 µU/mL (Fisher and Polk 1989; Thorpe-Beeston et al. 1992). Fetal levels of thyroid hormone also rise throughout pregnancy, reflecting both the maturation of the hypothalamic-pituitary-thyroid axis and increasing levels of thyroid hormone–binding proteins.

The role of maternal thyroid hormones in fetal development remains controversial (Porterfield and Hendrich 1993). Earlier studies suggested that only small amounts of maternal thyroid cross the placenta (Roti et al. 1983). However, studies examining thyroid hormone levels in newborns with thyroid agenesis or organification defects have indicated that some maternal thyroid hormone does cross the placenta (Vulsma et al. 1989). These infants, who were incapable of any endogenous thyroid hormone production, had T_4 levels approximately 40% of normal. Thus, maternal thyroid may be of some importance in fetal development.

Thyroid hormone receptors are present in fetal brain during the first trimester, several weeks before fetal thyroid function begins (Bernal and Pekonen 1984; Porterfield and Hendrich 1993). It is possible that these receptors are binding other ligands or are simply "waiting" for fetal thyroid to appear. However, there is evidence (mostly from nonhuman models) that thyroid hormone, presumably from the maternal circulation, is important in early development of the central nervous system (CNS). The presence of maternal thyroid hormone in the developing fetal brain may also play an important role in the success of early thyroid replacement in infants with congenital hypothyroidism. These hypothyroid infants may receive sufficient exogenous thyroid hormone for CNS development from maternal sources during gestation and from thyroid hormone therapy postpartum.

Thyroid Function at Birth

Just before birth, TSH concentration is about 10–15 µU/mL. However, at birth, TSH levels rise dramatically, sometimes reaching 70 µU/mL (Fisher and Odell 1969). This increase in TSH is thought to be the result of "cold shock" as the fetus emerges from the warm uterine environment. The normal postpartum increase in TSH is followed by rises in T_4 and free T_4 (Figure 1–5). The final maturation of the hypothalamic-pituitary-thyroid axis appears to be a late event in fetal development. Premature infants have a smaller postpartum rise in TSH (and consequently lower thyroid hormone levels) than do term infants. These relatively lower rates of increase may persist for weeks (Fisher and Klein 1981; Thorpe-Beeston et al. 1992).

T_3 metabolism is somewhat more complicated. In the prenatal state, levels of reverse T_3 exceed those of T_3. Postpartum, 5'-deiodinase activity increases, resulting in both the increased formation of T_3 from T_4 and the increased deiodination of reverse T_3. The result is an increase in T_3 concentration postpartum, accompa-

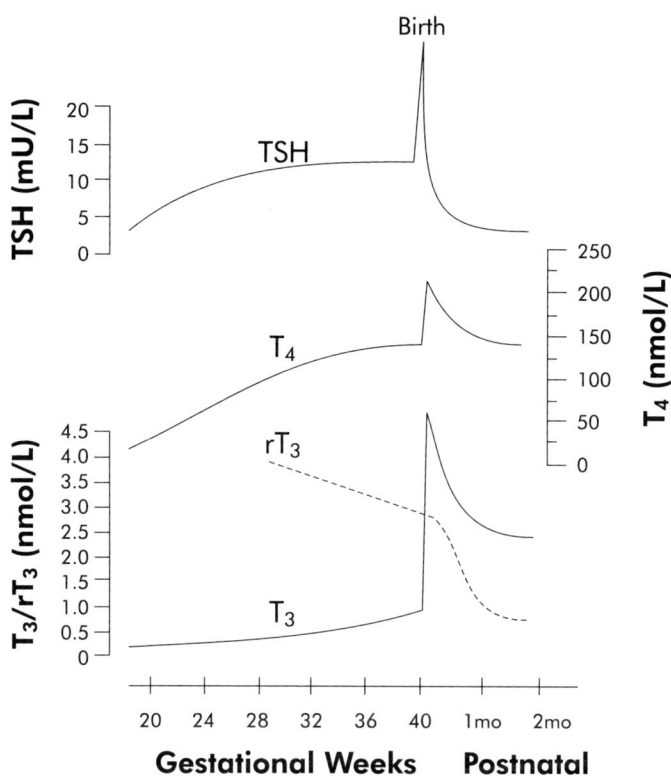

Figure 1–5. Fetal and neonatal thyroid development.
Top panel. Thyroid-stimulating hormone (TSH) levels rise throughout the second and third trimesters of pregnancy. There is a sharp rise in TSH levels within minutes of birth (see text), with a rapid return to normal neonatal levels. **Bottom panel.** Thyroxine (T_4) levels, paralleling those of TSH, rise steadily throughout the second and third trimesters, due both to the action of TSH and to increasing levels of thyroid hormone binding proteins. During fetal development, the concentrations of reverse triiodothyronine (rT_3) exceed those of T_3. However, after birth, T_3 levels rise dramatically, with a fall in reverse T_3. This is most likely due to the increase in 5'-deiodinase activity, which deiodinates T_4 to give T_3, as well as metabolizing reverse T_3.
Source. Reprinted from Fisher DA, Polk DR: "Thyroid Disease in the Fetus, Neonate, and Child," in *Endocrinology*, 3rd Edition, Vol 1. Edited by DeGroot LJ, Besser M, Burger HG, et al. Philadelphia, PA, WB Saunders, 1995, p. 784. Used with permission.

nied by a decrease in the reverse T_3 level. Postpartum levels of both T_4 and T_3 are typically higher than levels in adults (see Figure 1–5), and thyroid hormone requirements in hypothyroid neonates are substantially higher than in adults on a micrograms per kilogram basis (discussed below). These findings suggest that thyroid hormone metabolism is also higher in the postpartum period.

Thyroid Function Testing

Using a variety of immunoassay techniques, the concentrations of thyroid hormones (both bound and free), TSH, and thyroid-binding proteins can be measured. The ease and accuracy of these tests have made it possible to implement widespread screening programs to identify infants with congenital hypothyroidism. In addition to measuring hormone levels, one can identify a number of antithyroid antibodies, including antibodies that activate the TSH receptor in Graves' disease. These thyroid function tests—combined with imaging studies (ultrasound and thyroid scans), functional studies (thyroid uptake and biological indices of thyroid function), and fine-needle biopsies—enable clinicians to diagnose and thyroid disorders accurately and to treat them successfully.

Total and Free Thyroid Hormone Measurement

Total and free concentrations of T_4 and T_3 can be measured in serum, in amniotic fluid, and from blood samples obtained in utero from the umbilical vein (cordocentesis) (Hare and Ludomirsky 1994). As discussed above, more than 99.5% of T_4 and T_3 circulates bound to thyroid hormone–binding proteins. Thus, measurements of total T_4 and T_3 levels are affected by both the level of thyroid hormones and the amount of binding protein present. Measurements of free (unbound) thyroid hormone levels (e.g., free T_4), in contrast, are not affected by differences in binding proteins. Free thyroid hormone levels therefore provide a more clinically relevant measure of thyroid hormone levels, particularly during pregnancy. Several methods are available for measuring free thyroid hormone levels, with equilibrium dialysis remaining the "gold standard." However, it is an expensive and a somewhat cumbersome technique. Free thyroid hormone levels can also be determined indirectly by measuring the availability of thyroid hormone binding sites (e.g., using a T_3 resin uptake) and applying this value as a correction factor to the measured amount of total hormone. The resulting value is known as the *free thyroid index*. Automated methods for direct measurement of free thyroid hormone levels have recently been developed that are reliable and cost-effective. Most clinical laboratories rely on one of the latter two methods for the routine measurement of free thyroid hormone concentrations.

Measurement of Thyroid-Stimulating Hormone

The measurement of TSH remains the single best way to assess a patient's thyroid status. The TSH concentration responds to changes in levels of circulating thyroid hormone in a log-linear manner. Thus, even small changes in thyroid hormone levels can result in large fluctuations in TSH. As TSH assays have become more sensitive over the past 20 years, their clinical usefulness has also improved. Although today's TSH assays have normal values in the range of 0.5–5.0 mU/L, the first generation of TSH assays were unable to detect levels lower than 2.0 mU/L. With these earlier assays, it was possible to diagnose hypothyroidism on the basis of an elevated TSH concentration. However, the inability to obtain accurate measurements of TSH levels below 2.0 mU/L made it difficult to separate clinically euthyroid patients from those with mild thyrotoxicosis.

TSH assays in use today have much greater sensitivity—some as low as 0.005 mU/L. With these assays, TSH levels can now be used to identify groups of patients who were previously difficult to categorize, such as those with mild degrees of thyrotoxicosis or those being overreplaced with thyroxine. The newer assays also make it possible to adjust thyroxine replacement doses to fit specific clinical situations, such as suppressing TSH concentrations in patients with thyroid cancer without rendering them thyrotoxic.

Because these assays can identify almost all patients as hypothyroid, euthyroid, or thyrotoxic, TSH measurements can also be used to screen patients for thyroid disease in a cost-effective manner (Danese et al. 1996). Finally, the TSH assay is particularly useful during pregnancy, when estrogen-mediated increases in thyroxine-binding globulin often make measurements of total T_4 and T_3 difficult to interpret.

Neonatal Thyroid Screening

The incidence of congenital primary hypothyroidism is about 1 in 4,200 live births; the incidence of pituitary and hypothalamic hypothyroidism is about 1 in 68,200 (Fisher et al. 1979). Prior to the initiation of screening programs, the average IQ in this group of patients was below 80. Prospective studies have shown that the prompt diagnosis and treatment of congenital hypothyroidism generally results in normal mean IQ scores (Rovet et al. 1984) (Figure 1–6). These dramatic responses have led to the widespread implementation of neonatal screening programs (discussed in Chapter 3).

However, it is important to note that detailed studies by Rovet (Rovet et al. 1984, 1992) suggest that subtle developmental abnormalities persist despite early thyroid hormone replacement.

Infants who are identified as likely to be hypothyroid (TSH >40 mU/L) are given thyroxine replacement therapy pending the results of retesting. Infants with TSH levels between 20 and 40 mU/L are typically retested before therapy is initiated. It is worth noting that shorter lengths of stay for childbirth have resulted in earlier screening for hypothyroidism. Because the TSH levels are highest in the first 24 hours of life, there may be some increase in the number of infants misidentified as hypothyroid (on the basis of an elevated TSH value) on initial screening.

Other Measurements of Thyroid Function

Routine thyroid function testing assumes that the hypothalamic-pituitary portion of the thyroid axis is working properly.

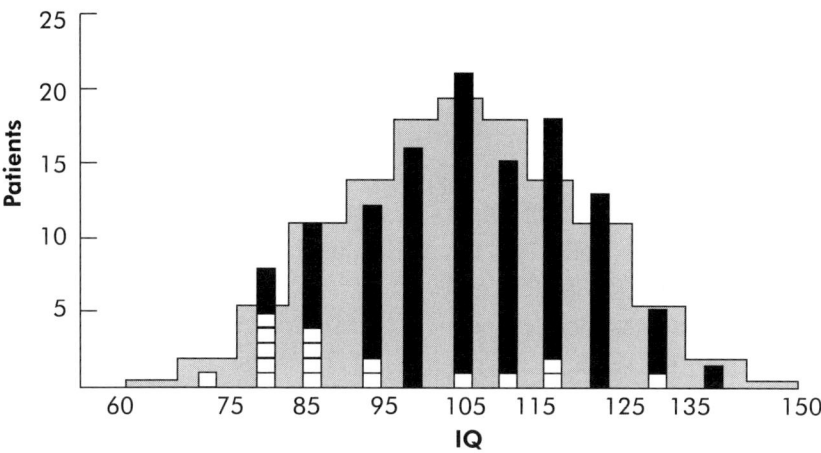

Figure 1–6. Effects of congenital hypothyroidism (with and without adequate thyroid hormone replacement) on Stanford-Binet IQ scores in 117 children with neonatal hypothyroidism. *Open squares* represent children who did not receive adequate thyroid hormone replacement, and *closed squares* indicate those who received full replacement. The normal distribution of IQ scores is shown in the shaded background.
Source. Reprinted from Klein RZ, Mitchell ML: "Hypothyroidism in Infants and Children," in *Werner and Ingbar's The Thyroid: A Fundamental and Clinical Text*, 7th Edition. Edited by Braverman LE, Utiger RD. Philadelphia, PA, Lippincott-Raven, 1996, p. 985. Used with permission.

However, there are several causes of pituitary (secondary) hypothyroidism, as well as hypothalamic (tertiary) hypothyroidism. In cases of pituitary hypothyroidism, such as panhypopituitarism, TSH levels are either low or inappropriately normal. Measuring only TSH in these patients would mistakenly lead to the diagnosis of thyrotoxicosis. However, if both TSH and free T_4 are measured, the diagnosis is easier to make. Hypothalamic hypothyroidism presents an additional level of complexity, because patients with this disorder may have significantly decreased levels of thyroid hormones with only a minimal elevation in TSH concentration. Interestingly, TSH bioactivity in these patients is low but increases after administration of TRH (Beck-Peccoz et al. 1985).

Nuclear Medicine Testing

Nuclear medicine testing in thyroid disease is useful for defining thyroid anatomy (e.g., are both lobes of the thyroid present?), assessing function (e.g., is a nodule hot or cold?), or quantifying thyroid activity (e.g., how much iodine is taken up by the thyroid in 24 hours?). Current techniques result in minimal radiation exposure (both whole body and thyroidal) and can be safely performed in both infants and children. Typically, ^{99}Tc is used to assess anatomy and the presence or absence of functioning tissue in a thyroid scan. Quantification of thyroid function is usually done with ^{131}I and is expressed as the percentages of an administered ^{131}I dose remaining in the thyroid after 4 and 24 hours. In some centers, both studies are done using a single dose of ^{123}I. However, ^{123}I is expensive and has a short half-life, making the combination of a ^{131}I uptake test and a ^{99}Tc scan a more cost-effective alternative. Theoretically, it is possible to perform a scan using ^{131}I. However, the amount of ^{131}I that must be administered to obtain quality images of the thyroid causes the thyroid gland to receive a significant radiation exposure.

Thyroid Abnormalities in Pregnancy

Primary Disorders of Fetal Thyroid Function

Most cases of primary fetal hypothyroidism can be divided into three major groups: iodine deficiency, thyroid dysgenesis or dysfunction, and hypothalamic-pituitary disorders. *Iodine deficiency* is by far the most common of these causes, and congenital hypothyroidism secondary to iodine deficiency (endemic goiter) remains a worldwide health problem (Delange 1996). In iodine-replete areas of the world, congenital hypothyroidism is most often due to *thyroid dysgenesis*. Thyroid dysgenesis may be complete (thyroid agenesis) or partial (lingual thyroid or thyroid hypoplasia). Fetal *thyroid dysfunction* may be due to synthetic defects, such as abnormal forms of thyroglobulin, or defects in the enzymatic pathways leading to thyroid hormone synthesis. There have also been reports of mutant forms of TSH that are biologically inactive

(Dacou-Voutetakis et al. 1990; Hayashizaki et al. 1990); researchers have also found resistance to TSH action resulting from defects in TSH-receptor signal transduction (Sunthornthepvarakui et al. 1995; Utiger 1995). A variety of hypothalamic and pituitary disorders have been associated with congenital hypothyroidism due to deficiencies of TSH or TRH.

Disorders of Fetal Thyroid Function Secondary to Maternal Thyroid Abnormalities

As discussed above, maternal thyroid hormones may play a role in early brain development. However, their effect on subsequent fetal development appears to be limited. Because only small amounts of thyroid hormone cross the placenta, abnormal levels of maternal thyroid hormones rarely alter fetal thyroid homeostasis. However, some causes of maternal thyroid dysfunction may also result in either hypothyroidism or thyrotoxicosis in the fetus. These include drugs (e.g., thionamides), antibodies (stimulating and/or blocking), and radioactive iodine.

Fetal *hypothyroidism* secondary to maternal thyroid disease is most often due to thionamide therapy, radioactive iodine treatment, or antibodies blocking the TSH receptor. Thionamide therapy with either propylthiouracil (PTU) or methimazole has been successfully used for many years in the treatment of maternal Graves' disease during pregnancy. Although PTU is used more frequently in the United States, there are no convincing data to support the superiority of one thionamide over another in the treatment of maternal Graves' disease. It is frequently noted that PTU, but not methimazole, blocks the peripheral conversion of T_4 to T_3. However, this effect is rarely of clinical significance and occurs only with higher doses of PTU (Saberi et al. 1975).

Methimazole has been implicated as a cause of aplasia cutis (circumscribed areas of hair loss on the scalp) in newborns, but this association may be spurious (Van Dijke et al. 1987; Mandel et al. 1994). Because thionamides cross the placenta, thionamide therapy can result in both maternal and fetal hypothyroidism. Fortunately, the dosages of thionamides typically used in pregnancy (300–450 mg of PTU daily) are associated with transient neonatal hypothyroidism in only about 1% of women receiving thionamide treatment. An even more rare complication of thionamide therapy is the development of a fetal goiter.

Neonatal hypothyroidism may also be caused by maternal antibodies that bind to, and block, both the maternal and fetal TSH receptors. Patients with these blocking antibodies typically have hypothyroidism with a small thyroid gland (nongoitrous myxedema). However, in some patients, both stimulating and blocking antibodies are present, complicating the clinical picture for both mother and fetus (Zakarija et al. 1986). Finally, administration of radioactive iodine therapy to a pregnant woman can result in fetal thyroid ablation, with subsequent hypothyroidism. This complication occurs only if functioning fetal thyroid tissue is present at the time the radioactive iodine is administered.

Neonatal *thyrotoxicosis* is usually the result of maternal Graves' disease. In this disorder, maternal TSH receptor–stimulating antibodies (also known as thyroid-stimulating immunoglobulins, or TSI) cross the placenta, resulting in fetal hyperthyroidism. It is important to note that the antibodies that cause Graves' disease may persist long after the disease has been successfully treated in the mother. Although these antibodies may no longer cause maternal thyrotoxicosis, they can result in fetal hyperthyroidism. TSI levels should therefore be measured in all pregnant patients with current or prior Graves' disease. Patients with levels of TSI greater than 5 times normal should have their pregnancies closely monitored for fetal hyperthyroidism (Tamaki et al. 1988). Fetal thyrotoxicosis typically presents with fetal tachycardia or an estimated fetal weight lower than expected. In cases of suspected fetal thyrotoxicosis, the mother should be given low doses of thionamides, which will cross the placenta and reduce the synthesis of fetal thyroid hormones.

Thyroid Disease in the Neonate and Child

Neonatal Thyroid Disease

Most cases of *congenital hypothyroidism* are not apparent on initial clinical evaluation and are instead identified by neonatal screening. Profoundly hypothyroid newborns may have prolonged gestation and macrosomia. Jaundice is frequently present and may take days to resolve. Other physical findings include abdominal distention, an umbilical hernia, and a large posterior fontanel. Once a child is diagnosed with congenital hypothyroidism, prompt initiation of therapy is critical. Delays of as little as 6 weeks may compromise intellectual development, although most children treated within 3 months of birth have normal or near-normal intelligence.

Treatment of congenital hypothyroidism consists of thyroxine replacement therapy. Newborns require much larger doses of thyroxine than adults (on a per-kilogram basis). The usual starting dosage in a newly diagnosed child is 50 µg per day. For a 4,000-g infant, 50 µg daily is 12.5 µg/kg. In contrast, a typical adult replacement dosage is 1.6 µg/kg. Hypothyroid newborns should be observed closely, and their dosage of thyroxine should be adjusted to keep the serum TSH level within the normal range. It is also important to follow the growth curves of these infants to ensure that they are having a clinical as well as a biochemical response to thyroxine replacement therapy.

Neonatal thyrotoxicosis is most frequently caused by the placental transfer of TSI from mother to child. As discussed above, clinical signs of *maternal* Graves' disease may or may not be present. Like congenital hypothyroidism, neonatal Graves' disease is uncommon, occurring in about 2% of women with active Graves' disease during their pregnancies. Infants with neonatal thyrotoxicosis typically have tachycardia, low birth weight, and marked irritability. They may also have microcephaly with ventricular enlargement on CNS imaging.

Antithyroid therapy may be needed for several weeks. Thionamides, β-blockers, nonradioactive iodine, and corticosteroids can all be used to treat this form of neonatal hyperthyroidism. Because neonatal Graves' disease is the result of maternal antibodies (which have a limited half-life in the neonate), the hyperthyroidism usually resolves during the first few months of life. Thus, the use of ablative doses of radioactive iodine is generally contraindicated.

There have been case reports of neonatal hyperthyroidism due to mutations that continuously activate the fetal TSH receptor (Van Sande et al. 1995). This disorder is analogous to activating mutations of the TSH receptor seen in some patients with autonomously functioning thyroid adenomas (Parma et al. 1993). Patients in the latter group develop a somatic mutation of the TSH receptor gene, leading to the development of a toxic adenoma; the rest of the gland remains normal. In contrast, this form of thyrotoxicosis in infants probably results from a mutation early in embryological development and may therefore affect the entire thyroid gland.

Acquired Thyroid Disease

Hypothyroidism. The differential diagnosis of hypothyroidism in infants and children is similar to that in adults. In iodine-deficient regions, endemic goiter remains the most common cause of hypothyroidism. In iodine-replete regions, the most common cause is autoimmune thyroid disease (Hashimoto's thyroiditis). Much less common are pituitary and hypothalamic causes. These include pituitary and hypothalamic tumors, congenital abnormalities of midline CNS structures, and genetic defects in pituitary function. There are also a variety of iatrogenic causes of hypothyroidism, including drugs (e.g., thionamides and lithium), thyroidectomy, and thyroid irradiation. Thyroid irradiation is typically due to external beam radiotherapy for malignancy but may also result from radioactive fallout (see below). Iatrogenic central hypothyroidism may result from the treatment of hypothalamic or pituitary disorders with surgery or irradiation.

During childhood, the clinical manifestations of hypothyroidism vary with age, and have been well described by Foley (1996). During the first 2–3 years of life, children with acquired hypothyroidism present with symptoms similar to those seen in infants with congenital hypothyroidism. The most obvious of these are slowing of linear growth and failure to reach developmental milestones. Hypothyroidism appearing later in childhood usually presents with a slowing of linear growth, poor school performance, and goiter. Rarely, affected children will have skeletal abnormalities (stippled epiphyses) or precocious puberty. The latter sign occurs only in primary hypothyroidism, and it has been postulated that it is due to stimulation of FSH receptors by high levels of TSH (Anasti et al. 1995). As children enter adolescence, the symptoms and signs of hypothyroidism are similar to those seen in adults.

Although newborns with congenital hypothyroidism are treated with relatively large doses of thyroxine (see above), children with acquired hypothyroidism can be treated with more conventional doses. As in adults, the goal of therapy is to keep the TSH within the normal range. TSH cannot be used to monitor therapy in patients with central hypothyroidism. This group of patients is best followed up with free T_4 and close monitoring of clinical status, including growth.

Thyrotoxicosis. The most common cause of thyrotoxicosis in children is Graves' disease, but even this occurs rarely, with less than 0.5% of children developing the disease. Thyrotoxicosis secondary to thyroiditis can also occur in children, but it is probably less common than Graves' disease. More exotic causes of thyrotoxicosis, such as McCune-Albright syndrome (Weinstein et al. 1991) and TSH-secreting pituitary tumors (Gesundheit et al. 1989), have also been reported.

The symptoms and signs of Graves' disease are similar in children and adults. Most children will present with tachycardia and anxiety and will have a goiter on physical examination. There may also be an acceleration in linear growth accompanied by an inappropriate advancement in bone age. As in adults, the diagnosis of thyrotoxicosis in children is based on elevated levels of thyroid hormones in the setting of suppressed TSH. The diagnosis of Graves' disease can be confirmed by measuring TSI or by demonstrating increased radioactive iodine uptake by the thyroid gland.

Children with Graves' disease are usually treated medically, with the hope that their disease will eventually remit. Radioactive iodine ablation and surgery are also therapeutic options but are less frequently used. Medical therapy is based on the use of thionamides and β-blockers. More than two-thirds of children treated with thionamides will have a therapeutic response. These patients usually continue medical therapy for a number of years, after which the thionamide therapy is slowly tapered. Remission rates vary substantially but are probably between one-third and one-half. Agranulocytosis can occur in patients receiving thionamides and must be ruled out during acute illnesses, particularly when patients have a fever or complain of a sore throat.

Other Forms of Childhood Thyroid Disease. Thyroid cancer does occur in the pediatric age group but is uncommon. A notable exception has been the unfortunate rise in the incidence of thyroid cancer among children exposed to radioactive fallout following the 1986 accident at the Chernobyl nuclear power plant in the former Soviet Union (Baverstock et al. 1992; Kazakov et al. 1992). As in adults, thyroid cancer in children typically presents as a solitary thyroid nodule or, less frequently, an enlarged cervical lymph node. Treatment of thyroid cancer is essentially the same in adults and children. However, many authors believe that thyroid cancer in children, even when widely metastatic, has a better prognosis than the adult form of the disease.

More than 100 families have now been reported with a variety of mutations of the thyroid hormone receptor that result in resistance to the action of thyroid hormone. This disorder, known as resistance to thyroid hormone (RTH), has widely varying clinical manifestations. A single patient may have signs of both hypothyroidism (such as short stature) and thyrotoxicosis (such as tachycardia). As discussed in subsequent chapters, attention-deficit/hyperactivity disorders are among the most common clinical manifestations associated with RTH (Hauser et al. 1993). Furthermore, mutations within specific regions of the thyroid hormone receptor appear to be associated with abnormalities of language development (Brucker-Davis et al. 1995). At present, there is no generally effective therapy for RTH. Some authors advocate treating patients with thyroid hormone while monitoring carefully for clinical thyrotoxicosis. However, most of the evidence supporting this approach is anecdotal.

Conclusion

Normal fetal development, particularly that of the central nervous system, depends on maintenance of the euthyroid state in utero. The role of maternal thyroid hormones in this process remains controversial, but they are probably important in CNS development during the first trimester. Mild abnormalities (either increases or decreases) in maternal thyroid hormone levels do not usually affect fetal thyroid homeostasis. However, the underlying causes of maternal thyroid dysfunction, such as TSI, may also affect fetal thyroid function. In addition, infants and children can develop a variety of thyroid disorders that result in both hypothyroidism and thyrotoxicosis.

Fortunately, thyroid dysfunction can be accurately diagnosed and successfully treated in infants and children. In some cases, it is also possible to diagnose and treat thyroid dysfunction in utero. In the case of congenital hypothyroidism, screening and treatment programs have been remarkably successful in preventing lifelong disabilities.

References

Anasti JN, Flack MR, Froehlich J, et al: A potential novel mechanism for precocious puberty in juvenile hypothyroidism. J Clin Endocrinol Metab 80:276–279, 1995

Baverstock K, Egloff B, Pinchera A, et al: Thyroid cancer after Chernobyl (letter). Nature 359:21–22, 1992

Beck-Peccoz P, Amr S, Menezes-Ferreira MM, et al: Decreased receptor binding of biologically inactive thyrotropin in central hypothyroidism: effect of treatment with thyrotropin-releasing hormone. N Engl J Med 312:1085–1090, 1985

Bernal J, Pekonen F: Ontogenesis of the nuclear 3,5,3'-triiodothyronine receptor in the human fetal brain. Endocrinology 114:677–679, 1984

Boler J, Enzmann F, Folkers K, et al: The identity of chemical and hormonal properties of the thyrotropin releasing hormone and pyroglutamyl-histidyl-proline amide. Biochem Biophys Res Commun 37:705–710, 1969

Brucker-Davis F, Skarulis MC, Grace MB, et al: Genetic and clinical features of 42 kindreds with resistance to thyroid hormone: the National Institutes of Health Prospective Study. Ann Intern Med 123:572–583, 1995

Burgus R, Dunn TF, Desiderio D, et al: [Molecular structure of the hypothalamic hypophysiotropic TRF factor of ovine origin: mass spectrometry demonstration of the PCA-His-Pro-NH_2 sequence]. Comptes Rendus Hebdomadaires Des Seances De L'Academie Des Sciences. D: Sciences Naturelles 269:1870–1873, 1969

Carr FE, Kaseem LL, Wong NC: Thyroid hormone inhibits thyrotropin gene expression via a position-independent negative L-triiodothyronine-responsive element. J Biol Chem 267:18689–18694, 1992

Dacou-Voutetakis C, Feltquate DM, Drakopoulou M, et al: Familial hypothyroidism caused by a nonsense mutation in the thyroid-stimulating hormone β-subunit gene. Am J Hum Genet 46:988–993, 1990

Danese MD, Powe NR, Sawin CT, et al: Screening for mild thyroid failure at the periodic health examination: a decision and cost-effective analysis. JAMA 276:285–292, 1996

Delange FM: Endemic cretinism, in Werner and Ingbar's The Thyroid: A Fundamental and Clinical Text, 7th Edition. Edited by Braverman LE, Utiger RD. Philadelphia, PA, Lippincott-Raven, 1996, pp 756–767

Dracopoli NC, Rettig WJ, Whitfield GK, et al: Assignment of the gene for the β subunit of thyroid-stimulating hormone to the short arm of human chromosome 1. Proc Natl Acad Sci U S A 83:1822–1826, 1986

Dunn JT: Thyroglobulin: chemistry and biosynthesis, in Werner and Ingbar's The Thyroid: A Fundamental and Clinical Text. Edited by Braverman LE, Utiger RD. Philadelphia, PA, Lippincott-Raven, 1996, pp 85–95

Fiddes JC, Goodman HM: Isolation, cloning and sequence analysis of the cDNA for the α-subunit of human chorionic gonadotropin. Nature 281:351–356, 1979

Fisher DA, Klein AH: Thyroid development and disorders of thyroid function in the newborn. N Engl J Med 304:702–712, 1981

Fisher DA, Odell WD: Acute release of thyrotropin in the newborn. J Clin Invest 48:1670–1677, 1969

Fisher DA, Polk DH: Development of the thyroid. Baillieres Clin Endocrinol Metab 3:627–657, 1989

Fisher DA, Polk DR: Thyroid disease in the fetus, neonate, and child, in Endocrinology, 3rd Edition, Vol 1. Edited by DeGroot LJ, Besser M, Burger HG, et al. Philadelphia, PA, WB Saunders, 1995

Fisher DA, Dussault JH, Foley TP Jr, et al: Screening for congenital hypothyroidism: results of screening one million North American infants. J Pediatr 94:700–705, 1979

Foley TP: Congenital hypothyroidism, in Werner and Ingbar's The Thyroid: A Fundamental and Clinical Text. Edited by Braverman LE, Utiger RD. Philadelphia, PA, Lippincott-Raven, 1996, pp 988–999

Gesundheit N, Petrick PA, Nissim M, et al: Thyrotropin-secreting pituitary adenomas: clinical and biochemical heterogeneity: case reports and follow-up of nine patients. Ann Intern Med 111:827–835, 1989

Hare JY, Ludomirsky A: Cordocentesis: direct access to the fetal circulation for evaluating fetal well-being and thyroid function. Curr Opin Obstet Gynecol 6:440–444, 1994

Hauser P, Zametkin AJ, Martinez P, et al: Attention-deficit hyperactivity disorder in people with generalized resistance to thyroid hormone. N Engl J Med 328:997–1001, 1993

Hayashizaki Y, Hiraoka Y, Tatsumi K, et al: Deoxyribonucleic acid analyses of five families with familial inherited thyroid stimulating hormone deficiency. J Clin Endocrinol Metab 71:792–796, 1990

Kazakov VS, Demidchik EP, Astakhova LN: Thyroid cancer after Chernobyl (letter) [see comments]. Nature 359:21, 1992

Klein RZ, Mitchell ML: Hypothyroidism in infants and children, in Werner and Ingbar's The Thyroid: A Fundamental and Clinical Text, 7th Edition. Edited by Braverman LE, Utiger RD. Philadelphia, PA, Lippincott-Raven, 1996

Koller KJ, Wolff RS, Warden MK, et al: Thyroid hormones regulate levels of thyrotropin-releasing-hormone. Proc Natl Acad Sci U S A 84:7329–7333, 1987

Laurent E, Mockel J, Van Sande J, et al: Dual activation by thyrotropin of the phospholipase C and cyclic AMP. Mol Cell Endocrinol 52:273–278, 1987

Mandel SJ, Brent GA, Larsen PR: Review of antithyroid drug use during pregnancy and report of a case. Thyroid 4:129–133, 1994

Parma J, Duprez L, Van SJ, et al: Somatic mutations in the thyrotropin receptor gene cause hyperfunctioning thyroid adenomas. Nature 365:649–651, 1993

Pierce JG, Parsons TF: Glycoprotein hormones: structure and function. Annu Rev Biochem 50:465–495, 1981

Porterfield SP, Hendrich CE: The role of thyroid hormones in prenatal and neonatal neurological development—current perspectives. Endocr Rev 14:94–106, 1993

Raspé E, Dumont JE: Robert Feulgen Lecture 1991. Control and role of major signalling cascades of the thyrocyte. Prog Histochem Cytochem 26:1–29, 1992

Roti E, Gnudi A, Braverman LE: The placental transport, synthesis and metabolism of hormones and drugs which affect thyroid function. Endocr Rev 4:131–149, 1983

Rovet JF, Westbrook DL, Ehrlich RM: Neonatal thyroid deficiency: early temperamental and cognitive characteristics. J Am Acad Child Psychiatry 23:10–22, 1984

Rovet JF, Ehrlich RM, Sorbara DL: Neurodevelopment in infants and preschool children with congenital hypothyroidism: etiological and treatment factors affecting outcome. J Pediatr Psychol 17:187–213, 1992

Saberi M, Sterling FH, Utiger RD: Reduction in extrathyroidal triiodothyronine production by propylthiouracil in man. J Clin Invest 55:218–223, 1975

Sap J, Munoz A, Damm K, et al: The c-erb-A protein is a high-affinity receptor for thyroid hormone. Nature 324:635–640, 1986

Segerson TP, Kauer J, Wolfe HC, et al: Thyroid hormone regulates TRH biosynthesis in the paraventricular nucleus of the rat hypothalamus. Science 238:78–80, 1987

Shepard TH: Onset of function in the human fetal thyroid: biochemical and radioautographic studies from organ culture. J Clin Endocrinol Metab 27:945–958, 1967

Shupnik MA, Chin WW, Habener JF, et al: Transcriptional regulation of the thyrotropin subunit genes by thyroid hormone. J Biol Chem 260:2900–2903, 1985

Sunthornthepvarakui T, Gottschalk ME, Hayashi Y, et al: Brief report: resistance to thyrotropin caused by mutations in the thyrotropin-receptor gene. N Engl J Med 332:155–160, 1995

Tamaki H, Amino N, Aozasa M, et al: Universal predictive criteria for neonatal overt thyrotoxicosis. Am J Perinatol 5:152–158, 1988

Thorpe-Beeston JG, Nicolaides KH, McGregor AM: Fetal thyroid function. Thyroid 2:207–217, 1992

Utiger RD: Thyrotropin-receptor mutations and thyroid dysfunction (editorial). N Engl J Med 332:183–185, 1995

Van Dijke CP, Heydendael RJ, De Kleine MJ: Methimazole, carbimazole, and congenital skin defects. Ann Intern Med 106:60–61, 1987

Van Sande J, Parma J, Tonacchera M, et al: Somatic and germline mutations of the TSH receptor gene in thyroid. J Clin Endocrinol Metab 80:2577–2585, 1995

Vulsma T, Gons MH, de Vijlder JJ: Maternal-fetal transfer of thyroxine in congenital hypothyroidism due to a total organification defect or thyroid agenesis. N Engl J Med 321:13–16, 1989

Weinberger C, Thompson CC, Ong ES, et al: The c-erb-A gene encodes a thyroid hormone receptor. Nature 324:641–646, 1986

Weinstein LS, Shenker A, Gejman PV, et al: Activating mutations of the stimulatory G protein in the McCune-Albright syndrome. N Engl J Med 325:1688–1695, 1991

Yamada M, Radovick S, Wondisford FE, et al: Cloning and structure of human genomic DNA and hypothalamic cDNA encoding human prepro thyrotropin-releasing hormone. Mol Endocrinol 4:551–556, 1990

Zakarija M, McKenzie JM, Hoffman WH: Prediction and therapy of intrauterine and late-onset neonatal hyperthyroidism. J Clin Endocrinol Metab 62:368–371, 1986

Chapter 2

Thyroid Hormone and Development: Brain and Peripheral Tissues

Christoph A. Meier, M.D.

Although thyroid hormones are necessary for life in adults, the most dramatic effects of these hormones are seen during development. In many species, thyroid hormones regulate the secretion of growth hormone during ontogeny. Their presence is required for the induction of metamorphosis in amphibians and for normal neonatal brain development in mammals and birds. The role of thyroid hormones in regulating metamorphosis and the spatially and temporally distinct expression of thyroid hormone receptors (TRs) during this process is reviewed elsewhere (Baker and Tata 1990; Chatterjee and Tata 1992; Kawahara et al. 1991; Tata 1994; Tata et al. 1993). In this chapter, the effects of thyroid hormones on the developing brain are reviewed; this is followed by a summary of current knowledge of thyroid hormone action at the molecular level. Finally, the molecular aspects of the syndrome of resistance to thyroid hormone—an example of inhibition of thyroid hormone action at the nuclear level resulting in functional derangements of the central nervous system—are discussed.

Effects of Thyroid Hormones on Brain Development

Synthesis, Uptake, and Local Deiodination of Thyroid Hormones

Production of thyroid hormones by the human thyroid gland begins between weeks 9 and 12 of gestation. The hormones are transported into the cerebrospinal fluid (CSF) through the choroid plexus (Fisher et al. 1976; Pontecorvi and Robbins 1989; Porterfield and Hendrich 1993; Robbins and Lakshmanan 1992). Because the choroid plexus is a site for the production of transthyretin, it was hypothesized that this thyroid hormone–binding protein might contribute to the uptake of L-thyroxine (T_4) into the CSF and possibly the brain cells (Chanoine and Braverman 1992; Southwell et al. 1992). However, experiments in mice involving targeted disruption of both transthyretin alleles resulted in animals with no evidence of tissue hypothyroidism (including brain), indicating that transthyretin is not essential for T_4 uptake into the CSF (Palha et al. 1994).

Whereas the thyroid gland secretes its hormone mainly in the form of the virtually inactive T_4, this prohormone is deiodinated in various organs to its active derivative L-triiodothyronine (T_3). The main organs of T_4-to-T_3 conversion are the liver and kidney, expressing the type I selenocysteine–containing monodeiodinase (Beckett and Arthur 1994; Larsen and Berry 1994; Mandel et al. 1992; St. Germain 1994). However, less than 25% and 10% of the nuclear T_3 is locally produced in liver and kidney, respectively, reflecting the fact that most of the T_3 is released into the systemic circulation (Figure 2–1) (Silva and Larsen 1986). This is in contrast to the pituitary gland and brain, where 50%–80% of the T_3 reaching the nuclear receptor is derived from local deiodination by the type II deiodinase (Farwell et al. 1993; Larsen et al. 1981). The type II deiodinase was recently cloned and was found to share a limited but significant degree of homology with the type I deiodinase, while also containing a selenocysteine (Davey et al. 1995). The selenium moiety is essential for enzymatic activity, and it is likely to explain the altered thyroid function tests and decreased cerebral T_3 supply in severe selenium deficiency (Beckett and Arthur 1994; Chanoine et al. 1992a, 1992b). Type I and type II deiodinase differ in their regulation by endogenous and exogenous molecules. Most important, the type II enzyme is downregulated by T_4, possibly preventing the local overproduction of T_3 in the brain in states of elevated T_4 levels (Escobar-Morreale et al. 1995).

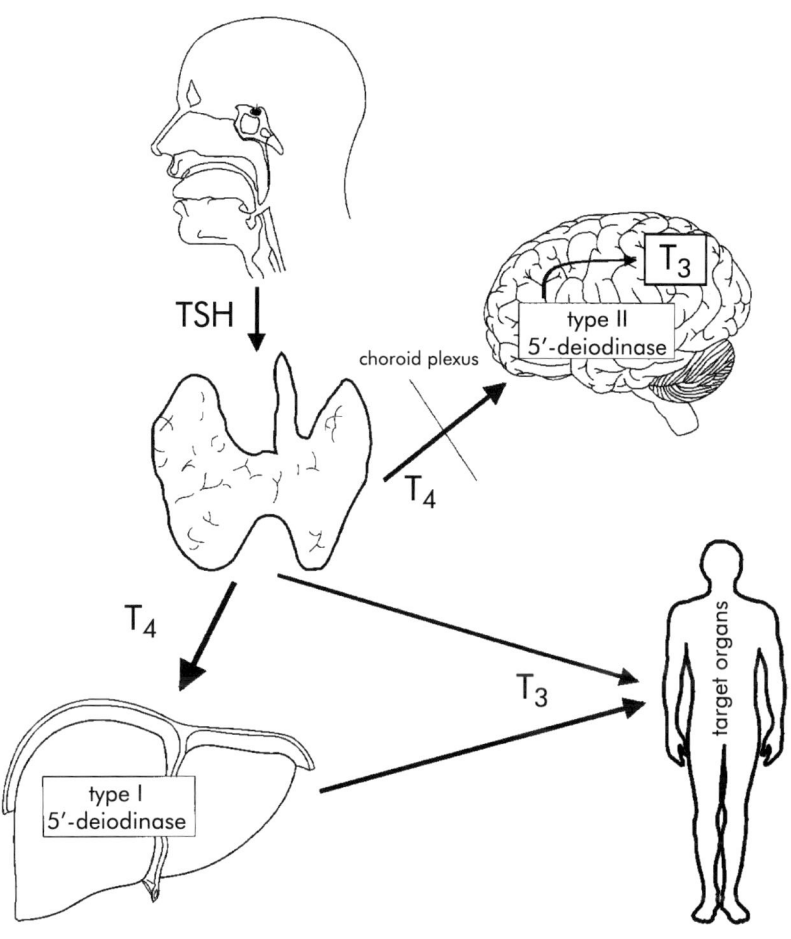

Figure 2–1. Metabolism of thyroid hormones. Under the influence of thyroid-stimulating hormone (TSH) produced by the pituitary gland, the thyroid gland secretes thyroid hormones, the majority being the prohormone thyroxine (T_4). T is deiodinated in the liver and, to a lesser degree, the kidney by the type I deiodinase to yield the active hormone triiodothyronine (T_3), which is released back into the circulation to reach the various target organs. In contrast, the brain is the only organ capable of producing the majority of its T_3 supply locally by means of the type II deiodinase.

In addition to the thyroid hormones produced by the fetus, maternal hormone is able to cross the placenta and contributes to the fetal hormone levels, as reviewed in detail elsewhere (Burrow et al. 1994; Maruo et al. 1992; Morreale de Escobar et al. 1993).

Time Course of Thyroid Hormone Effects on the Developing Brain

During the first 9–12 weeks of gestation in the human, the fetal total T_4 concentration is very low (<10 nM) and is entirely derived from placental transfer. During this first phase of brain development, the cerebral neurogenesis and migration are largely believed to be independent of thyroid hormones. However, as discussed below, it is quite possible that the unliganded TR, whose expression precedes the beginning of fetal thyroid function, exerts a silencing function on the expression of certain genes.

Subsequently, the second phase of brain development, beginning after week 12, is characterized by neuronal differentiation, axonal outgrowth, synaptogenesis, and gliogenesis as well as cerebellar neurogenesis (Porterfield and Hendrich 1993). It is extremely difficult to experimentally define the exact role of thyroid hormones during this period, because the transplacental supply from the mother ensures the presence of some hormone even in fetuses with thyroid agenesis (Vulsma et al. 1989). Nevertheless, the findings in experimental cell culture models discussed below strongly support a role of thyroid hormones in regulating neuronal migration, differentiation, and apoptosis; neurite outgrowth; synaptogenesis; oligodendrocytic differentiation; and myelin synthesis.

The importance of thyroid hormones for neurological development was best established for the postnatal period and lasting 1–2 years, since the protective influence of the maternal hormone supply is no longer present. This third period is marked by continued neuronal differentiation, axonal outgrowth, and synaptogenesis and gliogenesis in all parts of the brain. However, it is worth mentioning that forebrain neurogenesis and migration are essentially completed by the time of birth, whereas the majority of neuronal proliferation in the cerebellum takes place postnatally

(Porterfield and Hendrich 1993). Clinically, this is reflected in the abnormal development of the central nervous system found in children with untreated congenital hypothyroidism as discussed elsewhere in this book.

Thyroid Hormone Effects on Brain Cells in Vivo and in Vitro

In thyroid hormone deficiency the cerebral and cerebellar anatomy is deranged at the microscopic level but not at the macroscopic level. In brain tissue from cretins this is reflected by the histologic finding of smaller neurons, decreased myelinization, and gliosis. Similar morphologic features are found in the central nervous system of hypothyroid rats. Cell migration, neuritic outgrowth, synaptogenesis, and myelinogenesis are all delayed, whereas the proliferation of glial cells and the death of neurons are accelerated (Bernal and Nunez 1995). This results in a distorted cytoarchitecture and lamination of the cortex as well as aberrant gliosis. However, so far very few molecular mechanisms have been defined by which thyroid hormones influence the processes mentioned above. Nevertheless, effects of thyroid hormones on the expression of microtubular and myelin-associated proteins, as well as neurotropins, have been studied in some detail.

Axonal and dendritic polarity and the outgrowth of neurons are determined by the cytoskeleton, which is partly composed of microtubules constructed of tubulin polymers. The microtubules are capable of undergoing posttranslational modifications (acetylation, detyrosination), a process referred to as *maturation.* These modifications are thought to be important for the binding to microtubule-associated proteins (MAPs), such as *tau* in axons and MAP2 in dendrites. These proteins are implicated in the regulation of the rate of tubulin polymerization and assembly, and they mediate the attachment of the microtubulins to specific subcellular compartments, resulting in differential sprouting of the afferent dendritic and efferent axonal projections. Thyroid hormones were shown to differentially regulate the messenger RNAs (mRNAs) of the various tubulin and MAP isoforms, providing a possible link to the effects of T_3 on the cytoarchitecture of the developing brain and to the retardation of neuritic outgrowth in hypothyroidism (Aniello et al. 1991a, 1991b). Thyroid hormones are capable of modulating the level of maturation (differential splicing) of the tubulin and MAP mRNAs. However, thyroid hormones determine the timing rather than being an absolute requirement for these effects to occur, thereby complicating the analysis of the precise molecular mechanisms involved. Hence, it remains currently unknown whether the expression of tubulins and MAPs is directly regulated by thyroid hormones at the transcriptional or the posttranscriptional level (Bernal and Nunez 1995).

Other brain genes regulated by thyroid hormones have been described in oligodendrocytes and neurons but not in astrocytes. Specifically, oligodendrocytes produce myelin, which is composed of myelin basic protein (MBP), proteolipid protein (PLP), and myelin-associated glycoprotein (MAG) (Baas et al. 1994a, 1994b). Although all three gene products are induced by thyroid hormones in a time-specific and site-specific manner, a TR binding site (T_3-response element [TRE]) on the regulatory promoter region of target genes has been identified only for the MBP gene (Farsetti et al. 1991, 1992; Rodriguez-Peña et al. 1993). A response element for heterodimers between TRs and the peroxisome proliferator–activated receptor (PPAR) in the PLP promoter has been reported (Bogazzi et al. 1994), but the existence of PPAR:TR heterodimers remains controversial (Juge-Aubry et al. 1995). Three types of neuronal proteins subject to thyroid hormone regulation have been well studied so far: the PCP-2 and RC3 (neurogranin) genes in cerebellum and cerebrum, respectively, and the neurotropins (Bernal and Nunez 1995). The PCP-2 gene product is of unknown function and its promoter structure was demonstrated to contain a functional TRE, implying that the regulation by thyroid hormones is at the transcriptional level (Zou et al. 1994). However, as for virtually all other thyroid hormone–regulated brain genes, it is the timing of expression, rather than the absolute level, that is controlled by thyroid hormones. The RC3 gene is expressed in the cortex and hippocampus, and it codes for a protein kinase C substrate; hence it has been speculated that it is involved in long-term potentiation. In contrast to the MBP and PCP-2 proteins described above, the RC3 gene is unique in two aspects: 1) its expression is absolutely dependent on thyroid hormones, and it is therefore not normalized spontaneously after a certain lag period, and 2) by virtue of the property just described, it represents the only brain gene known to be regulated by thyroid hormones in adult animals (Iniguez et al. 1992). Finally, some of the effects of thyroid hormones on brain development may be mediated through the control of the expression of growth factors. Nerve growth factor and neurotropin-3 were both shown to be regulated by thyroid hormones through a yet-unknown mechanism (Black et al. 1992; Lindholm et al. 1993).

Molecular Basis of Thyroid Hormone Action

Although the number of brain genes known to be regulated by thyroid hormones is still relatively small, and the number of TREs identified in the promoter regions of these genes is even smaller, the molecular details involved in thyroid hormone–mediated transcriptional control are fairly well characterized. The principle of action of thyroid hormones is very similar to that of the steroids, vitamin D, and retinoic acid (Mangelsdorf et al. 1995). The hormone enters the cytoplasm and nucleus, where it binds to a receptor protein capable of directly binding to the regulatory region of target genes (Figure 2–2). Most nuclear receptors, however, do not bind as single molecules (monomers) to DNA, but rather as dimers (homodimers) or complexed with other members of the nuclear receptor family (heterodimers). The binding of liganded receptor dimers is thought to stabilize the transcription initiation complex, leading to the recruitment and activation of RNA polymerase type II, thereby resulting in an increased rate of mRNA synthesis.

The Nuclear Hormone Receptor Superfamily

With the cloning of the receptor genes for retinoids, vitamin D, and the steroid and thyroid hormones, it became apparent that they all

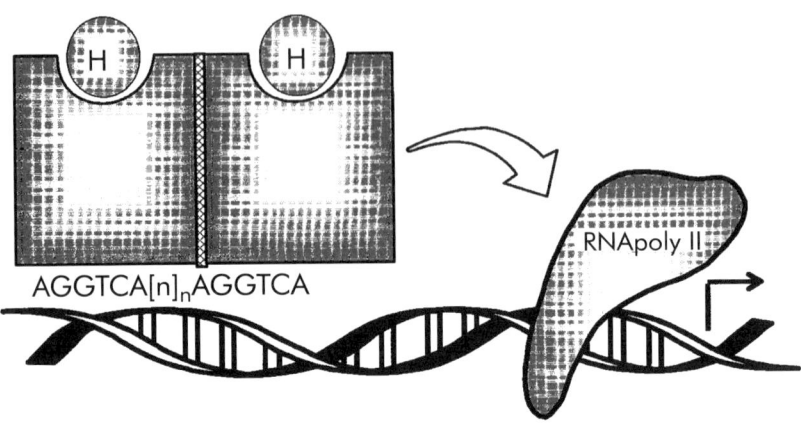

Figure 2–2. Principle of action of retinoid, steroid, and thyroid hormones (H). The specific nuclear hormone receptor proteins bind to well-defined target sequences (hormone response elements consisting of two similar half-sites) in the regulatory region of target genes. The receptors generally bind as homodimers (steroid receptors) or heterodimers (retinoid, thyroid hormone receptors) to DNA and are thereby able to alter the activity of the RNA polymerase II (RNApoly II) (mRNA synthesis).

share similar structural domains (Evans 1988). A highly variable amino-terminal region is followed by the DNA-binding domain (DBD), which contains two zinc fingers involved in contacting the consensus DNA-binding motif AGGTCA. A hinge region involved in the activation of transcription links the DBD to the ligand-binding domain (LBD), whose role is to mediate not only specific ligand binding but also dimerization with other nuclear proteins. Owing to the conserved structure of the nuclear hormone receptors from *Drosophila* (ecdysone receptor) to mammals, it has been speculated that the various members of this receptor superfamily arose from gene duplication of a common ancestor gene (Laudet et al. 1992).

How is the regulatory specificity encoded, given that TRs,

retinoic acid receptors (RARs and RXRs), vitamin D receptors (VDRs), and PPAR bind to the same AGGTCA site? First, the AGGTCA consensus motif is somewhat variable, and it has been shown that the adjacent flanking sequences also contribute to the binding specificity of these receptors. Second, and most important, these receptors usually bind to DNA as a heterodimer with the 9-*cis*-retinoic acid receptor RXR (Mangelsdorf and Evans 1995). The spacing of the two binding sites is then crucial to determine the binding specificity, as illustrated in Figure 2–3 (Umesono and Evans 1989; Umesono et al. 1991). Indeed, many naturally occurring hormone response elements have been shown to be compatible with this concept.

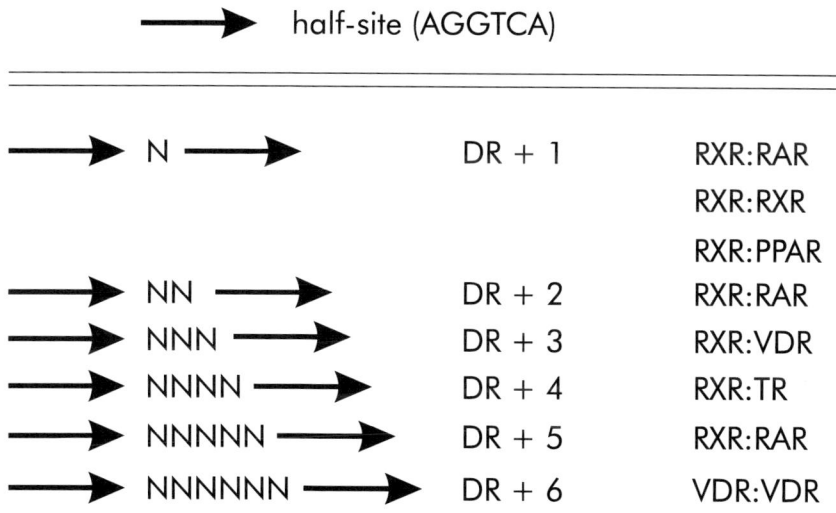

Figure 2–3. Target gene specificity for retinoid (RAR, RXR), vitamin D (VDR), thyroid hormone (TR), and peroxisome proliferator–activated receptors (PPAR). The receptors bind to DNA as homodimers or heterodimers, where each receptor binds tandem repeats of the consensus half-site AGGTCA (direct repeat, DR), and RXR typically occupies the upstream position. However, the various receptor homodimers and heterodimers have different spacing requirements between the two repeats (DR + N) for DNA binding to occur.

Thyroid Hormone Receptors

Two genes encode for four subtypes of thyroid hormone receptors (Figure 2–4). The TRα gene on human chromosome 17 can be alternatively spliced to yield the TRα1 and TRα2 isoforms, whereas the TRβ gene on chromosome 3 is differentially spliced into the TRβ1 and TRβ2 isoforms (Lazar 1993). Functionally, the TRα1, TRβ1, and TRβ2 receptors are similarly active in in vitro systems, although subtle differences have been described (Darling et al. 1993; Schueler et al. 1990; Tomura et al. 1995). In addition, in a model using the neuronal cell line Neuro-2a, TRβ1, but not the α1 isoform, was able to induce differentiation in a T_3-dependent manner (Lebel et al. 1994). Similarly, in vivo the spatial, temporal, and hormonal regulation of expression differs for each of the various subtypes. Whereas the TRα1 and TRβ1 mRNAs are present at similar levels in most brain regions except in the hippocampus (where the TRβ1 expression is limited to the CA1 field), the TRα1 form is expressed much earlier, before the fetus is able to produce thyroid hormones

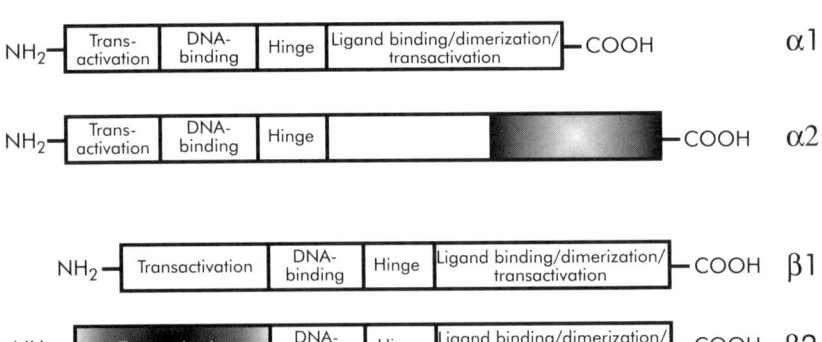

Figure 2–4. TR subtypes. The two human thyroid hormone receptor (TR) genes can be alternatively spliced to yield four TR subtypes, differing in the amino- or carboxy-terminal part. Whereas $TRα_1$, $TRβ_1$, and $TRβ_2$ are functional TRs, the $TRα_2$ protein does not bind T_3 and inhibits thyroid hormone action.

(Bradley et al. 1989; Falcone et al. 1994; Wills et al. 1991). In addition, the TRβ1 and TRβ2 forms were shown to be expressed selectively and strongly during early inner-ear development (Bradley et al. 1994). The TRβ1 is markedly induced postnatally, possibly through a positive-feedback regulation involving positive TREs in the promoter region of the gene (Suzuki et al. 1994). The function of TRα1 receptors preceding the fetal production of thyroid hormones remains enigmatic. However, as previously stated, it is conceivable that the unliganded TRs have a modulatory effect on T_3- and retinoid-regulated gene expression. This concept has been well illustrated in the pheochromocytoma-derived PC12 cell culture model, in which unliganded TRα1 resulted in the repression of neuron-specific genes and an inhibition of nerve growth factor–induced differentiation (Munoz et al. 1993). In contrast, unliganded TRα1 was able to induce the *trkB* mRNA, which codes for a neurotropin receptor in neuronal N2a cells (Pastor et al. 1994).

The TRβ2 isoform, differing only in the amino-terminal from its splicing variant TRβ1, was originally thought to be restricted to the pituitary, where its expression is negatively regulated by thyroid hormones (Hodin et al. 1989). However, the mRNA for this isoform was recently shown to be present not only in the inner ear area, but also in the hypothalamic, hippocampal, and caudate regions, although no protein has been detected thus far (Bradley et al. 1992; Schwartz et al. 1994).

Finally, the TRα2 isoform differs markedly from TRα1 by having a different exon spliced into the ligand-binding domain, thereby eliminating the T_3-binding and transcriptional activity of this protein (Katz et al. 1992). This nonfunctional TRα2 (also termed c-erbAα2) is expressed in virtually every organ, including the brain. In vitro studies have demonstrated that the TRα2 protein is capable of significantly inhibiting the activity of the bona fide TRs as discussed below.

Thyroid Hormone–Regulated Target Genes

In view of the pleiotropic actions of thyroid hormones, surprisingly few directly regulated target genes have been identified, among them MBP, thyrotropin, malic enzyme, and myosin heavy chain. However, this limited number is most likely a reflection of the inadequacy of the current technology to identify differentially expressed genes, rather than of the true number of thyroid hormone–regulated genes. As indicated above, VDRs, RARs, RXRs, and TRs tend to bind most efficiently to two AGGTCA half-sites arranged in tandem (direct repeats, DRs) with variable spacing between the two repeats. TRα1 and TRβ1 were shown to preferentially bind as heterodimers with RXR to a DR with the two sites spaced by four nucleotides (DR+4), where RXR occupies the upstream position. Although RXR increases the binding affinity of TR for DNA, the ligand for RXR (9-*cis* retinoic acid) does not modulate TR activity under most circumstances (Forman et al. 1995b; Hallenbeck et al. 1993; Rosen et al. 1992). For TRs, however, other tandem arrangements of the half-sites have also been described, in which the two repeats are oriented in opposite directions, such as in the palindromic (TREpal) or inverted palindromic (TRE-IR) arrangement illustrated in Figure 2–5. Although the TREpal element is not found in nature except as part of a complex binding site in the rat growth hormone promoter, the TRE-IR element is present in the MBP gene (Farsetti et al. 1992). This IR element has the unique features of TRs binding as TR:TR homodimers in the absence of T_3, which are dissociated in favor of RXR:TR heterodimers in the presence of ligand (Yen et al. 1992a) (see Figure 2–8, upper panel). This finding indicates that RXR:TR, rather than TR:TR, may be the transcriptionally active complex.

The precise molecular details of T_3-induced transcriptional activation have remained unclear, because DNA binding of unliganded receptors does not increase transcription and even decreases basal transcription of target gene (Fondell et al. 1993; Yen et al. 1995). The latter phenomenon of basal repression of transcription by TRs is believed to be important in mediating gene silencing—for example, during development, when the expression of TRs precedes the production of thyroid hormone. Given these observations, it was of considerable interest to identify additional proteins (coactivators and corepressors) associated with TRs in a ligand-dependent manner that mediate an activating or inhibitory signal, respectively, to the transcriptional machinery (see Figure 2–5). The corepressor proteins are able to interact with unliganded TRs, thereby silencing basal transcriptional activity. However, once T_3 is bound to the TR, the corepressor dissociates and allows one or several coactivator proteins to interact with the TR. This latter interaction is currently thought to be essential for building a bridge of protein:protein interactions relaying the T_3-induced *trans*-activation signal to the basic transcriptional machinery, including the RNA polymerase II. The first coactivator proteins for TRs and estrogen receptors were recently identified, including *Trip1*, p140, and p160 (Cavailles et al. 1994; Halachmi et al. 1994; Lee et al. 1995). These factors are characterized by their ligand-

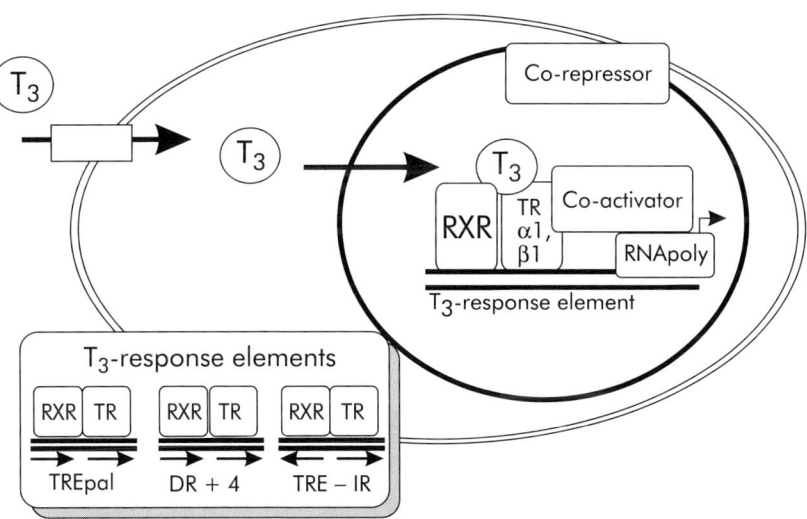

Figure 2–5. Current model of thyroid hormone action. The retinoic acid receptor–thyroid hormone receptor (RXR:TR) heterodimer binds to a T_3-response element (TRE) consisting of two half-sites arranged as palindromes (TREpal), direct repeats (DR+4), or inverted repeats (TRE-IR). On binding of ligand, the corepressor inhibiting transcription dissociates and a coactivator protein binds to the TR, leading to mRNA synthesis by mRNA polymerase II.

dependent ability to associate with the respective nuclear receptor and increase transcription for a variety of nuclear receptors (Chen and Evans 1995; Hörlein et al. 1995). Recently, it became apparent that different transcription factors (including the coactivators for nuclear receptor) from various intracellular signaling pathways can all interact with the same protein, termed CREB [cAMP–response element binding protein]-binding protein (CBP)/p300 (Figure 2–6). Thus it appears that this large 300-kd nuclear protein might serve as a central integrator and mediator of the transcriptional response to various hormonal stimuli, thereby offering another potential point for crosstalk. In addition to the proteins in-

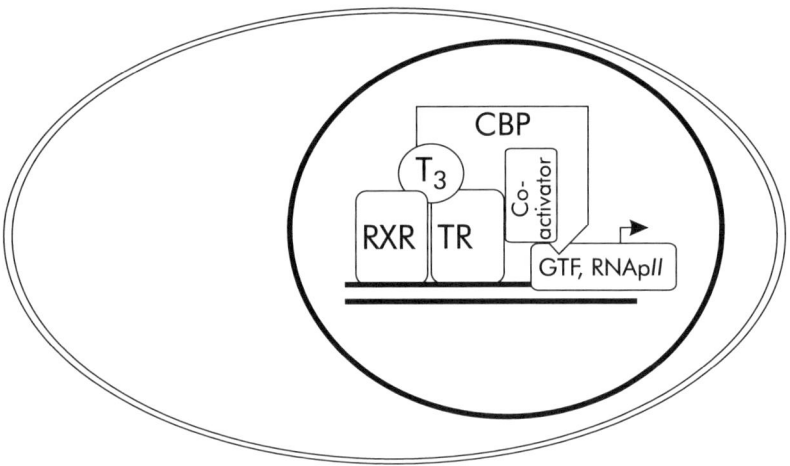

Figure 2–6. Interaction of thyroid hormone receptors (TRs) with coactivator proteins. The liganded TRs are able to recruit various coactivator proteins, such as SRC-1. The TR (as well as some coactivators) is able to interact with the large integrator protein CBP/p300. The CREB-binding protein (CBP) is also a cofactor for other hormonal signaling pathways, such as the the cAMP–response element binding protein (CREB). This multiprotein compex is then able to stabilize or destabilize the assembly of the basal transcriptional machinery consisting of general transcription factors (GTFs) and RNA polymerase *II* (RNAp*II*), thereby resulting in an increased or decreased transcription rate, respectively.

volved in the activation pathway, two distinct corepressors were cloned, the nuclear receptor corepressor (N-CoR) and the silencing mediator for RARs and TRs (SMRT), forming the new family of thyroid hormone– and retinoic acid–associated corepressors (TRACs). The N-CoR is a 270-kd protein without significant homology to any other known protein. It contains two repressor domains required for dimerizing with the hinge region (the juncture between the DNA- and ligand-binding domains) of TR. The SMRT protein has similar functional characteristics, but its molecular mass is smaller (168 kd). Both corepressors are ubiquitously expressed in the nuclei at low levels. The definitive physiological and possibly clinical relevance of these factors clearly remains to be demonstrated. However, it can be speculated that corepressors might serve an important role in gene silencing (e.g., during neuronal development), as well as in adding specificity to the sometimes promiscuous receptor:DNA interactions. In addition, it seems possible that the balance of coactivators to corepressors could not only modulate the sensitivity of a given target organ to a particular hormone but also lead to situations of conditional crosstalk among different nuclear receptors under circumstances in which one of these shared cofactors becomes limiting (Yen and Chin 1994).

Modulation of Thyroid Hormone Action

Thyroid hormone action in brain and other tissues depends not only on the availability of ambient or locally produced T_3 but also on the cellular sensitivity to the hormone. The latter property is likely to depend on a variety of factors, such as the number of TRs and the ratio of functional (TRα1, TRβ1, and TRβ2) to inhibitory (TRα2) isoforms. In addition, the local concentrations of free coactivators, corepressors, and RXRs probably influence the cellular response to T_3.

Three examples of the modulation of cellular T_3 responsiveness have been characterized in some detail (Figure 2–7): 1) the inhibitory effect of TRα2, which seems to compete for accessory proteins and, in its phosphorylated state, for binding to TREs (Katz et al.

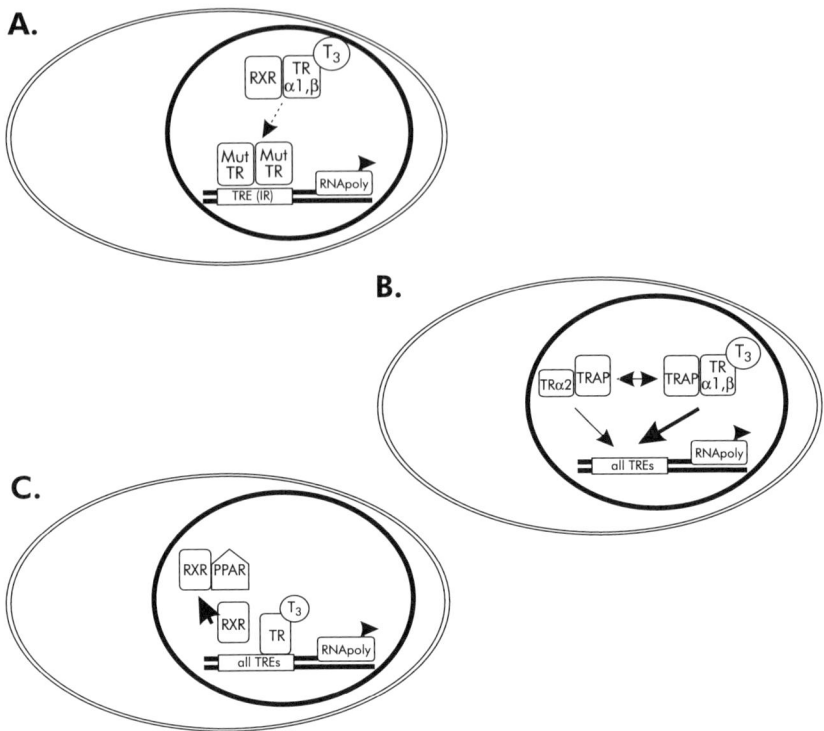

Figure 2–7. Modulatory inhibition of thyroid hormone action at the nuclear level. **A.** Mutant TRβ1 from kindreds with the syndrome of resistance to thyroid hormone (RTH) competes with normal thyroid hormone receptors (TRs) for binding to DNA. **B.** The nonfunctional splicing variant TRα2 competes for DNA binding as well as for TR-associated proteins (TRAPs) such as retinoic acid receptors (RXRs) and possibly coactivators and other transcription factors. **C.** Peroxisome proliferator–activated receptors (PPARs) inhibit TR action by competing for limited numbers of RXRs.

1995; Liu et al. 1995; Meier-Heusler et al. 1995); 2) the dominant negative mutant TRs from patients with resistance to thyroid hormone (see below); and 3) PPARs competing for limited numbers of RXRs (Juge-Aubry et al. 1995). PPARs are nuclear receptors activated by fatty acids, arachidonic acid, and prostaglandins of the PG J2 series (Forman et al. 1995a; Kliewer et al. 1995). These receptors are pivotal for mediating adipose tissue differentiation and fatty acid metabolism; one of their three isoforms is expressed in most tissues, including the brain, where its function is completely unknown (Braissant et al. 1996; Kainu et al. 1994). However, PPARs are able to downregulate thyroid hormone action drastically in vitro and in vivo by competing for RXRs (Chu et al. 1995; Juge-Aubry et al. 1995; Meier-Heusler et al. 1995). To increase the regulatory complexity of the nuclear signaling network, the relative affinity of TRs or PPARs for RXRs or other cofactors is likely to be regulated through receptor phosphorylation, providing the possibility for crosstalk with membrane-bound signaling systems (Bhat et al. 1994; Sugawara et al. 1994).

Molecular Basis of Resistance to Thyroid Hormone

The importance of molecular mechanisms resulting in a modulation of thyroid hormone action are best illustrated by the in vivo consequences of a dominant negative regulator of thyroid hormone action in the syndrome of resistance to thyroid hormone (RTH) (Refetoff et al. 1993). In this rare autosomal dominant disease, one allele of the TRβ gene is mutated to yield a partially or completely inactive TR that is capable of inhibiting the normal TRα1 and TRβ1 through a dominant negative mechanism (Chatterjee et al. 1991; Meier et al. 1992, 1993; Yen et al. 1992b). Clinically this is correlated with the observation that only patients with a mutant, but not those with a completely deleted, TRβ allele exhibit the phenotype of RTH, which is discussed in detail in Chapter 5 (Takeda et al. 1992). This inhibition by mutant TRs requires DNA binding and heterodimerization with RXRs to be preserved; hence it mainly involves competing with the normal TRs for binding to TREs and possibly for binding to limited amounts of cofactors (Nagaya and Jameson 1993; Nagaya et al. 1992; Yen et al. 1992b). Interestingly, the dominant negative property of the mutant TRs is most pronounced on TREs of the IR type, resulting from the combined effects of the mutant TR homodimers, which 1) compete for DNA binding, and 2) once bound to the TRE-IR are not able to bind

T_3 and to dissociate (Figure 2–8) (Meier et al. 1993; Zavacki et al. 1993). It can hence be speculated that the MBP-TRE containing an inverted repeat is particularly susceptible to the dominant negative effect of mutant TRβ.

Although dozens of different phenotypes and mutations in the TR genes have been described, a good correlation between the genotype and phenotype remains elusive. This is most apparent in families in which the same TRβ mutation results in markedly different clinical manifestations (Brucker-Davis et al. 1995). This implies that polymorphisms in other proteins, such as RXR, coactivators, or corepressors, may contribute to the expression of thyroid hormone effects in vivo (Weiss et al. 1993).

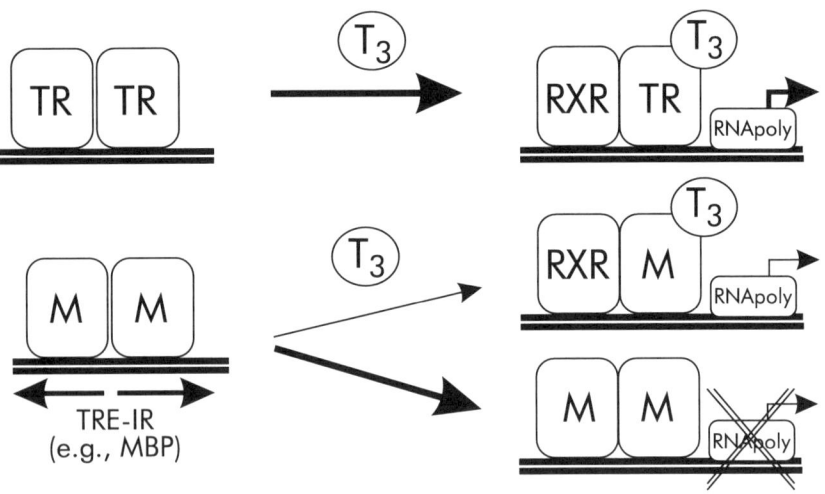

Figure 2–8. Model of the dominant negative action of mutant TRβ in the syndrome of resistance to thyroid hormone (RTH). First, the mutant thyroid hormone receptors (TRs) compete for DNA binding, thereby inhibiting TR action on all known types of T_3 response elements (TREs)—palindromes (TREpal), direct repeats (DR+4), and inverted palindromes (TRE-IR). However, on the TRE-IR this effect is even more pronounced, because the normal TR homodimer dissociates after binding T_3, whereas the mutant TRs are deficient in T_3 binding and stay bound to the TRE, thereby blocking access by functional TRs.

Summary and Conclusions

Thyroid hormones are essential for the embryonal and postnatal development of the brain. Only a few of thyroid hormone–regulated genes and proteins involved in the maturation of the brain have been identified so far—among them certain microtubule and associated proteins, as well as myelin basic protein and neurotropins. Some of these genes were shown to be directly regulated by thyroid hormones at the transcriptional level where T_3 binds to specific DNA-binding nuclear receptor proteins, the TRs. The ligand-activated TR bound to DNA response elements in the promoter region of these target genes is subsequently able to recruit various coactivator proteins, thereby assembling a DNA-bound multiprotein complex resulting in transcriptional activation or inhibition. The diversity of proteins involved in mediating T_3 action also provides multiple opportunities for interference from other signaling pathways—for example, by competition for limited amounts of cofactors. The physiological relevance of such protein interactions in vivo resulting in the modulation of thyroid hormone action in target tissues is best illustrated by the autosomal dominant genetic human disorder of resistance to thyroid hormones, in which a transcriptionally silent TR mutant is able to induce hormone resistance by inhibiting the activity of the normal TRs encoded by the nonmutant alleles. The presence of other "dominant negative" regulators of thyroid hormone action—such as TRα2 and PPARs in many thyroid hormone–responsive tissues, including the brain—suggests that target cells have the ability to adapt their physiological responses to relatively constant serum levels of thyroid hormones.

References

Aniello F, Couchie D, Bridoux AM, et al: Splicing of juvenile and adult *tau* mRNA variants is regulated by thyroid hormone. Proc Natl Acad Sci U S A 88:4035–4039, 1991a

Aniello F, Couchie D, Gripois D, et al: Regulation of five tubulin isotypes by thyroid hormone during brain development. J Neurochem 57: 1781–1786, 1991b

Baas D, Bourbeau D, Carre JL, et al: Expression of alpha and beta thyroid receptors during oligodendrocyte differentiation. Neuroreport 5: 1805–1808, 1994a

Baas D, Fressinaud C, Ittel ME, et al: Expression of thyroid hormone receptor isoforms in rat oligodendrocyte cultures: effect of 3,5,3'-triiodo-L-thyronine. Neurosci Lett 176:47–51, 1994b

Baker BS, Tata JR: Accumulation of proto-oncogene c-erb-A–related transcripts during *Xenopus* development: association with early acquisition of response to thyroid hormone and estrogen. EMBO J 9:879–885, 1990

Beckett GJ, Arthur JA: The iodothyronine deiodinases and 5'-deiodination. Baillieres Clin Endocrinol Metab 8:285–304, 1994

Bernal J, Nunez J: Thyroid hormones and brain development. Eur J Endocrinol 133:390–398, 1995

Bhat MK, Ashizawa K, Cheng SY: Phosphorylation enhances the target gene sequence-dependent dimerization of thyroid hormone receptor with retinoid X receptor. Proc Natl Acad Sci U S A 91:7927–7931, 1994

Black MA, Pope L, Lefebvre FA, et al: Thyroid hormones precociously increase nerve growth factor gene expression in the submandibular gland of neonatal mice. Endocrinology 130:2083–2090, 1992

Bogazzi F, Hudson LD, Nikodem VM: A novel heterodimerization partner for thyroid hormone receptor-peroxisome proliferator-activated receptor. J Biol Chem 269:11683–11686, 1994

Bradley DJ, Young WS III, Weinberger C: Differential expression of alpha and beta thyroid hormone receptor genes in rat brain and pituitary. Proc Natl Acad Sci U S A 86:7250–7254, 1989

Bradley DJ, Towle HC, Young WS III: Spatial and temporal expression of alpha- and beta-thyroid hormone receptor mRNAs, including the beta 2-subtype, in the developing mammalian nervous system. J Neurosci 12:2288–2302, 1992

Bradley DJ, Towle HC, Young WS III: Alpha- and beta-thyroid hormone receptor (TR) gene expression during auditory neurogenesis: evidence for TR isoform-specific transcriptional regulation in vivo. Proc Natl Acad Sci U S A 91:439–443, 1994

Braissant O, Foufelle F, Scotto C, et al: Differential expression of peroxisome proliferator-activated receptors (PDARs): tissue distribution of PPAR α, β, and γ in the adult rat. Endocrinology 137:354–366, 1996

Brucker-Davis F, Skarulis MC, Grace MB, et al: Genetic and clinical features of 42 kindreds with resistance to thyroid hormone: the National Institutes of Health Prospective Study. Ann Intern Med 123:572–583, 1995

Burrow GN, Fisher DA, Larsen PR: Maternal and fetal thyroid function. N Engl J Med 331:1072–1078, 1994

Cavailles V, Dauvois S, Danielian PS, et al: Interaction of proteins with transcriptionally active estrogen receptors. Proc Natl Acad Sci U S A 91:10009–10013, 1994

Chanoine JP, Braverman LE: The role of transthyretin in the transport of thyroid hormone to cerebrospinal fluid and brain. Acta Med Austriaca 19 (suppl 1):25–28, 1992

Chanoine JP, Safran M, Farwell AP, et al: Effects of selenium deficiency on thyroid hormone economy in rats. Endocrinology 131:1787–1792, 1992a

Chanoine JP, Safran M, Farwell AP, et al: Selenium deficiency and type II 5′-deiodinase regulation in the euthyroid and hypothyroid rat—evidence of a direct effect of thyroxine. Endocrinology 131:479–484, 1992b

Chatterjee VKK, Tata JR: Thyroid hormone receptors and their role in development. Cancer Surv 14:147–167, 1992

Chatterjee VKK, Nagaya T, Madison LD, et al: Thyroid hormone resistance syndrome—inhibition of normal receptor function by mutant thyroid hormone receptors. J Clin Invest 87:1977–1984, 1991

Chen JD, Evans RM: A transcriptional co-repressor that interacts with nuclear hormone receptors. Nature 377:454–457, 1995

Chu RY, Madison LD, Lin YL, et al: Thyroid hormone (T_3) inhibits ciprofibrate-induced transcription of genes encoding b-oxidation enzymes: cross talk between peroxisome proliferator and T_3 signaling pathways. Proc Natl Acad Sci U S A 92:11593–11597, 1995

Darling DS, Carter RL, Yen PM, et al: Different dimerization activities of alpha and beta thyroid hormone receptor isoforms. J Biol Chem 268:10221–10227, 1993

Davey JC, Becker KB, Schneider MJ, et al: Cloning of a cDNA for the type II iodothyronine deiodinase. J Biol Chem 270:26786–26789, 1995

Escobar-Morreale HF, Obregón MJ, Del Rey FE, et al: Replacement therapy for hypothyroidism with thyroxine alone does not ensure euthyroidism in all tissues, as studied in thyroidectomized rats. J Clin Invest 96:2828–2838, 1995

Evans RM: The steroid and thyroid hormone receptor superfamily. Science 240:889–895, 1988
Falcone M, Miyamoto T, Fierrorenoy F, et al: Evaluation of the ontogeny of thyroid hormone receptor isotypes in rat brain and liver using an immunohistochemical technique. Eur J Endocrinol 130:97–106, 1994
Farsetti A, Mitsuhashi T, Desvergne B, et al: Molecular basis of thyroid hormone regulation of myelin basic protein gene expression in rodent brain. J Biol Chem 266:23226–23232, 1991
Farsetti A, Desvergne B, Hallenbeck P, et al: Characterization of myelin basic protein thyroid hormone response element and its function in the context of native and heterologous promoter. J Biol Chem 267: 15784–15788, 1992
Farwell AP, Dibenedetto DJ, Leonard JL: Thyroxine targets different pathways of internalization of type II iodothyronine 5'-deiodinase in astrocytes. J Biol Chem 268:5055–5062, 1993
Fisher DA, Dussault JH, Sack J, et al: Ontogenesis of hypothalamic-pituitary-thyroid function and metabolism in man, sheep, and rat. Recent Prog Horm Res 33:59–116, 1976
Fondell JD, Roy AL, Roeder RG: Unliganded thyroid hormone receptor inhibits formation of a functional preinitiation complex—implications for active repression. Genes Dev 7:1400–1410, 1993
Forman BM, Tontonoz P, Chen J, et al: 15-Deoxy-delta^{12,14}-prostaglandin J$_2$ is a ligand for the adipocyte determination factor PPARgamma. Cell 83:803–812, 1995a
Forman BM, Umesono K, Chen J, et al: Unique response pathways are established by allosteric interactions among nuclear hormone receptors. Cell 81:541–550, 1995b
Halachmi S, Marden E, Martin G, et al: Estrogen receptor–associated proteins: possible mediators of hormone-induced transcription. Science 264:1455–1458, 1994
Hallenbeck PL, Phyillaier M, Nikodem VM: Divergent effects of 9-cis-retinoic acid receptor on positive and negative thyroid hormone receptor-dependent gene expression. J Biol Chem 268:3825–3828, 1993
Hodin RA, Lazar MA, Wintman BI, et al: Identification of a thyroid hormone receptor that is pituitary-specific. Science 244:76–79, 1989
Hörlein A, Näär AM, Heinzel T, et al: A transcriptional co-repressor that interacts with nuclear hormone receptors. Nature 377:397–404, 1995

Iniguez MA, Rodriguez-Peña A, Ibarrola N, et al: Adult rat brain is sensitive to thyroid hormone—regulation of RC3/neurogranin messenger RNA. J Clin Invest 90:554–558, 1992

Juge-Aubry CE, Gorla-Bajszczak A, Pernin A, et al: Peroxisome proliferator–activated receptor mediates cross-talk with thyroid hormone receptor by competition for retinoid X receptor. J Biol Chem 270:18117–18122, 1995

Kainu T, Wikström A-C, Gustafsson J-Å, et al: Localization of the peroxisome proliferator-activated receptor in the brain. Neuroreport, 5:2481–2485, 1994

Katz D, Berrodin TJ, Lazar MA: The unique C-termini of the thyroid hormone receptor variant, C-erbA alpha$_2$, and thyroid hormone receptor alpha$_1$ mediate different DNA-binding and heterodimerization properties. Mol Endocrinol 6:805–814, 1992

Katz D, Reginato MJ, Lazar MA: Functional regulation of thyroid hormone receptor variant TRa2 by phosphorylation. Mol Cell Biol 15:2341–2348, 1995

Kawahara A, Baker BS, Tata JR: Developmental and regional expression of thyroid hormone receptor genes during *Xenopus* metamorphosis. Development 112:933–943, 1991

Kliewer SA, Lenhard JM, Willson TM, et al: A prostaglandin J$_2$ metabolite binds peroxisome proliferator-activated receptor gamma and promotes adipocyte differentiation. Cell 83:813–819, 1995

Larsen PR, Berry MJ: Type I iodothyronine deiodinase: unexpected complexities in a simple deiodination reaction. Thyroid 4:357–362, 1994

Larsen PR, Silva JE, Kaplan MM: Relationship between circulating and intracellular thyroid hormones: physiological and clinical implications. Endocr Rev 2:87–102, 1981

Laudet V, Hänni C, Coll J, et al: Evolution of the nuclear receptor gene superfamily. EMBO J 11:1003–1013, 1992

Lazar MA: Thyroid hormone receptors—multiple forms, multiple possibilities. Endocr Rev 14:184–193, 1993

Lebel JM, Dussault JH, Puymirat J: Overexpression of the beta$_1$ thyroid receptor induces differentiation in neuro-2a cells. Proc Natl Acad Sci U S A 91:2644–2648, 1994

Lee JW, Ryan F, Swaffield JC, et al: Interaction of thyroid-hormone receptor with a conserved transcriptional mediator. Nature 374:91–94, 1995

Lindholm D, Castren E, Tsoulfas P, et al: Neurotropin-3 induced by tri-iodothyronine in cerebellar granule cells promotes Purkinje cell differentiation. J Cell Biol 122:443–450, 1993

Liu R-T, Suzuki S, Miyamoto T, et al: The dominant negative effect of thyroid hormone receptor splicing variant a2 does not require binding to a thyroid response element. Mol Endocrinol 9:86–95, 1995

Mandel SJ, Berry MJ, Kieffer JD, et al: Cloning and in vitro expression of the human selenoprotein, type I iodothyronine deiodinase. J Clin Endocrinol Metab 75:1133–1139, 1992

Mangelsdorf DJ, Evans RM: The RXR heterodimers and orphan receptors. Cell 83:841–850, 1995

Mangelsdorf DJ, Thummel C, Beato M, et al: The nuclear receptor superfamily: the second decade. Cell 83:835–839, 1995

Maruo T, Katayama K, Matuso H, et al: The role of maternal thyroid hormones in maintaining early pregnancy in threatened abortion. Acta Endocrinol 127:118–122, 1992

Meier CA, Dickstein BM, Ashizawa K, et al: Variable transcriptional activity and ligand binding of mutant $beta_1$ 3,5,3'-triiodothyronine receptors from four families with generalized resistance to thyroid hormone. Mol Endocrinol 6:248–258, 1992

Meier CA, Parkison C, Chen A, et al: Interaction of human beta-1 thyroid hormone receptor and its mutants with DNA and retinoid-X receptor-beta: T_3 response element dependent dominant negative potency. J Clin Invest 92:1986–1993, 1993

Meier-Heusler SC, Zhu X, Juge-Aubry C, et al: Modulation of thyroid hormone action by mutant thyroid hormone receptors, c-erbAα2 and peroxisome proliferator-activated receptor: evidence for different mechanisms of inhibition. Mol Cell Endocrinol 107:55–66, 1995

Morreale de Escobar G, Obregon MJ, Calvo R, et al: Effects of iodine deficiency on thyroid hormone metabolism and the brain in fetal rats: the role of the maternal transfer of thyroxin. Am J Clin Nutr 57:280S–285S, 1993

Munoz A, Wrighton C, Seliger B, et al: Thyroid hormone receptor/c-erbA—control of commitment and differentiation in the neuronal chromaffin progenitor line-PC12. J Cell Biol 121:423–438, 1993

Nagaya T, Jameson JL: Thyroid hormone receptor dimerization is required for dominant negative inhibition by mutations that cause thyroid hormone resistance. J Biol Chem 268:15766–15771, 1993

Nagaya T, Madison LD, Jameson JL: Thyroid hormone receptor mutants that cause resistance to thyroid hormone—evidence for receptor competition for DNA sequences in target genes. J Biol Chem 267: 13014–13019, 1992

Palha JA, Episkopou V, Maeda S, et al: Thyroid hormone metabolism in a transthyretin-null mouse strain. J Biol Chem 269:33135–33139, 1994

Pastor R, Bernal J, Rodriguez-Peña A: Unliganded c-erbA/thyroid hormone receptor induces *trkB* expression in neuroblastoma cells. Oncogene 9:1081–1089, 1994

Pontecorvi A, Robbins J: The plasma membrane and thyroid hormone entry into cells. Trends Endocrinol Metab 1:90–94, 1989

Porterfield SP, Hendrich CE: The role of thyroid hormones in prenatal and neonatal neurological development—current perspectives. Endocr Rev 14:94–106, 1993

Refetoff S, Weiss RE, Usala SJ: The syndromes of resistance to thyroid hormone. Endocr Rev 14:348–399, 1993

Robbins J, Lakshmanan M: The movement of thyroid hormones in the central nervous system. Acta Med Austriaca 19 (suppl 1):21–25, 1992

Rodriguez-Peña A, Ibarrola N, Iniguez MA, et al: Neonatal hypothyroidism affects the timely expression of myelin-associated glycoprotein in the rat brain. J Clin Invest 91:812–818, 1993

Rosen ED, Odonnell AL, Koenig RJ: Ligand-dependent synergy of thyroid hormone and retinoid X-receptors. J Biol Chem 267:22010–22013, 1992

Schueler PA, Schwartz HL, Strait KA, et al: Binding of 3,5,3'-triiodothyronine (T_3) and its analogs to the in vitro translational products of c-erb A protooncogenes: differences in the affinity of the alpha- and beta-forms for the acetic acid analog and failure of the human testis and kidney alpha-2 prod. Mol Endocrinol 4:227–234, 1990

Schwartz HL, Lazar MA, Oppenheimer JH: Widespread distribution of immunoreactive thyroid hormone beta$_2$ receptor (TR beta$_2$) in the nuclei of extrapituitary rat tissues. J Biol Chem 269:24777–24782, 1994

Silva JE, Larsen PR: Regulation of thyroid hormone expression at the prereceptor and receptor levels, in Thyroid Hormone Metabolism. Edited by Henneman G. New York, Marcel Dekker, 1986, pp 441–500

Southwell BR, Tu GF, Duan W, et al: Cerebral expression of transthyretin: evolution, ontogeny and function. Acta Med Austriaca 19 (suppl 1): 28–31, 1992

St. Germain DL: Iodothyronine deiodinases. Trends Endocrinol Metab 5:36–42, 1994

Sugawara A, Yen PM, Apriletti JW, et al: Phosphorylation selectively increases triiodothyronine receptor homodimer binding to DNA. J Biol Chem 269:433–437, 1994

Suzuki S, Miyamoto T, Opsahl A, et al: Two thyroid hormone response elements are present in the promoter of human thyroid hormone receptor beta$_1$. Mol Endocrinol 8:305–314, 1994

Takeda K, Sakurai A, DeGroot LJ, et al: Recessive inheritance of thyroid hormone resistance caused by complete deletion of the protein-coding region of the thyroid hormone receptor-beta gene. J Clin Endocrinol Metab 74:49–55, 1992

Tata JR: Autoregulation and crossregulation of nuclear receptor genes. Trends Endocrinol Metab 5:283–290, 1994

Tata JR, Baker BS, Machuca I, et al: General review—autoinduction of nuclear receptor genes and its significance. J Steroid Biochem Mol Biol 46:105–119, 1993

Tomura H, Lazar J, Phyillaier M, et al: The N-terminal region (A/B) of rat thyroid hormone receptors $\alpha 1$, $\beta 1$, but not $\beta 2$ contains a strong thyroid hormone-dependent transactivation function. Proc Natl Acad Sci U S A 92:5600–5604, 1995

Umesono K, Evans RM: Determinants of target gene specificity for steroid/thyroid hormone receptors. Cell 57:1139–1146, 1989

Umesono K, Murakami KK, Thompson CC, et al: Direct repeats as selective response elements for the thyroid hormone, retinoic acid, and vitamin D_3 receptors. Cell 65:1255–1266, 1991

Vulsma T, Gons MH, de Vijlder JJ: Maternal-fetal transfer of thyroxine in congenital hypothyroidism due to a total organification defect or thyroid agenesis. N Engl J Med 321:13–16, 1989

Weiss RE, Marcocci C, Bruno-Bossio G, et al: Multiple genetic factors in the heterogeneity of thyroid hormone resistance. J Clin Endocrinol Metab 76:257–259, 1993

Wills KN, Zhang X, Pfahl M: Coordinate expression of functionally distinct thyroid hormone receptor alpha isoforms during neonatal brain development. Mol Endocrinol 5:1109–1119, 1991

Yen PM, Chin WW: Minireview: molecular mechanisms of dominant negative activity by nuclear hormone receptors. Mol Endocrinol 8:1450–1454, 1994

Yen PM, Darling DS, Carter RL, et al: Triiodothyronine (T_3) decreases binding to DNA by T_3-receptor homodimers but not receptor-auxiliary protein heterodimers. J Biol Chem 267:3565–3568, 1992a

Yen PM, Sugawara A, Refetoff S, et al: New insights on the mechanism(s) of the dominant negative effect of mutant thyroid hormone receptor in generalized resistance to thyroid hormone. J Clin Invest 90:1825–1831, 1992b

Yen PM, Wilcox EC, Hayashi Y, et al: Studies on the repression of basal transcription (silencing) by artificial and natural human thyroid hormone receptor-β mutants. Endocrinology 136:2845–2851, 1995

Zavacki AM, Harney JW, Brent GA, et al: Dominant negative inhibition by mutant thyroid hormone receptors is thyroid hormone response element and receptor isoform specific. Mol Endocrinol 7:1319–1330, 1993

Zou LL, Hagen SG, Strait KA, et al: Identification of thyroid hormone response elements in rodent PCP-2, a developmentally regulated gene of cerebellar Purkinje cells. J Biol Chem 269:13346–13352, 1994

Part II

Clinical Studies of Thyroid Diseases in Infancy and Childhood

Chapter 3

Overview of Newborn Screening for Congenital Hypothyroidism

Kenneth Pass, Ph.D.

The goal of newborn screening is early identification of children at increased risk for selected metabolic or genetic diseases so that medical treatment can be promptly initiated to avert metabolic crises and prevent irreversible neurological and developmental sequelae. Babies are screened during the first few days of life using blood collected from a heel-stick onto special paper. Not all of the more than 300 gene disorders linked to specific biochemical defects are amenable to newborn screening, most being either too rare to be of public health concern or lacking any effective therapeutic intervention. However, today every state in the nation provides screening for phenylketonuria (PKU) and congenital hypothyroidism (CH) through a newborn screening program (Council of Regional Networks for Genetics Services [CORN] Newborn Screening Committee 1995). Screening efforts for these two disorders have established the scope of benefits that can be achieved through newborn screening, whereby early identification and treatment have the potential to change the course of the infant's life. On the basis of pilot studies, the availability of funds, and the abilities and limitations of screening technology, organizations across the nation have selected the conditions most suitable for inclusion in screening programs for their populations. As with any laboratory test, both false-negative and false-positive results are possible. Thus it is important to remember that screening test results provide insufficient information on which to base a diagnosis or treatment (Levy 1990). This chapter describes the development and practice of newborn screening, with emphasis on congenital hypothyroidism.

Historical Background

"Mental retardation is perhaps the greatest single source of human suffering." So begins Pearl Buck in the foreword to a 1963 monograph on phenylketonuria (Buck 1963). She continues, "Since there are relatively few cases of phenylketonuria among the mentally retarded, the argument has sometimes been made that the expense of universal testing of babies is not practical. The argument is now logically defeated." Those words, written more than 30 years ago, still ring with truth. Witness the provision of newborn screening for PKU and hypothyroidism to every newborn child in the United States (CORN Newborn Screening Committee 1995), the adoption of this public health program by every one of the "developed nations," and its high priority in the nations moving into this group (Levy 1990).

Newborn screening as it is known today can be traced to a persistent mother in Norway at the end of the 19th century (Lyman 1963). Her unrelenting efforts to find the reason for the peculiar behavior of her two children led her to the biochemist and physician Asbjörn Fölling. Fölling observed that urine from these children turned green when ferric chloride was added. Through painstaking analytical work, and the use of more than 20 L of urine collected by the dutiful mother, Fölling identified the substance in the urine as phenylpyruvic acid. From that observation, he theorized that a disturbance in metabolism of phenylalanine (phe) might be responsible for the mental retardation in the two children. Surveys organized by Fölling in local nursing homes and a local school for the retarded uncovered eight more individuals with a positive urine test. Fölling published his findings in 1934 (Fölling 1934), and thus was laid the first brick in the structure known today as newborn screening.

Fölling had shown that a simple color change in urine could be used to detect individuals with PKU. Early attempts at screening involved testing urine for these ketones using ferric chloride—a test that became known as the "wet diaper test." But a test without a concomitant therapy was less than useful. Nearly a half century later, Bickel devised a simple dietary therapy for PKU that prevented the effects of the condition from appearing (Bickel 1954).

Thus by 1961 there was a method for detecting PKU and a means for treating the condition (i.e., lowering the phe level). Early trials with the diaper test, particularly those conducted in California (Poole 1963), revealed an unacceptably high rate of false-negative results. In addition, it was impractical to design a large-scale screening program using urine, or a wet diaper, as the specimen source. These technical failures (as well as two personal tragedies) led Dr. Robert Guthrie, a physician-microbiologist in Buffalo, New York, to develop the dried blood specimen and the analytical test procedures that are used today throughout the world in newborn screening (Guthrie 1992).

Dr. Guthrie organized the first trials for screening newborns for PKU, with a goal of testing one million infants using the dried blood specimen and the bacterial inhibition assay (BIA). In the early 1960s he coordinated a 29-state pilot study of 400,000 newborns, which proved so successful in identifying infants affected with PKU that many states instituted screening programs immediately. The results of those trials proved conclusively that infants could be screened for PKU shortly after birth using a specimen that was easy to obtain, safe to handle, and easily transportable (Guthrie and Whitney 1964). The BIA provides a semiquantitative measurement of the phe in a dried blood specimen, thereby identifying newborns who have elevated levels of phe and thus are at risk for PKU.

From Dr. Guthrie's efforts has grown a system of programs to ensure that every newborn baby in the United States—over 4 million annually—receives a screen for PKU and hypothyroidism. Many newborn screening programs, mostly sponsored by state public health departments, also test for other congenital conditions such as sickle cell disease, biotinidase deficiency, homocystinuria, maple syrup urine disease (MSUD) (branched-chain ketonuria), galactosemia, and congenital adrenal hyperplasia

(CORN Newborn Screening Committee 1995).

In 1992, more than 1,500 infants were identified with one of these conditions and referred for medical care. Since the adoption of newborn screening in 1963, more than 4,200 infants with PKU have been identified and placed under care (CORN Newborn Screening Committee 1995). Many of them are now productive members of society. Certainly, as Pearl Buck said, "The argument [against screening] is now logically defeated." Newborn screening is a routine part of medical care, providing important information for pediatricians, even in the absence of one of the screened conditions (American Academy of Pediatrics 1992). Perhaps more important—certainly so, according to Dr. Guthrie—the specimen used for this test is a dried blood specimen collected by heel-stick from the newborn baby at a few days of age.

In honor of Dr. Guthrie, who recently died, the specimen type he developed is now known as the Guthrie spot. The Guthrie spot has become the standard for all newborn testing programs throughout the world. It has proved to be reliable for tests measuring metabolites (phenylalanine), hormones (T_4), proteins (hemoglobin), and now DNA. The specimen has been used in other ways also, ranging from police work (drug testing) to farming (genotyping of cattle).

When newborn screening programs were initiated, New York was one of the first states to provide testing for all its newborns, with legislation enacted in 1964 (New York Public Health Law 2500-a) initiating newborn screening for PKU in 1965. After several amendments to this law, the New York Newborn Screening program today includes eight disorders: PKU, MSUD, homocystinuria, galactosemia, sickle hemoglobin, congenital hypothyroidism, HIV-1 antibodies, and biotinidase deficiency. Since 1965, more than eight million newborns have been screened by the New York Newborn Screening Program, with over 6,000 infants diagnosed with one of these congenital conditions after initial detection by screening.

New York's screening profile is among the most comprehensive in the United States and requires reporting of over 2.1 million test results each year. The eight disorders now included in the screening profile of the New York Newborn Screening Program have an incidence ranging from 1:2,100 to 1:339,000, but all share the feature of not being readily diagnosed at birth without the specialized testing offered by the Newborn Screening Program.

A recent review by Thomas Carter, former director of the New York screening program, summarizes the program and discusses the disorders constituting the profile (Carter and Willey 1986). Disorders that are now a part of other screening programs in the United States and that are being considered for possible addition to the New York program include congenital adrenal hyperplasia and cystic fibrosis. With some minor exceptions, all of these conditions meet the requirements presented by the World Health Organization (WHO) for newborn screening programs (WHO Scientific Group 1968). Each is a definable medical condition, has an accepted laboratory test, is amenable to therapeutic intervention, and occurs at sufficiently high frequency to warrant public health intervention. The fulfillment of these requirements, which led to the addition of thyroid testing to newborn screening programs, is described in the following section.

Newborn Thyroid Screening

Hypothyroidism results from an inadequate supply of the thyroid hormone thyroxine (T_4). Approximately 1 of every 4,000 newborn infants has hypothyroidism. Left untreated, hypothyroidism will result in growth impairment and mental retardation. Congenital hypothyroidism (CH) is caused by a biochemical defect that reduces thyroid hormone secretion and consequently causes a deficiency in circulating T_4. Fewer than 10% of cases are genetically determined (Fisher 1978). This deficiency in thyroid hormone can result from the absence of a thyroid gland, incomplete or ectopic gland development, thyroid inflammation resulting from autoimmune disorders, hereditary defects in thyroid hormone synthesis, or an inability to synthesize T_4 because of dietary iodine deficiency (Fisher 1978). Infants with CH may appear clinically normal up to 6 months of age, but they are unable to produce adequate amounts of T_4 for normal organ function and brain development. Laboratory tests are the only reliable means of diagnosing CH in the newborn infant. Some of the more commonly described clinical findings—jaundice, constipation, lethargy, feeding problems, large tongue, puffy face, distended abdomen, and umbilical hernia—are nonspecific for CH and are found in fewer than 30% of neonates with CH. Therefore, in the newborn, clinical signs and symptoms are not reliable indicators of CH (Levy 1990).

Goiter has been known since 3,000 B.C., when it was first described in Chinese writings, and depictions of cretinism can be seen in pre-Columbian sculptures dating from the fifth century (Hetzel 1971). However, it was not until the early 20th century that the relationship between adequacy of treatment of cretins and improved mental development was defined (Brunch and McCune 1944). It was even more recently that the importance of early treatment with thyroid hormone in preventing mental retardation due to thyroid deficiency was recognized (Raiti and Newns 1971). In the early 1970s it was reported that treatment of CH before 3 months of age was critical for maximum mental development (Klein et al. 1972). However, early treatment was not the norm, because CH was not usually diagnosed until well into the first year of life. At about the same time, the notion that adequate amounts of T_4 for fetal development were provided via placental transfer of maternal T_4 came into question. Fisher (Fisher et al. 1964) showed conclusively that this was not the case and that the fetal thyroid system in fact develops autonomously such that an athyrotic fetus demonstrates low serum T_4 and elevated serum thyrotropin (thyroid-stimulating hormone, TSH) in utero (Fisher et al. 1973). Thus there could be no protective effects from the maternal environment for a thyroid-deficient fetus.

Congenital hypothyroidism may be caused by a variety of defects in the biosynthesis of thyroid hormone (LaFranchi 1979). The presence of goiter is the hallmark of these defects, the condition being termed *goitrous hypothyroidism* or *goitrous cretinism.* This condition is reported by newborn screening programs in approximately 1 in 50,000 births. In most instances it is inherited as an autosomal recessive trait (LaFranchi 1979). Congenital hypothyroidism can also result from TSH deficiency, which is reported in approximately 1 in 110,000 births. This deficiency may occur in any of the conditions associated with the developmental defects of the pituitary or hypothalamus or in children with idiopathic hypopituitarism. In these cases challenge with thyrotropin-releasing hormone is necessary to rule out hypothalamic involvement (Behrman and Vaughn 1983).

Congenital hypothyroidism is more than twice as common in girls as in boys. The clinical signs and symptoms are usually absent or are so nonspecific or subtle that the majority of infants look completely normal at birth. There is a tendency for infants with congenital hypothyroidism to have prolonged gestation (20% > 42 weeks) and increased birth weight (33% > 90th percentile), although they are normal in birth length and head circumference (LaFranchi 1979).

Among infants with congenital hypothyroidism, the incidence of cardiac malformations is almost five times that of the general population. (Cassio et al. 1994) (Table 3–1). Other malformations frequently reported include esophageal atresia and cleft palate (Fernhoff et al. 1987; Grant and Smith 1988; New England Congenital Hypothyroidism Collaborative 1988; Siebner et al. 1992). Cassio (Cassio et al. 1994) offered the hypothesis that a common teratogenic insult to the embryological area shared by these tissues may be responsible for these observations and therefore suggested that the presence of any of these malformations should alert the clinician to the possibility of concomitant hypothyroidism.

These reports in the 1970s of treatment efficacy for CH and lack of clinical signs at birth, coupled with the difficulty of making a diagnosis of CH during the first few months of life (Van Gemund and DeAngulao 1997), set the stage for the initiation of newborn screening for CH. During this same time, radioimmunoassays (RIAs), then routinely available for serum thyroid studies, were improved in sensitivity so that the Guthrie spot could be used as a specimen (Dussault and Laberge 1973), thereby completing the requisites for the introduction of CH testing into newborn screening. Adding CH testing to the existing PKU newborn screening programs facilitated its introduction, so that within 5 years of pilot

Table 3–1. Congenital malformations associated with congenital hypothyroidism (CH)

Reference	CH infants	Malformations (all, %)	Cardiac malformations (%)
Majeed-Saidan et al. 1993	25	24.0	16.0
Fernhoff et al. 1987	100	23.0	13.0
Siebner et al. 1992	243	15.6	5.8
Cassio et al. 1994	235	9.4	3.4
Rosenthal et al. 1988	100	9.0	3.0
Lazarus and Hughes 1988	1538	8.0	2.3
Grant and Smith 1988	493	7.3	1.2

Source. Adapted from Cassio et al. 1994.

studies in Quebec (Dussault et al. 1975), almost all programs in the United States had added CH testing to their newborn screening profiles. Mandated screening for CH in New York was initiated in 1978 as RIAs for T_4 and TSH became available that were sufficiently sensitive and specific for use on Guthrie spots (Bellisario and Carter 1986). Many European and Asian programs also rapidly adopted CH testing.

Current Practices for Screening, Diagnosis, and Treatment

The assays initially available for use on the Guthrie spot were for T_4, and thus most programs in the United States used analysis of T_4 as the primary mechanism to screen for CH. However, it was soon recognized that infants with manifest athyrosis could have measurable levels of T_4 at birth typical of unaffected infants (Fisher 1986). These cases could be detected only using an assay for TSH. Thus, to maximize the effectiveness of screening programs, a two-tiered approach to screening was adopted in which the infants were first tested with a T_4 assay, and those with low T_4 levels were then tested for TSH level. A "positive" screen would result when T_4 level was low and TSH was elevated. This remains the primary mechanism used by most programs in the United States (CORN Newborn Screening Committee 1995). Unlike their counterparts in the United States, screening programs in Canada, Europe, and Asia adopted a strategy of initial testing for TSH with no testing for T_4. These programs have been quite successful, with no apparent differences in detection rates or false-positive reports from the T_4/TSH systems (Fisher et al. 1979). Initially, the ease of automating the T_4 assay proved the attraction for programs in the United States, which generally process larger numbers of specimens. Recently, with improvements in automation and improved sensitivity of the assay, several United States programs have adopted the TSH strategy (Foley and Torresani 1995).

Another possibility for hypothyroid screening was recently proposed: the use of free T_4 (FT_4) measurements. Whereas measurement of total T_4 in the Guthrie spot is widely used, it is recognized that a large number of false-positive reports will occur, requiring follow-up testing to confirm the initial findings. With the use of the newer and more sensitive TSH tests, this obstacle is largely overcome, but these tests cannot detect secondary or tertiary hypothyroidism. Analysis with FT_4 could possibly surmount both these problems, although it brings with it the handicap of transient low FT_4 values in premature and low–birth weight babies (Ashida et al. 1992). Thus the definitive newborn screening test for hypothyroidism remains elusive.

Regardless of the analyte chosen for assay, a critical function is determination of the "cutoff level," the value at which normal results become abnormal, requiring further follow-up testing. Most screening program use an algorithm that incorporates control values of the assay, comparison with the population mean (historical mean of the program), and clinical chemistry quality assessments. Screening programs differ in the mechanisms used, but they typically maintain their competency through proficiency testing programs such as that offered by the Centers for Disease Control and Prevention (Slazyk and Hannon 1993). Nevertheless, it is incumbent on the physician to know and understand the procedures used by the screening laboratory so that reported results can be properly interpreted.

Most newborn screening programs operate on a regional or state/province basis. An emphatic attention to details within a program ensures maximum efficiency, so that most children are now identified and diagnosed as soon after birth as possible. However, organizational efficiency varies widely among programs; the better organized programs are able to provide earlier treatment and have fewer missed diagnoses. Because of efforts to increase sensitivity, false-positive rates are often high, which can be associated with undue and long-lasting psychological distress (Bodegard et al. 1982).

In premature infants, there appears to be a physiological reduction in blood T_4 levels. This is not due to thyroxine-binding globulin (TBG) deficiency, and the TSH levels are not usually elevated. These patients need special follow-up to ensure that the T_4 concentration rises to the normal range as the infant matures, as occurs in all normal patients (LaFranchi 1979). Altogether, approximately

10% of infants identified by screening programs will demonstrate this transient type of hypothyroidism (Fisher et al. 1979). It has recently been reported that measurement of TSH binding inhibitory activity from the dried blood specimen can provide a mechanism to identify some of these infants, who would otherwise require complete clinical workup (Brown et al. 1993)

In addition to the timing of specimen collection (see below), other events during the perinatal period can have a profound influence on assessment of thyroid status in the newborn. Chief among these is perinatal exposure to iodine, either through the use of iodine-containing antiseptics on the breast-feeding mother or in care of the infant's umbilical cord (Francis et al. 1982). These effects are not unexpected, resulting almost surely from the antithyroid effects of excess iodine (the Wolff-Chaikoff effect) (Delange 1990). The effects are usually transient and pose no problem, except when one is trying to interpret newborn screening results, in which case these infants appear to be hypothyroid (Francis et al. 1982; Grüters et al. 1982). Subsequent testing at a later date will usually demonstrate normal thyroid values. Obviously, this problem can be completely prevented by selection of a non-iodine-based antiseptic for the neonatal period. However, the situation becomes somewhat more problematic, because contained within this false-positive group of infants whose thyroid physiology is temporarily disrupted are infants demonstrating the same initial screening results (low normal T_4 and mild elevation of TSH) but who remain mildly hypothyroid. Appropriate therapy for this group of infants is controversial (Harada et al. 1994). Tyfield could find no clinical sequelae in three children with mild hypothyroidism who received no hormone therapy (Tyfield et al. 1991). Others strongly recommend hormone replacement in children with mild hypothyroidism (Alm et al. 1984; Harada et al. 1995; LaFranchi et al. 1985).

Detection of CH does not depend on nutritional factors. The majority of hypothyroid infants are detected on the basis of the initial blood specimen even if it is collected within a few hours after birth. However, in the first 24 hours after birth, TSH values may be transiently elevated; the normal newborn demonstrates a TSH surge in the first hours of life as an adaptation to the extrauterine environment. Thus, the newborn specimen should be collected as late as possible after birth, but no later than 72 hours. As is true with other conditions, a blood transfusion may alter the test results. Therefore, the newborn screening specimen should always be collected before a blood transfusion, regardless of the infant's age.

It is important for primary physicians to be cognizant of these late-appearing forms of CH in order to make a clinical diagnosis immediately and to prevent subsequent impairment associated with a delay during infancy. The need is paramount for all screening programs to have an explicit policy that emphasizes to pediatricians and parents that signs suggestive of congenital hypothyroidism should never be ignored merely because the infant has "passed" the neonatal screening test (DeGroot et al. 1996; Fisher 1991). Not to be overlooked is the possibility of human error in failing to identify affected infants at the laboratory or hospital or the failure to test an infant who is transferred between hospitals during the neonatal period (DeGroot et al. 1996).

Confirmatory diagnosis of CH involves notification of the primary physician or the family by the screening laboratory or a designated representative. This must be accomplished as soon as possible. Diagnosis is based on a reduced serum T_4, elevated serum TSH, and low FT_4 index. Serum TBG measurement is useful in confirming athyrosis, since TBG is absent in these children. Although most newborns with CH appear normal at birth, there may be some with mild clinical symptoms and signs, such as jaundice, umbilical hernias, and constipation. The pattern is nonspecific and nondiagnostic. About 60% of children with CH have significantly delayed ossification, suggesting intrauterine hypothyroidism. Bone age, in fact, is often used as a marker for timing the onset of disease. In a number of centers, technetium scans or ultrasonography is used to confirm the type of hypothyroidism (Muir et al. 1988).

CH is treated with levothyroxine (L-T_4). The two available commercial preparations (Synthroid, Knoll Pharmaceutical Company; and Levothroid, Forest Pharmaceuticals) are interchangeable and do not differentially affect T_4 levels or TSH concentrations (Escalante et al. 1995). Early guidelines suggested initial doses of

8–10 mg/kg daily (Fish et al. 1987); present practice is to administer 10–16 mg/kg or 50 mg (Germak and Foley 1990) in order to allow serum T_4 to reach target levels sooner and reduce the incidence of subnormal intelligence (American Academy of Pediatrics 1993; Grüters et al. 1993). However, these levels are not used by all clinicians for fear of craniosynostosis and developmental abnormalities associated with hyperthyroidism (Touati et al. 1993), as well as persisting behavior problems (Rovet et al. 1987). Several studies are under way to determine the optimal dosage for normal intellectual and behavioral development in severely and moderately affected CH children (Campos et al. 1995; Dubuis et al. 1996). Although the issue of optimal therapy can be best addressed only by a clinical trial (Ehrlich 1995), the likelihood of such research receiving ethics approval or funding is low and so may never be done. At present, the Toronto protocol involves a dosage of 10 mg/kg daily to the nearest 25-, 37.5-, or 50-mg tablet, which allows for normalization of serum T_4 within 2 weeks. If by 3 months the T_4 is still less than 10 mg/dL (120 nmol/L) or the TSH is not normal, the dosage of L-T_4 is increased in 12.5- to 25-mg amounts until the desired values are reached. If symptoms of hyperthyroidism appear or TSH is suppressed too much, the dosage is reduced (Ehrlich 1995).

Optimally, it takes the neonate about 3–6 weeks from birth or about 1–2 weeks from the start of therapy to achieve euthyroidism (Germak and Foley 1990), which is defined as TSH levels in the high normal range. The duration reflects the severity of the disease, the exact age when treatment is initiated, and the dosage of replacement hormone. A high dosage usually achieves euthyroidism within 2 weeks, versus 4 weeks for a moderate dosage (Campos et al. 1995). The effects of this delay may be associated with certain selective neurocognitive impairments, the nature of which reflect brain regions with high T_4 requirements during this time. This insufficiency can be mildly offset by breast-feeding, because mother's milk is known to contain small amounts of T_4 (Bode et al. 1978; Hahn et al. 1986; Sack et al. 1979). Breast-feeding in CH is associated with slightly improved intellectual outcome (Rovet 1990).

Because some of the children identified by screening may have transient hypothyroxinemia due to maternal antibodies (LaFranchi

1979), it is important to identify these children by withdrawing medication at a later time (Davy et al. 1985). This is routinely done for the majority of children with CH. However, to ensure that their brains are protected during the critical period for brain damage, most programs recommend a 1-month trial off therapy and subsequent reevaluation at about age 3 years (Ehrlich and Rovet 1993).

With regard to later dosages of T_4, recommendations support gradually raising dosage levels until reaching adult levels of 88–125 mg when body proportions have increased to adult size. However, these levels are not based on empirical evidence and may be too high for certain aspects of cognitive functioning. Continuous monitoring of these pediatric patients is essential, especially during adolescence, when problems with compliance may arise in as many as 50% of teenagers with CH (New England Congenital Hypothyroidism Collaborative 1994).

The American Academy of Pediatrics (AAP) has issued basic recommendations for follow-up of abnormal newborn hypothyroid screening test results:

> Any infant with a low T_4 level and TSH concentration greater than 40 mU/L is considered to have primary hypothyroidism until proven otherwise. Such infants should be examined immediately and have confirmatory serum tests done to verify the diagnosis. Treatment with replacement L-thyroxine should be initiated before the results of the confirmatory tests are available. In cases in which the screening TSH concentration is only slightly elevated ... but less than 40 mU/L, another filter paper specimen should be obtained for a subsequent screening test. (American Academy of Pediatrics 1993)

In a recent update of its newborn "fact sheets," the AAP noted the contradiction among reports from large screening programs regarding outcomes following newborn identification of hypothyroid infants (American Academy of Pediatrics 1996). Although no one questions the efficacy of newborn screening for hypothyroidism, many reports have shown that children detected and treated still exhibit some degree of neuropsychological sequelae (Fuggle et al. 1991; Glorieux et al. 1983; Heyerdahl et al. 1991; Rovet et al. 1987; Virtanen et al. 1989). Several possibilities have been offered to explain this, including thyroid hormone deficiency during fetal life, severe neonatal hypothyroidism, insufficient or inappropriate hormone replacement during the first days and weeks of life, and late age at onset of therapy. Nevertheless, it is worth noting that, among the many factors considered for predictive purposes for subsequent IQ development, T_4 levels less than 50 µmol/L were predictive of a decline in IQ.

Beyond Newborn Congenital Hypothyroidism Screening

In the 1980s the usefulness of the Guthrie spot was demonstrated in a totally new application (Pass et al. 1989). Since 1987 every newborn in New York has been tested for antibodies to HIV using the Guthrie spot submitted for newborn screening. This project is part of the epidemiological study of acquired immunodeficiency syndrome (AIDS) in New York and is not an integral component of the routine newborn screening program of testing for congenital conditions. Before the Guthrie spot is tested for HIV antibodies, all identifiers are stripped from the specimen; a subset of information necessary for the epidemiological studies is reapplied to the record; and a new, anonymous identification number is assigned to the specimen. Thus, following HIV testing, only the new subset of demographic information is linked to the HIV test results. This study, which provides unbiased information on the entire childbearing population of New York, has allowed tracking of the AIDS epidemic and targeting of public health resources. [*Note:* In February 1997 New York instituted mandatory testing of all newborns for HIV-1 antibodies.]

Perhaps the most exciting development in newborn screening was the demonstration of the capability to extract DNA from the Guthrie spot, amplify the DNA by use of the polymerase chain reaction (PCR), and identify a suspect gene. The first report by McCabe in 1987 for the sickle cell mutation (McCabe et al. 1987) was followed quickly by others for cystic fibrosis (Spence et al.

1993), Duchenne muscular dystrophy (Naylor et al. 1992), thalassemia (Sutcharitchan et al. 1995), and PKU (McCabe 1994). Present technology does not permit broad-scale use of genotyping by screening programs; instead the procedures are used for confirmatory diagnosis and to eliminate unnecessary follow-up procedures. However, it is likely that future advances will allow this technology to supplant some, if not all, of the current metabolite assays that have been the mainstay of newborn screening programs.

A recent report by Mizejewski (Mizejewski et al. 1995) opens the possibility of a totally new application in newborn screening: the identification of a nonmetabolic condition with behavioral implications. Hauser (Hauser et al. 1993) had shown that certain children exhibiting behavior characterized as attention-deficit/hyperactivity disorder (ADHD)—a common childhood behavioral disorder affecting 3%–5% of the school-age population—were more likely to be found in families exhibiting the syndrome of resistance to thyroid hormone (RTH). RTH is an autosomal dominant disease characterized by pituitary and peripheral tissue insensitivity to thyroid hormone, clinically exemplified by elevated serum total T_4 and free T_4 concentrations coincident with inappropriately normal or elevated levels of TSH. Because studies of neonates with RTH indicate that the T_4 and TSH concentrations characteristic of RTH are present at birth (Weiss et al. 1990), development of a newborn screening method for RTH would allow early identification of these infants. These RTH infants represent a unique sample for prospectively studying the impact of ADHD symptomatology on children's emotional and social development. In a preliminary study (Mizejewski et al. 1995), it was demonstrated that it is feasible to identify newborns presumed positive for RTH from the newborn Guthrie spot. Specimens from approximately 60,000 newborns were obtained from the total T_4 and TSH analysis already in place for congenital hypothyroidism in the New York newborn screening program. Selected demographic data—including age, birth weight, and sex—were collected for all specimens. All other identifying information was deleted, and the specimens were renumbered and blinded to the study. A blood thyroid profile was generated on 600 specimens that exceeded the 99th percentile of total T_4 values in the screening program (test group). These 600 specimens were then compared with 600 specimens obtained from the 50th percentile of each day's respective assays (control group). The complete thyroid blood chemistry profile consisted of total T_4, FT_4, and TSH concentrations derived from the same blood spot specimen. All three thyroid parameters were quantitated by radioimmunoassay and tabulated for comparison. The study employed predominantly bloodspots from 2- to 5-day-old infants and avoided specimens from premature and transfused infants and from babies older than 14 days of age, since these conditions are known to alter thyroid serum profiles (Bellisario and Carter 1986).

As intended by the experimental design, the total T_4 mean of the test group was significantly higher than the mean of the control group, whereas the TSH and FT_4 means and variances were similar between the two groups. However, following probability analysis, 14 newborns were identified who had FT_4 concentrations greater than 2 standard deviations above the test group mean, together with the elevated total T_4 concentrations. Of these 14 newborns, seven demonstrated inappropriate TSH levels ranging from 10 to 27 µU/mL. This thyroid profile is compatible with a diagnosis of RTH and is similar to those of bloodspot specimens collected by the National Institutes of Health from individuals known to have RTH. Genetic studies for identification of mutations in the βTR gene and confirmation of the RTH diagnosis are currently under way. It was concluded that newborn infants with RTH could be identified from the Guthrie specimen on the basis of the following criteria: 1) an initial screen for elevated total T_4 exceeding the 90th percentile; 2) FT_4 exceeding a 2–standard deviation cutoff; and 3) an inappropriately nonsuppressed TSH concentration. These data serve to confirm that the thyroid profile triad employed with the Guthrie specimen can provide a logical screening protocol to detect individuals presumed positive for RTH.

A new medical care initiative—very early hospital discharge of infants—has recently affected all aspects of newborn screening, and notably that of CH testing. Until recently, most newborns were 48 hours of age or older when discharged from the hospital.

Among other important happenings during that first 48 hours of life, stabilization of the thyroid axis and maturation of liver enzyme systems provided a milieu from which an adequate Guthrie spot could be obtained. With many infants now being discharged at 24 hours of age or less, serious concerns arise about the suitability of the Guthrie spot taken at that time for newborn screening. Infants less than 24 hours of age are still within the postnatal TSH surge (and its effects) resulting from the birth process. These infants cannot provide a reliable sample for assessment of CH either by T_4/TSH testing or by TSH alone. This dependency on the timing of specimen collection has been recognized since the inception of CH testing (Fisher 1986) but has been largely ignored in the recent rush to reduce costs associated with hospitalization (Pass and Levy 1995). Recent New York and federal legislation requires insurance carriers to provide for at least 48 hours of hospitalization for mother and newborn.

In most instances, the screening program does not use the complete blood specimen collected from the infant. Because of this, screening programs are now being confronted with the issue of allocation of the remaining dried blood specimen following laboratory testing—that is, the residual spots. With the demonstration of DNA extraction from the Guthrie spot in 1986 (McCabe et al. 1987), the potential for use of molecular genetic techniques in the newborn screening laboratory has been realized. Whereas metabolites and proteins disappear with storage of the blood spots, DNA remains viable and available. Who then has "rights" to these residual specimens—the family of the child from whom the specimen was drawn, the medical researcher anxious to perfect a new procedure, or the manufacturer developing new products? There is no easy answer to this question. The Newborn Screening Committee of the federally sponsored Council of Regional Networks for Genetics Services (CORN) is currently addressing these issues and has recently published guidelines on storage of these specimens (Therrell et al. 1996).

The ability to identify specific genes following PCR expansion of the DNA in the dried blood specimen brings additional new and vexing issues to the newborn screening program. The technology allows identification—at birth—of infants with Huntington's disease, with markers for diabetes or Alzheimer's disease, with genes predisposing to emphysema or high cholesterol, and potentially with genes for behavioral disorders when those genes become known. This raises the difficult issue of which tests *should* be done, rather that which ones *can* be done. Because only one newborn screening program in the United States currently obtains parental consent prior to testing, utilization of DNA-based tests in newborn screening programs is problematic when compared with their use in other medical settings. Aside from DNA testing, present testing methods used by many newborn screening programs identify unaffected carriers of genetic disorders (sickle trait) through procedures designed for a different purpose (identification of sickle cell disease). How best to deal with these inadvertent test results was the subject of a national conference in 1995 and a subsequent report (Wethers and Pass, in review). A special task force of the Human Genome Project is examining many of these issues and has recently issued a preliminary report that has generated a great deal of controversy (Task Force on Genetic Testing 1996).

In conclusion, newborn screening has become an integral part of public health programs in the United States and elsewhere and has become a valuable guide for pediatricians in assessing an infant's health. No one can question its effectiveness in identifying infants with one of several congenital conditions at a time when therapeutic intervention can be most beneficial. Likewise, no one can predict the future course of newborn screening as the full array of molecular analyses is applied to the Guthrie spot.

References

Alm J, Larsson A, Lundberg K: Incidence of congenital hypothyroidism: retrospective study of neonatal laboratory screening versus clinical symptoms as indicators leading to diagnosis. BMJ 289:1171–1175, 1984

American Academy of Pediatrics, Committee on Genetics: Issues in newborn screening. Pediatrics 89:345–349, 1992

American Academy of Pediatrics, Section on Endocrinology and Committee on Genetics: Newborn screening for congenital hypothyroidism: recommended guidelines. Pediatrics 91:1203–1209, 1993

American Academy of Pediatrics, Committee on Genetics: Newborn screening fact sheets. Pediatrics 98:473–501, 1996

Ashida N, Ichihara K, Amino N, et al: A new cutoff method and its application in neonatal screening of free thyroxine for detection of hypothyroidism. Screening 1:89–97, 1992

Behrman IA, Vaughn RC: Nelson Textbook of Pediatrics, 12th Edition. Philadelphia, PA, WB Saunders, 1983

Bellisario R, Carter TP: Results of NYS newborn hypothyroid screening program, in Perinatal Genetics: Diagnosis and Treatment. Edited by Porter IH, Hatcher NH, Willey AM. San Diego, CA, Academic Press, 1986, pp 219–242

Bickel H: The effects of a phenylalanine-free and phenylalanine-poor diet in phenylpyruvic oligophrenia. Experimental Medicine and Surgery 12:114–117, 1954

Bode HH, Vanjonack WV, Crawford JD: Mitigation of cretinism by breast-feeding. Pediatrics 62:13–16, 1978

Bodegard G, Fyro K, Larsson A: Psychological reactions in 102 families with a newborn who has a falsely positive screening text for congenital hypothyroidism. Acta Paediatr Scand 304:1–21, 1982

Brown RS, Bellisario RL, Mitchell E, et al: Detection of thyrotropin binding inhibitory activity in neonatal blood spots. J Clin Endocrinol Metab 77:1005–1008, 1993

Brunch W, McCune DJ: Mental development of congenitally hypothyroid children. Its relation to physical development and adequacy of treatment. American Journal of Diseases of Children 67:205–224, 1944

Buck PS: Foreword, in Phenylketonuria. By Lyman FL. New York, Charles C Thomas, 1963

Campos SP, Sandberg DE, Barrick C, et al: Outcome of lower L-thyroxine dose for treatment of congenital hypothyroidism. Clin Pediatr 34:514–520, 1995

Carter TP, Willey A: Genetic Disease Screening and Management. New York, Alan R Liss, 1986

Cassio A, Tata L, Colli C, et al: Incidence of congenital malformations in congenital hypothyroidism. Screening 3:125–130, 1994

Council of Regional Networks for Genetics Services (CORN), Newborn Screening Committee: National Newborn Screening Report—1992. Atlanta, GA, Council of Regional Networks for Genetics Services, December 1995

Davy T, Daneman D, Walfish PG, et al: Congenital hypothyroidism: the effect of stopping treatment at 3 years. American Journal of Diseases of Children 139:1028–1030, 1985

DeGroot LJ, Larsen PR, Hennemann G: The Thyroid and Its Diseases, 6th Edition. New York, Churchill Livingstone, 1996

Delange F: The Wolff-Chaikoff effect in paediatrics, in Iodine Prophylaxis Following Nuclear Accidents. Edited by Rubery E, Smales E. Oxford, UK, Pergamon, 1990, p 83

Dubuis JM, Glorieux J, Richer F, et al: Outcome of severe congenital hypothyroidism: closing the developmental gap with early high dose levothyroxine treatment. J Clin Endocrinol Metab 81:222–227, 1996

Dussault JH, Laberge C: Thyroxine (T_4) determination in dried blood by radioimmunoassay: a screening method for neonatal hypothyroidism. Union Medicale du Canada 102:2062–2064, 1973

Dussault JH, Coulombe P, Laberge C, et al: Preliminary report on a mass screening program for neonatal hypothyroidism. J Pediatr 86:670–674, 1975

Ehrlich RM: Thyroxine dose for congenital hypothyroidism. Clin Pediatr 34:521–522, 1995

Ehrlich RM, Rovet JF: Congenital hypothyroidism. Contemporary Pediatrics (September):4–9, 1993

Escalante DA, Arem N, Arem R: Assessment of interchangeability of two brands of levothyroxine preparations with a third-generation TSH assay. Am J Med 98:374–378, 1995

Fernhoff PM, Brown Al, Elsas LJ: Congenital hypothyroidism: increased risk of neonatal morbidity results in delayed treatment. Lancet 1:490, 1987

Fish LH, Schwartz HL, Cavanaugh J, et al: Replacement dose, metabolism, and bioavailability of levothyroxine in the treatment of hypothyroidism. N Engl J Med 316:764–770, 1987

Fisher DA: Pediatrics aspects, in The Thyroid: A Fundamental and Clinical Text. Edited by Werner SC, Ingbar SH. New York, Harper & Row, 1978

Fisher DA: Background strategies and problems of newborn screening for congenital hypothyroidism, in Genetic Disease Screening and Management. Edited by Carter TP, Willey AM. New York, Alan R Liss, 1986, pp 133–154

Fisher DA: Clinical review 19—management of congenital hypothyroidism. J Clin Endocrinol Metab 72:523–529, 1991

Fisher DA, Lehman H, Lacky C: Placental transport of thyroxine. J Clin Endocrinol Metab 24:393–400, 1964

Fisher DA, Dussault JH, Lorin RW: Serum and thyroid gland triiodothyronine in the human fetus. J Clin Endocrinol Metab 36:397–400, 1973

Fisher DA, Dussault JH, Foley TP Jr, et al: Screening for congenital hypothyroidism: results of screening one million North American infants. J Pediatr 94:700–705, 1979

Foley TP, Torresani TE: Congenital hypothyroidism, in Early Hospital Discharge: Impact on Newborn Screening. Edited by Pass KA, Levy HL. Atlanta, GA, Council of Regional Networks for Genetics Services (CORN), 1995, pp 133–154

Fölling A: Phenylpyruvic acid as a metabolic anomaly in connection with imbecility. Zeitschrift Physiologische Chemie 227:169–174, 1934

Francis I, Weldon A, Connelly J: Effect of Betadine treatment to umbilical cords on screening tests for congenital hypothyroidism, in Neonatal Screening. Edited by Naruse H, Irie M. Amsterdam, Excerpta Medica, 1982, p 52

Fuggle PW, Grant DB, Smith J, et al: Intelligence, motor skills and behavior at 5 years in early treated congenital hypothyroidism. Eur J Pediatr 150:570–574, 1991

Germak J, Foley T: Longitudinal assessment of L-thyroxine therapy for congenital hypothyroidism. J Pediatr 117:211–219, 1990

Glorieux J, Dussault JH, Letarte J, et al: Preliminary results on the mental development of hypothyroid infants detected by the Quebec screening program. J Pediatr 102:19–24, 1983

Grant DB, Smith I: Survey of neonatal screening for primary hypothyroidism in England, Wales, and Northern Ireland 1982–4. BMJ 296:1355–1358, 1988

Grüters A, Allemand D, Heidemann P, et al: Thyroid function and iodine concentrations in newborns and their mothers after vaginal PVP-iodine treatment in obstetrics, in Neonatal Screening. Edited by Naruse H, Irie M. Amsterdam, The Netherlands, Excerpta Medica, 1982, p 54

Grüters A, Delange F, Grant D, et al: Guidelines for neonatal screening programmes for congenital hypothyroidism (Working Group on Congenital Hypothyroidism of the European Society for Pediatric Endocrinology). Eur J Pediatr 152:974–975, 1993

Guthrie R: The origin of newborn screening. Screening 1:5–15, 1992

Guthrie R, Whitney S: Phenylketonuria detection in the newborn infant as a routine hospital procedure. A trial of the phenylalanine screening method in 400,000 infants (Children's Bureau Publ No 419). Washington, DC, U.S. Government Printing Office, 1964

Hahn HB, Brown LO, Hillis A, et al: Breast feeding and neonatal screening for congenital hypothyroidism. Tex Med 82:46–47, 1986

Harada S, Ichihara N, Arai J, et al: Influence of iodine excess due to iodine-containing antiseptics on neonatal screening for congenital hypothyroidism in Hokkkaido prefecture, Japan. Screening 3:115–123, 1994

Harada S, Ichihara N, Arai J, et al: Later manifestations of congenital hypothyroidism predicted by slightly elevated thyrotropin levels in neonatal screening. Screening 3:181–192, 1995

Hauser P, Zametkin AJ, Martinez P, et al: Attention-deficit hyperactivity disorder in people with generalized resistance to thyroid hormone. N Engl J Med 328:997–1001, 1993

Hetzel BS: The history of endemic cretinism, in Endemic Cretinism. Edited by Hetzel BS, Pharoah POD. Monograph Series No 2, Institute of Human Biology, Papua, New Guinea. New South Wales, Surrey Beatty and Sons, 1971, pp 5–8

Heyerdahl S, Kase BF, Lie SO: Intellectual development in children with congenital hypothyroidism in relation to recommended thyroxine treatment. J Pediatr 118:850–857, 1991

Klein AH, Meltzer S, Kenny FN: Improved prognosis of congenital hypothyroidism tested before age 3 months. J Pediatr 81:962–975, 1972

LaFranchi SH: Hypothyroidism. Pediatr Clin North Am 26:33–51, 1979

LaFranchi SH, Hanna CE, Krainz PL, et al: Screening for congenital hypothyroidism with specimen collection at two time periods: results of the Northwest Regional Screening Program. Pediatrics 76:734–740, 1985

Lazarus JH, Hughes IA: Congenital abnormalities and congenital hypothyroidism. Lancet 2:52, 1988

Levy HL: Neonatal screening for metabolic disorders, in Prevention of Developmental Disabilities. Edited by Pueschel SM, Mulick JA. Baltimore, MD, Paul H Brooks, 1990

Lyman FL: Phenylketonuria. New York, Charles C Thomas, 1963

Majeed-Saidan MA, Jouce B, Khan M, et al: Congenital hypothyroidism: the Riyadh Military Hospital experience. Clin Endocrinol 38:191–196, 1993

McCabe ERB: DNA techniques for screening of inborn errors of metabolism. Eur J Pediatr 153:S84–S85, 1994

McCabe ER, Huang SZ, Seltzer WK, et al: DNA microextraction from dried blood spots on filter paper blotters: potential applications to newborn screening. Hum Genet 75:213–216, 1987

Mizejewski GJ, Morris JE, Hauser P, et al: A strategy for newborn screening for resistance to thyroid hormone: possible relevance to attention deficit hyperactivity disorder. Screening 4:61–70, 1995

Muir A, Daneman D, Daneman A, et al: Thyroid scanning, ultrasound, and serum thyroglobulin in determining the origin of congenital hypothyroidism. American Journal of Diseases of Children 142:214–216, 1988

Naylor EW, Hoffman EP, Paulus-Thomas J, et al: Neonatal screening for Duchenne/Becker muscular dystrophy: reconsideration based on molecular diagnosis and potential therapies. Screening 1:99–104, 1992

New England Congenital Hypothyroidism Collaborative: Congenital concomitants of infantile hypothyroidism. J Pediatr 122:244–251, 1988

New England Congenital Hypothyroidism Collaborative: Correlation of cognitive test scores and adequacy of treatment in adolescents with congenital hypothyroidism. J Pediatr 124:383–387, 1994

Pass KA, Levy HL (eds): Early Hospital Discharge: Impact on Newborn Screening. Atlanta, GA, Council of Regional Networks for Genetics Services (CORN), 1995

Pass KA, Schedlbauer LM, Berns D: Utilization of the newborn specimen for HIV seroprevalence studies, in Placental-Mediated Disorders: Detection, Treatment and Management. Edited by Bellisario R, Mizejewski G. New York, Alan R Liss, 1989

Poole BD: Testing for phenylketonuria. J Pediatr 62:955–959, 1963

Raiti S, Newns GA: Cretinism: early diagnosis and its relation to mental development. Arch Dis Child 46:692–694, 1971

Rosenthal M, Addison GM, Price D: Congenital hypothyroidism: increased incidence in Asian families. Arch Dis Child 63:790–797, 1988

Rovet JF: Does breast-feeding protect the hypothyroid infant whose condition is diagnosed by newborn screening? American Journal of Diseases of Children 144:319–323, 1990

Rovet J, Ehrlich R, Sorbara D: Intellectual outcome in children with fetal hypothyroidism. J Pediatr 110:700–704, 1987

Sack J, Frucht HO, Amado O, et al: Breast milk thyroxine and not cow's milk may mitigate and delay the clinical picture of neonatal hypothyroidism. Acta Paediatr Scand 277:54–56, 1979

Siebner R, Merlob P, Kaiserman I, et al: Congenital anomalies concomitant with persistent primary congenital hypothyroidism. Am J Med Genet 44:57–63, 1992

Slazyk WE, Hannon WH: Quality assurance in the newborn screening laboratory, in Laboratory Methods for Neonatal Screening. Edited by Therrell BL. Washington, DC, American Public Health Association, 1993, p 23

Spence WC, Paulus-Thomas J, Orenstein DM, et al: Neonatal screening for cystic fibrosis: addition of molecular diagnosis to increase specificity. Biochemical Medicine and Metabolic Biology 49:200–211, 1993

Sutcharitchan P, Saiki R, Fucharoen S, et al: Reverse do-blot detection of Thai beta-thalassanemia mutations. Br J Haematol 90:809–816, 1995

Task Force on Genetic Testing: Interim Principles of the Task Force on Genetic Testing. Baltimore, MD, NIH-DOE Working Group on Ethical, Legal, and Social Implications of Human Genome Research, 1996

Therrell DB, Harrison WH, Pass KA, et al: Guidelines for the retention, storage, and use of residual dried blood spot samples after newborn screening analysis: statement of the Council of Regional Networks for Genetic Services. Biochem Mol Med 57:116–124, 1996

Touati G, Leger J, Toublanc J, et A.F.D.P.H.E.: An initial dosage of 8 µg/kg is appropriate for the vast majority of infants with congenital hypothyroidism (CH). Leo, France, 1993

Tyfield LA, Abusrewil SSA, Jones SR, et al: Persistent hyperthyrotropinaemia since the neonatal period in clinically euthyroid children. Eur J Pediatr 150:308–312, 1991

Van Gemund JJ, DeAngulao MSL: The effects of early hypothyroidism on IQ, school performance, and electroencephalogram pattern in children, in Normal and Abnormal Development of the Brain and Behavior. Edited by Stoelinga CBA, Van Der Werff Ten Bosch JJ. Leiden, The Netherlands, Leiden University Press, 1997, pp 299–313

Virtanen M, Santavuori P, Hirvonen E, et al: Multivariate analysis of psychomotor development in congenital hypothyroidism. Acta Paediatr Scand 78:405–408, 1989

Weiss RE, Balzano S, Scherberg NH, et al: Neonatal detection of generalized resistance to thyroid hormone. JAMA 264:2245–2250, 1990

Wethers D, Pass KA: Disposition of sickle carrier results in newborn screening programs. Am J Public Health (in review)

World Health Organization (WHO) Scientific Group: Technical Report. Screening for Inborn Errors of Metabolism. Series No 401. Geneva, Switzerland, World Health Organization, 1968

Chapter 4

Behavioral and Cognitive Abnormalities Associated With Congenital Hypothyroidism

Joanne Rovet, Ph.D.

Until as recently as 1988, congenital hypothyroidism (CH) was considered one of the most serious and devastating illnesses of childhood. Affected children, often referred to as "cretins," were extremely short with distinctive facial dysmorphology and characteristic neurological and hearing impairments (Figure 4–1). These children were also retarded intellectually, and CH was among the

---

The research on our patients with congenital hypothyroidism has represented a massive undertaking lasting more than 15 years. I am most appreciative of my long and fruitful collaboration with Dr. Robert Ehrlich, who provided the medical expertise and clinical wisdom to our understanding of this population. I am also grateful to Donna Sorbara, who originally recruited the patients and then tested them for many years; to Deborah Altmann, who took over and maintained close contact with the patients in the sample; to Jeannine Pinnsonneault-Uscales, Lindsay Ireland, and Minna Hockenberry for data analysis; and to Lori Brnjac for the pubertal assessments. Miguel Alvarez, on his two visits to Canada from Cuba, gave the project new inspiration and sought to answer new questions; Elizabeth Donner, Wynsome Walker, Kathy Petric, Sandra Cole, and Michal Leneman were summer students whose projects also set this research in new directions. Nancy Lobaugh provided helpful comments on an earlier draft of this paper. Above all, I wish to thank the many children and their parents and siblings who so willingly gave of their time in order to see us each year, a few of whom are still coming. This work has been continuously funded by grants from the Ontario Ministry of Health, the Ontario Ministry of Community and Social Services, and the Ontario Mental Health Foundation. A Health and Welfare Canada Scholarship in the early years of the project allowed me to do this research.

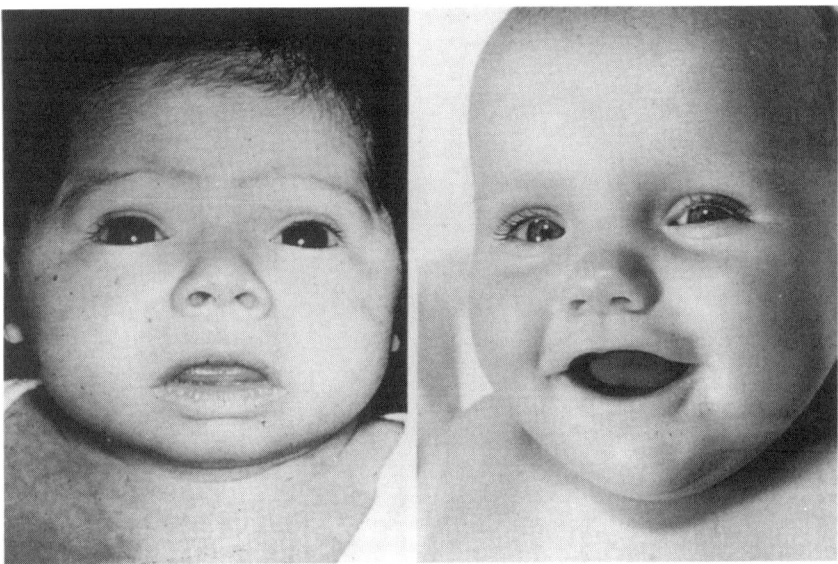

Figure 4–1. Two children with congenital hypothyroidism. *(left)* Child diagnosed clinically. *(right)* Child diagnosed by newborn screening.

leading causes of childhood mental retardation (Crome and Stern 1972). Although treatment with replacement hormone was effective in curbing progression of the disease, it was often begun quite late in infancy owing to the delayed presentation of clinical symptoms. This meant that by the time a child received therapy, widespread irreversible brain damage had occurred.

In the late 1970s and early 1980s, programs for screening newborns for CH were implemented throughout North America, Europe, Australia, and Japan and also parts of the developing world (see Pass, Chapter 3 in this volume). Newborn screening allowed for much earlier treatment of CH because diagnosis preceded the appearance of clinical symptoms. As a result of screening, mental retardation from cretinism was virtually eliminated from the developed world. However, there may be a relatively benign disorder that results from thyroid hormone (TH) deficiency during fetal development and a brief period in early life. This disorder has specific implications for treatment, management, and outcome. A large number of prospective studies on children detected by screening and treated very early in life have shown persisting subtle deficits (Fuggle et al. 1991; Heyerdahl et al. 1991; New England Congenital Hypothyroidism Collaborative 1994; Rovet 1990). However, the clinical profile of this "new" disorder is not well understood; suffice it to say that the children are not retarded and they grow and develop normally.

Since 1981, I have been collaborating with Dr. Robert Ehrlich, a pediatric endocrinologist at the Hospital for Sick Children (HSC) in Toronto. Together, we have conducted one of the world's largest and longest prospective investigations involving a substantial single series of children with CH. The children in our study represented the first wave of cases identified by the province of Ontario's newborn screening program. They resided in the greater metropolitan Toronto area, which represents about 40% of the total newborn population in the province of Ontario. These children were followed up on a regular basis at our hospital for medical intervention and neuropsychological evaluation. The majority, who are now into or past adolescence, were also tested once in puberty, marking the final stage in the assessment protocol. More recently, I have begun a second investigation, in collaboration with Dr. Nancy Lobaugh, which involves a new younger cohort of children with CH. The purpose of this study is to examine the attentional skills of children with CH and compare them with the skills of children with attention-deficit disorder and control subjects. Just beginning is a third study with Drs. Feig, Daneman, Astzalos, Perlman, and Kelly to study memory and attentional skills in infants who may have been thyroid hormone deficient at different stages of pregnancy as a result of having CH, being born to a mother who was hypothyroid during pregnancy or hyperthyroid and treated with antithyroid drugs, or being born preterm (and thus lacking the maternal thyroid hormone complement in the third trimester).

This chapter presents an overview of disease characteristics and physical and psychological manifestations of early-treated congenital hypothyroidism. It draws on my experience with the various groups of children with CH my colleagues and I have seen, as well as a broad and expanding body of literature on this topic. A description of thyroid-related brain effects and the critical aspects of timing of TH deficiency precedes this discussion. The chapter concludes with a discussion of critical and outstanding issues related to the care, management, and study of these children.

Thyroid Physiology and Pathophysiology

The two hormones produced by the thyroid gland are thyroxine (T_4) and triiodothyronine (T_3), which are regulated by negative feedback with the hypothalamus and pituitary (see Lash, Chapter 1; and Meier, Chapter 2 in this volume). These hormones travel via binding proteins in the bloodstream to tissues such as the liver, skeleton, heart, and brain. Although T_4 is produced in far greater quantity than T_3, T_3 is the active hormone, so T_4 must be converted to T_3 at the target tissue sites. This is accomplished by deiodinase enzymes, which function in a coordinated and developmentally regulated system to ensure that requisite levels of T_3 are provided at critical stages of development (Silva and Larsen 1982). The functions of T_3 in regulating specific genetic activities are well described elsewhere (see Meier, Chapter 2 in this volume).

Primary sporadic congenital hypothyroidism is caused by a deficiency in the production of thyroid hormone (TH) at the level of the thyroid gland. It can occur if the gland is missing (athyrosis), inadequately developed (hypoplasia), or improperly located owing to the gland's failure during embryogenesis to descend from its primordial location at the base of the tongue (ectopia). Primary sporadic CH can also be caused by an inborn error of thyroid hormone metabolism, which is often associated with goiter (dyshormonogenesis), and unique mutations at different stages of processing in thyroid follicles (Bikker et al. 1994, 1995; Veenboer and de Vijlder 1993). One frequent genetic defect is the result of a deficiency in thyroid peroxidase production (Pop et al. 1995). There are also secondary and tertiary forms of hypothyroidism at the level of the hypothalamus or pituitary, respectively (see Lash, Chapter 1 in this volume).

Maternal-Fetal Thyroid Hormone Relationships

It is now known that the fetus receives some TH contribution from the maternal thyroid system (Morreale de Escobar et al. 1989; Thorpe-Beeston et al. 1991; Vulsma et al. 1989). Because the fetal system matures slowly and is not fully functional until the third trimester, the fetus depends to varying degrees on the maternal thyroid supply (Burrow et al. 1994). This is the primary supply of fetal TH during early pregnancy because the fetal system is not yet functional. If the maternal supply is insufficient, the fetus—particularly the fetal brain—may be affected. For example, children of mothers who were severely hypothyroid during pregnancy have been shown to be at increased risk of brain damage and subsequent neurocognitive impairment (Bachrach and Burrow 1985; Man et al. 1991). Similar, but milder, results have been observed for the offspring of mothers who were hyperthyroid during pregnancy and treated with antithyroid drugs, which cross the placenta and turn off the fetal thyroid (Cheron et al. 1991; Eisenstein et al. 1992). Once the developing fetal thyroid becomes activated, this will partially or totally overcome any maternal deficit, but selective impairments from milder brain damage may still occur (DeGroot et al. 1996).

If the fetus is hypothyroid, especially because of athyrosis, it is totally dependent on the maternal supply of TH throughout pregnancy, which may not fully compensate it at later stages of gestation when the fetal need is greater. The maternal contribution has been estimated at approximately 33%–50% of normal (Vulsma et al. 1989). The insufficiency associated with fetal hypothyroidism may contribute to brain damage in regions that have a high need for TH during late gestation. Infants who are hypothyroid and whose mothers are also hypothyroid owing to iodine insufficiency have the most serious form of the disease, known as neurological cretinism (Boyages and Halpern 1993; Delange et al. 1989) (see also Lash, Chapter 1 in this volume). In addition to mental retardation, children who lack both sources of TH have impaired neurological development and deafness, suggestive of brain damage both early and late in pregnancy (Boyages et al. 1988).

In the normal state, the fetal supply of TH is its main source, but this can be supplemented by the maternal thyroid at times of increased need. This occurs via transplacental passage of maternal T_4 and conversion of T_4 to T_3 in the placenta by deiodinase enzymes. The deiodinase system is developmentally regulated to supply the fetal brain with the required amounts of thyroid hormones as they are needed (Ekins et al. 1989; Emerson 1991; Glinoer et al. 1990; Silva and Larsen 1982). When fetal function is normal and the requirements are low, the net flux from mother to fetus is limited (Larsen 1996). Infants born prematurely, however, do not receive maternal supplementation through the womb and must rely totally on their own glands in what would have been the latter months of pregnancy (Larsen 1996). Indeed, it is now recognized that persisting cognitive problems in otherwise healthy premature infants (Hack et al. 1994) may arise from the unavailability of sufficient TH for the brain's needs during this time (Lucas et al. 1988, 1996; Meijer et al. 1992; Vulsma and Kok 1996). Hypothyroxinemia in premature infants is an issue of recent interest and debate (Frank et al. 1996; Reuss et al. 1996) and has been the stimulus for at least one clinical trial of TH supplementation to premature infants (van Wassenaer et al. 1993, 1997). Although one research group has studied the long-term effects on IQ of low T_3 concentrations in preterm infants (Lucas et al. 1996), the long-term effect of prematurity (or postmaturity; see Lash, Chapter 1 in this volume) in congenitally hypothyroid children has (to this author's knowledge) never been studied as a distinct issue.

Thyroid Hormone Deficiency and Brain Development

Animal Studies

An extensive body of literature exists on the role of thyroid hormone in brain development and brain function from studies of laboratory animals, primarily the rat (Porterfield and Hendrich 1993; Porterfield and Stein 1994). The research has shown that TH is involved in a number of critical neurodevelopmental processes, including cell division and neurogenesis (Shapiro 1966), axon and dendrite formation (Legrand 1984), neuronal migration (Potter et al. 1982), synaptogenesis (Madeira and Paula-Barbarosa 1993; Nicholson and Altman 1972), and myelination (Rosman et al. 1972). TH affects the formation of both gray and white matter. Regions particularly affected by TH deficiency include the striatum, hippocampus, cerebellum, and cortex, which are underlying substrates for neurocognitive processing. There are two ways that TH affects white matter production: 1) by controlling production of glial cells, the procurers of myelin (Lauder and Krebs 1986), and 2) by regulating two genes that control myelin formation, namely myelin basic protein and myelin-associated glycoprotein (Farsetti et al. 1991, 1992; Munoz et al. 1991). Rodriguez-Peña et al. (1993) showed that neonatal hypothyroidism affects the timely expression of myelin-associated glycoprotein in rat brain, resulting in a delay in the development of rostral regions such as cortex and hippocampus; treatment appears to reduce these effects, and recovery is greater in the caudal regions of rat brain. TH also regulates the transcription of tau and microtubule-associated proteins, which are associated with cytoskeleton development in axons and dendrites (Nunez 1986) and facilitate neuronal migration (Fellous et al. 1979), respectively.

Four nuclear receptors for TH have been identified, two with α-subunits and two with β-subunits. Bradley et al. (1989) have shown that these receptors are differentially distributed in various brain regions. Whereas α_2 is ubiquitous, α_1 is restricted to the olfactory bulbs and cerebellum, β_2 to the pituitary and hypothalamus, and β_1 to cortex, hippocampus, caudate nucleus, and cerebellum, which are structures involved in cognitive processing. This fact has implications for cognitive dysfunction in individuals with resistance to thyroid hormone, who have a defect in the thyroid βreceptor (see Hauser, Chapter 5 in this volume). Different TH receptors have also been localized in different structures of the ear (Bradley et al. 1994; Corey and Breakefield 1994), as well as in brain structures comprising auditory pathways (Li and Boyages 1995).

The different TH receptors have also been shown to vary temporally in their periods of peak receptivity to TH (Strait et al. 1990), which suggests that there are different critical periods when TH is needed by various brain regions. More recently, Bradley et al. (1992) showed that there are different ontogenies of functional activity for TH receptors in different brain regions, which signifies the critical importance of the timing of TH deficiency. Bradley's findings have clear implications for permanent and highly circumscribed effects of missing thyroid hormone at a specific time for both brain and ear development.

TH is also involved in the development of different neurotransmitter systems (Hashimoto et al. 1994; Puymirat 1985; Virgili et al. 1991) and the later regulation of certain neurochemicals (Savard et al. 1983). Perinatal thyroid hormone deficiency affects striatal dopaminergic and basal forebrain cholinergic systems (Gould and Butcher 1989; Puymirat et al. 1983). Gould and Butcher, for example, found that a deficit in TH during early development led to morphological abnormalities in cell size and dendrite growth, which has implications for connectivity and the production of neurotransmitters affecting learning and memory. Animal research has shown that receptor sensitivity to central nervous system catecholamines is decreased in hypothyroidism, leading to a compensatory increase in catechol concentration (Klawans et al. 1974). In immature laboratory animals, hyperthyroidism is associated with increased synthesis and utilization of catecholamines and serotonin, as well as increased motor activity, whereas in mature animals, neurotransmitter changes are more subtle and have less effect on behavioral activity (Rastogi and Singhal 1976). In humans, maternal thyroendocrine pathology has been associated with increased incidence of schizophrenia in the offspring (MacSweeney et al. 1978), suggesting an effect of TH insufficiency on the developing dopaminergic system.

Human Studies

There are few studies of the neuroanatomic features associated with thyroid hormone deficiency. Because CH typically is not associated with increased mortality and because neuroimaging studies cannot readily be performed in this relatively young and otherwise healthy population, there is no direct evidence concerning brain structure in adequately and early-treated children with CH. Although obvious neuroanatomic differences should not be expected in children with CH who are treated early following screening, deficits that are more subtle and reflect qualitative changes in myelin formation might occur (Lobaugh et al. 1996), as well as changes in heavily myelinated regions such as the corpus callosum (see also Hauser, Chapter 5 in this volume).

Among late-treated CH patients who were diagnosed before the implementation of screening, only a few have been brought to autopsy or received neuroimaging. Histopathological studies have shown reduced brain size; poor development of cerebral and cerebellar cortex, basal ganglia, and thalamus; and abnormalities of the hippocampus (Benda 1941). Radiological studies reveal a generally normal brain appearance, but there are gliotic lesions of the globus pallidus and substantia nigra (DeGroot et al. 1996). One study using proton magnetic resonance spectroscopy on five older hypothyroid children showed mild cerebral atrophy in the frontal and parietal lobes, suggestive of delayed myelination, which normalized following therapy (Gupta et al. 1995). The authors suggested that treatment served to normalize the myelin maturation process. Alves et al. (1989) evaluated magnetic resonance imaging (MRI) changes in a 14-month-old girl diagnosed late with CH: on diagnosis, she showed decreased myelination in the frontal regions, which disappeared following hormone replacement. An MRI study by Rivkees and Hardin (1994) revealed delayed myelination in an 11-month-old child who received weekly (versus daily) dosing for CH and was markedly delayed and cretinoid in appearance. An autopsy shortly thereafter revealed microcephaly with no abnormalities in gray or white matter, cerebellum, or brain stem. Ectopic neurons were found in deep white matter adjacent to the lining of the cerebellum, suggesting a migrational defect.

With regard to brain function in early-treated hypothyroidism, Moschini et al. (1986) described their neurophysiological findings on 42 screened youngsters with CH. Electroencephalography revealed signs of minimal brain damage in a small percentage of promptly treated children: 7% showed focal patterns with slow waves. Visual evoked potential testing on the same sample revealed an increased latency in the P2 component of the visual evoked potential in 64%, which may correlate with problems in visual perception and attention.

Overall, there is a paucity of findings on humans, especially children, with thyroid hormone deficiency at a time when the brain is undergoing major development. To determine whether early thyroid deficiency has lasting effects and whether these correlate with persisting cognitive deficits (see below), further study is definitely required.

Overview of Congenital Hypothyroidism

Congenital hypothyroidism affects about 1 in 3,000–4,000 newborns in North America and Europe. CH affects more females than males, with a 2.5:1 preponderance. There is also considerable racial variability: In the United States, CH is six times as frequent in Caucasians as in African Americans (Brown et al. 1981), whereas it is about 40% higher in Hispanics than in Caucasians; for Native Americans it is even higher than in Hispanics (Hollowell et al., in press). CH is also more prevalent among children of Indo-European origin and less prevalent in Japanese (Hollowell et al., in press).

CH occurs if the thyroid gland is absent, ectopic, or hypoplastic (see above). Thyroid aplasia represents the most severe form of the disease, whereas the ectopic form is generally most common. Dyshormonogenesis with or without goiter is the cause of CH in up to 20% of cases. About 5% of children with CH and with normal thyroid glands have a defect at the level of the hypothalamus or pituitary (see Lash, Chapter 1 in this volume). There is considerable racial and ethnic variation in the distribution of the different etiologies: the ectopic thyroid is the predominant cause of CH in Finland, France, Germany, Australia, and Japan; dysplastic glands are more common among Hispanics in California; and in Kuwait and Saudi Arabia, due to the high incidence of consanguinity, dyshormonogenesis is most common (DeGroot et al. 1996).

Transient hypothyroxinemia may occur in a small proportion of children owing to the blocking action of maternal thyroid antibodies, which cross the placenta (Larsen 1996). Altered levels of

TH at birth can also be caused by environmental toxins such as polychlorinated biphenyls (PCBs), furans, and dioxins (Juarez de Ku and Meserve 1994: Juarez de Ku et al. 1994; Koopman-Esseboon et al. 1994; Pluim et al. 1993; see also Bhatara et al., Chapter 8 in this volume). Although animal studies have shown that maternal substance abuse affects fetal TH production (Hernandez et al. 1992), this finding has not been replicated in human infants (Hannigan et al. 1995). Prematurity is now considered a form of fetal hypothyroidism (Vulsma and Kok 1996), which may have associated neurological and developmental abnormalities.

Diagnosis and Treatment of Congenital Hypothyroidism

Screening for CH involves assessing either for low levels of T_4 or for elevations of thyroid-stimulating hormone (TSH) (see Pass, Chapter 3 in this volume) or both (LaFranchi et al. 1985). The program in Ontario screens for TSH. T_4 screening has the advantage of detecting secondary and tertiary forms of hypothyroidism as well as thyroid binding deficiencies. TSH screening, on the other hand, can detect children with compensated or subclinical hypothyroidism who produce low-normal levels of T_4 at birth owing to overstimulation of the pituitary. According to DeGroot et al. (1996), screening serum TSH may be the better indicator because it can identify children with ectopic and hypoplastic etiologies whose glands produce enough hormone to pass the initial screening test but progressively lose functional capacity and eventually give out or vanish several months after birth (Delange et al. 1989). Some T_4 screening programs recommend a second test at 3–4 months, usually to coincide with a well baby visit (Levine and Therrell 1978), which should identify these youngsters. The fact that different screening programs may detect children with different etiologies may have implications for the results of prospective studies.

Following a positive screening test, the primary physician or the family itself is notified by the screening laboratory or a delegated representative. Confirmatory diagnosis requires further thyroid function tests and is based on a reduced serum T_4 concentration, an elevated serum TSH level, and a low free thyroxine index. Serum thyroglobulin measurement is useful in confirming athyrosis (since thyroglobulin is absent in these children), and a thyroid scan will establish a diagnosis of thyroid ectopy. Although most children appear normal as neonates, some will have nonspecific clinical symptoms such as jaundice, umbilical hernias, and constipation. Technetium scans and ultrasonography are useful in determining etiology, whereas a bone scan serves to establish the timing of the onset of disease.

CH is treated with levothyroxine (Synthroid, Knoll Pharmaceutical Company) (see Pass, Chapter 3 in this volume). Current guidelines of the American Academy of Pediatrics (1993) recommend a relatively high starting dosage of 10–16 µg/kg or 50 µg in order to allow serum T_4 to reach target levels sooner and to reduce the incidence of subnormal intelligence; however, these levels are still controversial, and the issue of proper starting dosage has not been adequately resolved (Ehrlich 1995). Because the recommended levels are quite high and have never been assessed for adverse behavioral effects, several groups are conducting studies to determine the optimal dosage and examine the possibility of using different dosages depending on the severity of CH at diagnosis (Campos et al. 1995; Dubuis et al. 1996). Although a clinical trial that also addresses long-term effects (Rovet and Ehrlich 1995) is the optimal approach for resolving the issue, it is unlikely that this research can be done (Ehrlich 1995).

If treatment is optimal, it takes about 3–6 weeks from birth (or 1–2 weeks from start of therapy) to achieve euthyroidism (Germak and Foley 1990). The exact duration reflects disease severity, age when treatment is initiated, and dosage of replacement hormone. The effects of treatment delay are associated with selective neurocognitive impairments, the nature of which reflect the brain regions that have major TH requirements during this period of time (see below). Breast-feeding can mildly offset this insufficiency (Rovet 1990) because mother's milk contains small amounts of thyroxine (Bode et al. 1978; Hahn et al. 1986; Sack et al. 1979).

Recommendations for subsequent maintenance levels of thyroxine suggest gradually raising dosage levels until reaching adult dosage levels when body proportions reach adult size. However, because the proposed levels are not based on empirical evidence and may be too high for certain aspects of cognitive functioning (see below), it is important that patients be continuously monitored, especially during adolescence when problems with compliance may also arise (New England Congenital Hypothyroidism Collaborative 1994). To assess for transient hypothyroxinemia, it is important to identify such children at a time when the brain might be less vulnerable to a period of TH insufficiency. Davy et al. (1985) recommended withdrawing therapy for 1 month at 3 years of age to repeat thyroid function tests.

Growth and Development

Growth and development are normal in children with early-treated CH (Hulse et al. 1982). Aronson et al. (1990) showed that up to age 9, growth was within normal limits and projected adult height matched the parents'. Nevertheless, height was inversely correlated with factors reflecting the timing, duration, and severity of early hypothyroidism. Adequately treated CH was associated with slightly increased head circumference in childhood (Bucher et al. 1985).

There are no formal reports of pubertal and sexual development in this population. However, the children in my group's original cohort, who were evaluated physically at the time of psychological testing, demonstrated appropriate-for-age growth and development and no delays or abnormalities. Several mothers have reported severe premenstrual syndrome symptoms in adolescent females, but whether this exceeds normality is not clear and requires further study.

Psychometric Studies

General Intelligence

Most studies of children with CH use global indices of intelligence as the primary—and often the only—end point (e.g., Simons et al. 1994; see Rovet 1990 for a review). Because global IQ is a composite score based on many underlying abilities that reflect the involvement of multiple heterogeneous brain regions, IQ is a relatively crude measure to assess time-limited effects of inadequate TH supply. In the computed IQ, the subtle but significant effects of TH deficiency on selective neurocognitive domains could be masked by nonsignificant effects in other domains.

Across studies, the findings show a 5- to 10-point lowering of IQ in early-treated CH, although IQ is still within the normal range. The degree of IQ lowering depends on the initial severity of CH (Simons et al. 1994; Tillotson et al. 1994), cause of CH (Rovet et al. 1992), fetal duration (Rovet et al. 1987), and starting dosages of therapy (Rovet and Ehrlich 1995). In the New England follow-up study (New England Congenital Hypothyroidism Collaborative 1985, 1994), poor compliance with therapy was also associated with lower IQ. On the basis of a summary of 675 cases from seven studies in the literature, Derksen-Lubsen and Verkerk (1996) reported a 6.3-point IQ deficit compared to controls and a greater impact of disease than treatment variables as risk factors.

Fisher (1991) suggested that for each month that treatment is delayed, there is a 3- to 5-point loss in IQ. However, my group's experience with several clinically diagnosed patients indicates the effects are exponential, not linear, which may also explain why we fail to find correlations between treatment age and outcome in our screened CH sample. For example, in a pair of twin girls discordant for CH who were born in the Philippines (where newborn screening was unavailable at the time), diagnosis of CH in the affected child was made clinically when she was 3 months of age. We studied both girls when they were 3 and 6 years of age after they had immigrated to Canada. At age 6, the IQ differential between sisters was 65 points (>4 standard deviations). Similarly, the first Toronto patient identified by screening during preliminary investigations of the efficacy of laboratory methods for CH screening was not treated until she was 3 months of age; she is now severely retarded, as was the last patient to be identified clinically in the month prior to implementation of the provincial screening program. These findings suggest that every day that treatment is delayed is critical, especially if the thyroid gland is aplastic.

Specific Abilities

Because brain regions subserving various cognitive skills are different and are known to develop at different rates prenatally and postnatally, it is not surprising that early-treated CH is associated with a wide variety of neurocognitive deficits. The nature of these deficits depends on when exactly the hormone is missing during intrauterine and early postnatal life. In particular, there appear to be critical periods during fetal development and early life when there is an urgent need for TH to support adequate development of specific abilities (and presumably the development of their distinct underlying neurological substrates).

Research on affected children has shown that CH is associated with poorer motor skills (Fuggle et al. 1991; Kooistra et al. 1994; Rochiccioli et al. 1983), poorer visuomotor and visuospatial abilities (Rovet et al. 1992), delayed speech and language development (Gottschalk et al. 1994), and problems with attention and memory (Kooistra et al. 1996; Rovet and Alvarez 1996a, 1996b).

Neurodevelopmental profiles for motor, language, visuomotor, memory, and spatial abilities based on my group's research are presented in Figure 4–2. Shown are the results for both the entire group of children with CH and only those with the athyrotic etiology. The results are presented as difference scores relative to control values and for motor, language, visuomotor, memory, and spatial domains. Problems are evident in all domains studied.

In the motor domain, children with CH manifested problems from as early as 1 year of age to age 6, after which motor assessments were no longer done. Children with athyrosis appear to be more affected than the group as a whole. At age 6, neuromotor skills were assessed in detail using the Bruininks-Oseretsky Test of Neuromotor Proficiency. The results shown in Figure 4–3 indicate that skills involving the use of gross motor and mainly lower limb use (Rovet 1991a) are more problematic, both for children with athyrosis and for the group as a whole. Upper-limb coordination is much less affected, suggesting that TH insufficiency has *selective* effects on different aspects of the motor system, at least within the time interval that the children were hypothyroid (Rovet 1991a).

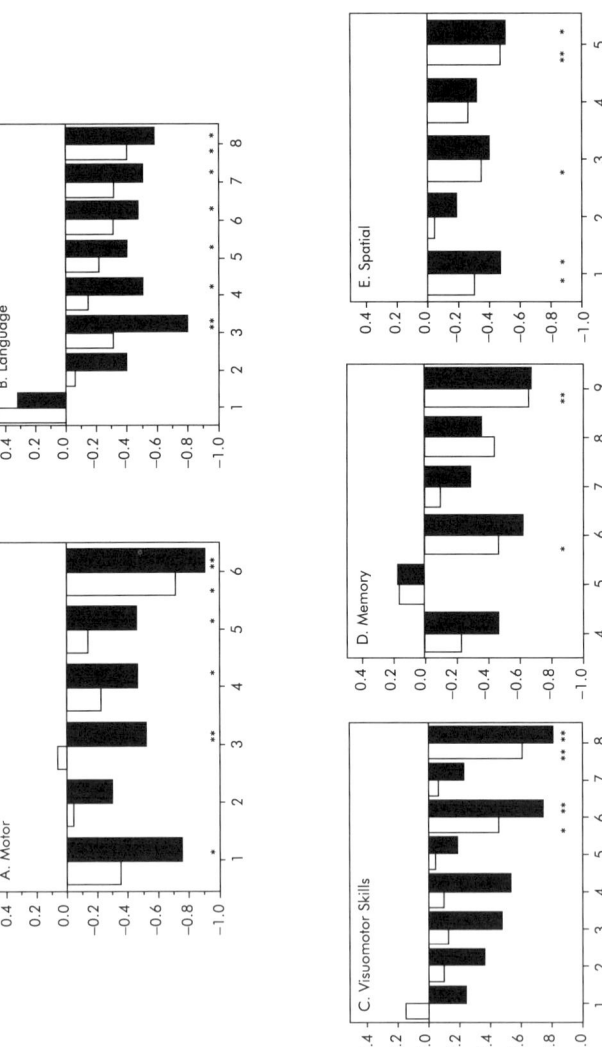

Figure 4–2. Neurodevelopmental profiles for motor, language, visuomotor, memory, and spatial abilities in children with congenital hypothyroidism (CH). *White bars* represent findings for total group with CH; *black bars* represent results for athyrotic group only. Results are expressed as differences from control subjects in standard deviation units. *$P < .05$; **$P < .01$.

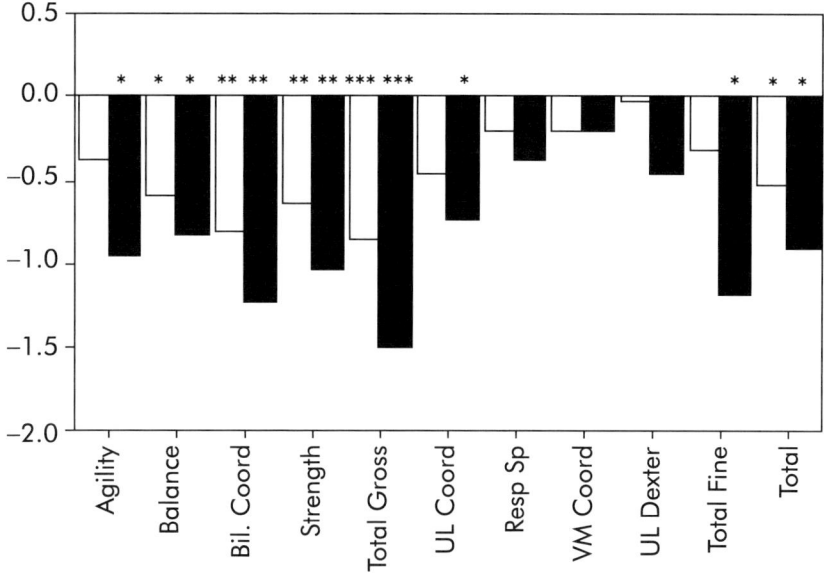

Figure 4–3. Results of the Bruininks-Oseretsky Test of Motor Proficiency (Bruininks 1978). *White bars* represent the total group with congenital hypothyroidism (CH); *black bars* represent the athyrotic group. Results are expressed as differences from controls in standard deviation units. Bil. Coord = Bilateral Coordination; UL Coord = Upper Limb Coordination; Resp Sp = Response Speed; VM Coord = Visuomotor Coordination; UL Dexter = Upper Limb Dexterity. *$P < .05$; **$P < .01$; ***$P < .001$.

Regarding language (Figure 4–2), it can be seen that delayed speech development is evident at about age 3, which anecdotally is when many parents seek consultation and neuropsychological evaluation; however, these deficits diminish, signifying catch-up later in childhood. Not all children are affected to the same degree, and in fact the majority are spared. Recent reanalysis of our findings to examine the incidence of expressive language delays at age 3 revealed mild to moderate deficits in 22%, with severe delays in only 4% (Rovet 1996a). For receptive language skills, 46% (versus 29% of control subjects) had mild to moderate deficits and none were severely affected.

Problems with visuomotor skills (Figure 4–2) appear to increase with age when greater demands are made on graphomotor production and task complexity increases. Difficulties on memory and spatial tasks are also evident.

Using multivariate correlational techniques, we also examined the contributions of different thyroid-related factors to specific abilities (Rovet et al. 1992). Our findings indicated associations between performance of motor tasks and prenatal hypothyroidism; between visuomotor skills and hypothyroidism in the first few weeks of life; and between auditory discrimination and hypothyroidism until 1–2 months after birth. Language skills, encompassing both expressive and receptive domains, were found to reflect both prenatal and postnatal hypothyroidism. Attentional skills were particularly sensitive to levels of circulating thyroid hormone at the time of testing (Rovet and Alvarez 1996a, 1996b), whereas memory reflected both early hypothyroidism and later hormone levels (Rovet and Ehrlich 1995).

Preliminary findings for our adolescent sample suggest that certain problems do persist, especially in the visuospatial domain, where deficits were first observed at age 2 (Rovet et al. 1992). A comparison of the first 38 patients with CH to reach adolescence and age-matched control subjects, who were tested with an extensive battery of neuropsychological tests, revealed that the CH group did significantly more poorly on all indices of spatial ability, as shown in Figure 4–4. They were also outscored by control subjects to a greater degree on Performance Intelligence Quotient (PIQ) tests (101 versus 114, $P < .001$) than on Verbal Intelligence Quotient (VIQ) tests (97.4 versus 105, $P = .03$). When the various visuospatial tests were subgrouped by type of spatial process, the most difficulty was observed on tasks of spatial location rather than object identity (Leneman and Rovet 1995), as shown in Figure 4–5. Because these types of tasks appear to tap different neuroanatomic pathways for processing "where" versus "what" information, respectively (Kosslyn et al. 1990), the present results suggest that a lack of TH in the perinatal period may differentially disrupt the development of the posterior parietal regions, which subserve these affected abilities (M. Leneman, L. Buchanan, and J. Rovet, "'What' and 'Where' Visuospatial Processing in Children With Congenital Hypothyroidism" (manuscript in preparation).

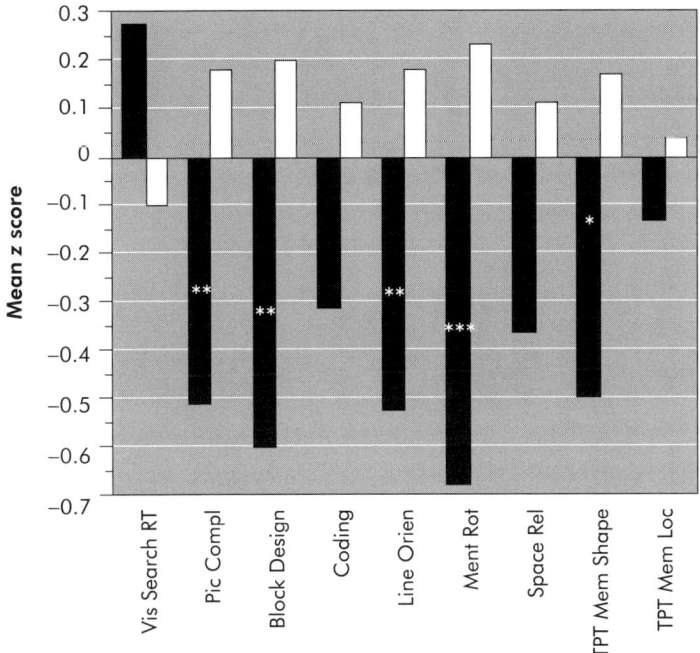

Figure 4–4. Performance of visuospatial processing tasks by adolescents with congenital hypothyroidism (CH) compared with control subjects. *Black bars* represent subjects with CH ($N = 38$); *white bars* represent control subjects ($N = 58$). Subjects with CH performed more slowly on the Visual Search task and made more errors than control subjects on the other tasks. Vis Search RT = Visual Search Reaction Time; Pic Compl = Picture Completion; Line Orien = Line Orientation; Ment Rot = Mental Rotation; Space Rel = Space Relations; TPT Mem Shape = Tactual Performance Test, Memory for Shapes Subtest; TPT Mem Loc = Tactual Performance Test, Memory for Locations Subtest.

Correlations computed between an index of disease severity and two kinds of visuospatial processing revealed a significant correlation for "where" ($P < .001$) but not "what" ($P > .05$) processes.

School Achievement

Academic progress has rarely been studied in children with CH. The New England Congenital Hypothyroidism Collaborative

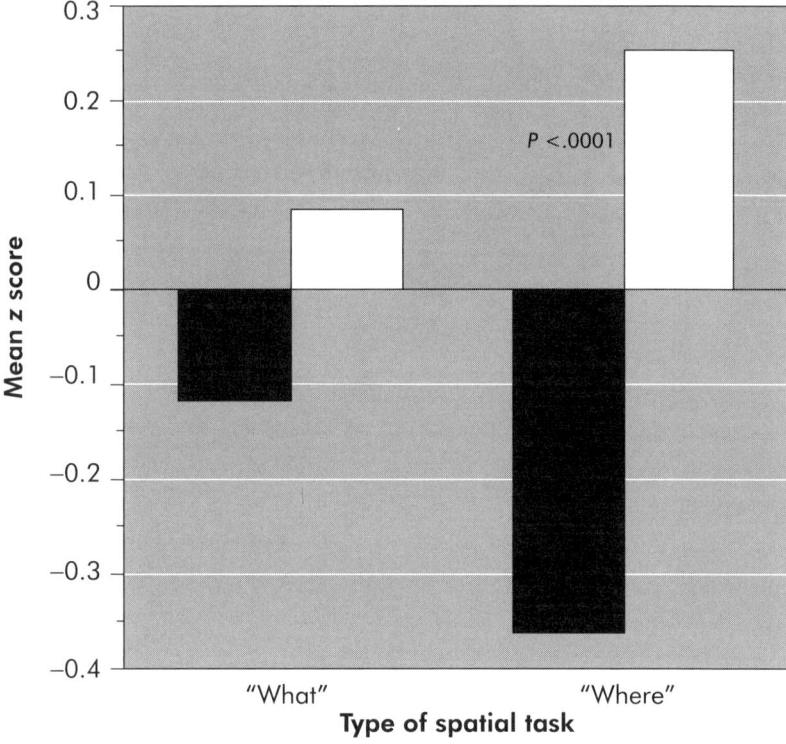

Figure 4–5. Comparison between adolescents with congenital hypothyroidism (CH) and control subjects on performance of "what" versus "where" spatial tasks. *Black bars* represent subjects with CH ($N = 38$); *white bars* represent control subjects ($N = 58$).

(1994) has reported average overall achievement. However, deficits in numerical skills have been observed by our group from as early as age 6. At age 7, reading performance was subnormal (<1 standard deviation) in 25% of subjects, and arithmetic performance was subnormal in 20%; these rates are somewhat higher than the rates for the general population.

As part of our research protocol, we conducted detailed psycho-educational evaluations on our sample during the third grade at school. All assessments were conducted during the spring semester to allow for a constant amount of teaching and experience with a teacher. Control subjects consisted of siblings and classmates. Using a screening test for learning disabilities, the Einstein, we found that children with CH had greater risk of arithmetic impairment but they did not differ from control subjects in reading impairment (Rovet et al. 1995) (see Figure 4–6). Approximately 45% of subjects with CH showed evidence of problems, in contrast to 23% of controls.

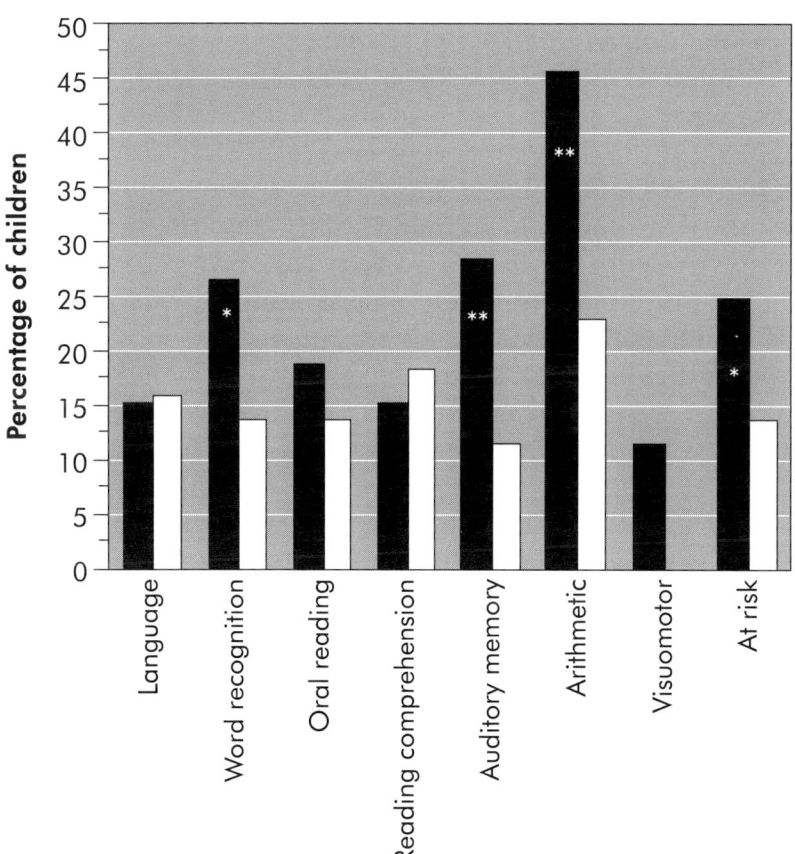

Figure 4–6. Results of learning disabilities screening test; proportion of children indicating problems on the Einstein Assessment of School-Related Skills (Gottesman and Cerullo 1988). *Black bars* represent subjects with congenital hypothyroidism (CH); *white bars* represent control subjects.

The results of more detailed testing showed that the children with CH were performing in grade 3 at about one-third of a grade below expectation, in contrast to control subjects, who were performing at grade level. This difference, although significant, is minimal in comparison with that of children with Turner's syndrome, for example, who by grade 6 are performing about two grades behind (Rovet 1996b). Detailed error analyses of the subjects' specific arithmetic performance were conducted in my laboratory by Kathy Petric, who did not find a specific arithmetic processing difficulty related to learning math facts or conducting math procedures (Petric and Rovet 1994). Similar studies were conducted when the children were in grade 6. By this grade, we found that some of the differences between the CH and control groups seemed to disappear, but it was not clear whether this reflected catch-up or the low ceiling (grade 6 level) of the arithmetic test they were given. With regard to reading, we observed that the CH group performed more poorly than control subjects at both the grade 3 and grade 6 levels on all measures of reading comprehension (Rovet et al. 1995), whereas their word decoding skills were unaffected. The only exception was children with CH who had hearing problems and showed problems with word decoding (see below).

The pattern of deficit in children with CH, which affects about 33% of the group, is suggestive of a mild nonverbal learning disability (Rovet 1995). Subtyping the children into different learning disability categories revealed children with CH were more likely to be arithmetic disabled than control subjects, as shown in Figure 4–7 (Rovet 1995).

With regard to actual school performance, parents reported that children with CH were less likely to be in gifted or advanced programs than control subjects and that they were slightly more likely to be receiving special education. However, they did not differ from control children without CH in their rates of grade retention. It is too soon to tell whether they will achieve the same levels of education as their siblings and how they will do vocationally. (Children clinically diagnosed with CH do very poorly in these areas.)

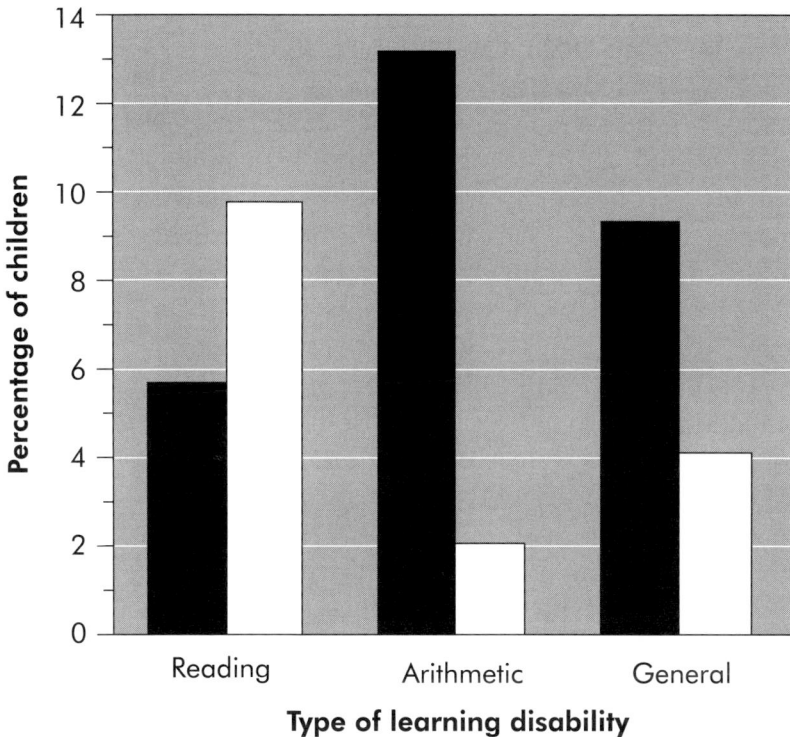

Figure 4–7. Proportion of grade 3 children with different kinds of learning disabilities. Results are based on the Wide Range Achievement Test—Revised (Jastak and Wilkinson 1984); cutoff scores are below the 10th percentile. *Black bars* represent subjects with congenital hypothyroidism (CH); *white bars* represent control subjects.

Hearing Problems

The disorder including thyroid hormone abnormalities and hearing problems known as Pendred's syndrome was characterized over a century ago (Pendred 1896) and involves both deafness and goiter (Fraser 1965). Similarly, hearing problems have been reported in endemic cretinism (DeLong et al. 1985) and resistance to thyroid hormone (Brucker-Davis et al. 1996; Refetoff et al. 1967; see also editorial by Forrest 1996). In children with late-treated CH, deafness or mild sensorineural hearing loss is not uncommon (Debruyne et al. 1983; Vandershueren-Lodewecykx et al. 1983). Similarly, in early-treated CH, as many as 20% of children have impaired hearing (Bellman et al. 1996; François et al. 1994), and problems in auditory processing have also been noted (Hébert et al. 1986). My group recently reported that children with CH have an increased incidence of hearing impairment, particularly a sensorineural hearing loss in the high frequency ranges. This is not surprising in light of studies with laboratory animals showing that thyroid hormone plays a significant role in the maturation of inner-ear structures (Deol 1976; Uziel et al. 1981; Withers et al. 1972) and the localization of thyroid β-receptors in the cochlea (Bradley et al. 1994) and brain structures comprising auditory pathways (Li and Boyages 1995). These receptors are involved in auditory ontogenesis (Corey and Breakefield 1994).

We examined the specific cognitive sequelae of hearing impairments in children with CH (Rovet et al. 1996). Our results revealed that sensorineural or conductive hearing loss had no effect on early and later speech and language development. However, impaired hearing was associated with poorer word recognition on reading tests and less adequate phonemic awareness ability.

We also examined the relationship between hearing impairment and indices of thyroid functioning at birth. Although there were no relationships with disease severity and duration, children with impaired hearing tended to have been treated about 1 week later, on average (day 22), than children with normal hearing (day 13); this suggests that the third week of life may be critical. However, recent reanalysis has revealed that this effect can be mostly attributed to one child who was treated beyond the second month of life. There was no association between cause of hypothyroidism and frequency or type of hearing problem.

Behavior Problems

Congenital hypothyroidism is generally associated with increased lethargy and passivity. In fact, one of the classic clinical features of late-treated CH is the "good baby" syndrome. There are few studies of the behavioral characteristics of early-treated children identified by newborn screening, because IQ appears to be the major end point (see above).

In a study of infant temperament my group conducted several years ago, 6-month-olds who were positively identified by newborn CH screening showed a significantly increased likelihood to have a difficult temperament (Rovet et al. 1989). This reflected their elevated scores on scales of arousal functions; however, their activity levels, persistence, and distractibility were not different than normal. The increase in difficult temperament at 6 months of age was found to be *positively* correlated with T_4 levels in the months preceding the assessment (i.e., 3–4 months of age) but not with T_4 levels at birth. In other words, a difficult temperament was associated with high levels of TH in infancy but not with severity of hypothyroidism at birth. We interpreted this finding as indicating that elevations in TH after birth (caused by excess hormone from therapy) served to advance the maturation of the hypothalamic-hypophyseal-adrenal axis for handling stress and sensitivity to stimulation. Atypical temperament characteristics at 8 years of age have also been described by Desjardins et al. (1987) in the Quebec cohort; these reflect increased levels of activity but milder than usual responses to stimulation and happier dispositions.

Several years ago, we examined whether an early screening diagnosis predisposed parents to increased protectiveness, creating a "vulnerable child" syndrome. This was determined retrospectively by correlating parents' scores on scales of family cohesiveness and enmeshment with their child's scores on behavior rating questionnaires. Contrary to expectations, parents who reported greater protectiveness rated their children as having fewer behavior problems (Rovet 1991b).

In our experience, significant behavior problems are seen infrequently among children with CH who are treated early. It is not known, however, whether the frequency differs from that of the normal population. The precipitating issues for behavior problems in children with CH appear to be similar to those in the general population: divorce, adoption, and sibling and peer problems. CH does not appear to be associated with an increased incidence of childhood psychopathology, including attention-deficit/hyperactivity disorder (ADHD). However, a limiting factor in our research has been that some of the more troubled families were among those who dropped out of our study early. We know of at least one child in our prospective study who was diagnosed with ADHD and successfully treated with methylphenidate. It is uncertain whether this is a comorbid or an associated problem. Informal observation of 7- to 12-year-old children with CH participating in our current thyroid and attention study suggests that their behavior and performance are somewhere between those of children with ADHD and children with neither disorder.

The behavior problems observed in children with juvenile acquired hypothyroidism following thyroxine therapy are rare in CH (see Rovet and Daneman, Chapter 6 in this volume), although several parents have reported that the children have difficulties focusing attention and increased jitteriness after a dosage increase (Ehrlich 1995). One toddler in our study demonstrated a paranoid reaction following a dosage increase, which abated when her dosage was lowered (see also Bhatara and McMillin, Chapter 7 in this volume).

Using parent and teacher rating scale data, my group studied whether children with CH are at increased risk of minor behavior problems. Our findings indicate that they do not differ from control subjects on any scale except attention, with which both parents and teachers agree the children have greater than normal difficulty (Rovet 1995). Figure 4–8 shows that hyperactivity is much less of an issue. In a previous report, we demonstrated a negative relationship between attention, which was measured by psychometric tests, and levels of circulating thyroxine: we found that attention was poorer when TH levels were higher (Rovet et al. 1993). The significance of this relationship is currently being investigated in detail in our laboratory.

Prompted by the work of Hauser et al. (1993) (see also Hauser, Chapter 5 in this volume), Miguel Alvarez, a visiting scientist in my laboratory from Cuba, and I examined how the combined effect of different levels of T_4 and TSH affected attention in children with

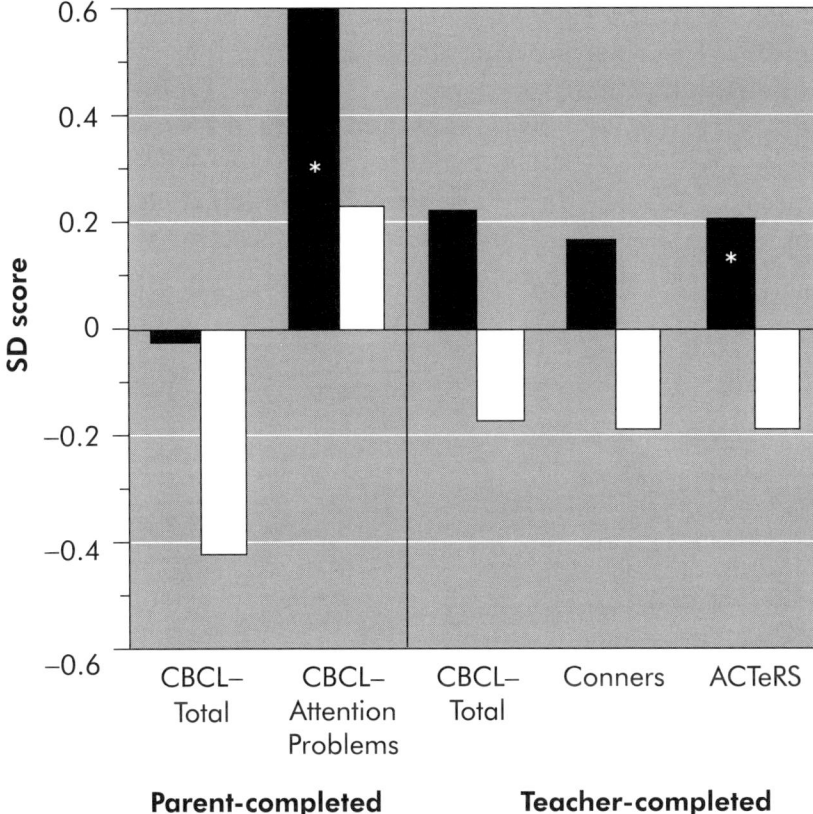

Figure 4–8. Results for Child Behavior Checklist (CBCL; Achenbach and Edelbrock 1983), Hyperactivity Index of the Conners Rating Scales (Conners 1990), and Attention-Deficit Disorder with Hyperactivity (ADD-H) Comprehensive Teachers Rating Scale (ACTeRS; Ullmann et al. 1991). *Black bars* represent subjects with congenital hypothyroidism (CH); *white bars* represent control subjects.

CH. We were concerned with determining the incidence of a hormonal profile suggestive of resistance to thyroid hormone (RTH) (i.e., high T_4/high TSH) in children with CH and how this differed from a hyperthyroid profile (high T_4/low TSH). In the first retrospective study, we subgrouped children according to their levels of T_4 and TSH at the time of testing. A comparison of those with normal levels and those with high T_4 values and TSH in the high, normal, or low ranges (see Figure 4–9) indicated that the subgroup with elevated T_4 and TSH levels (i.e., the RTH profile; see Rovet and Alvarez 1996a), which represented 9.3% of 7-year-olds in our sample, attended most poorly but had the lowest activity levels. In contrast, children with a hyperthyroid profile (T_4 elevated, TSH suppressed) showed no deficits on attention tests but were rated as

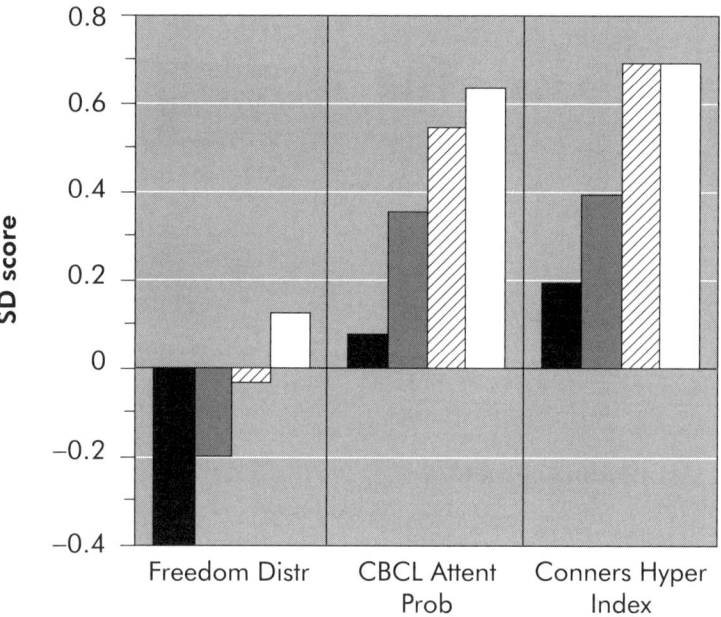

Figure 4–9. Mean attention and hyperactivity test scores in congenital hypothyroidism (CH) as a function of thyroxine (T_4) and thyrotropin (TSH) levels. *Black bars* represent the group with high T_4 and high TSH; *stippled bars* represent the group with high T_4 and normal TSH; *striped bars* represent the group with high T_4 and low TSH; and *white bars* represent the group with normal T_4 and varying TSH. Results are presented in standard deviation (SD) units. Freedom Distr = Wechsler (1974) Freedom from Distractibility factor; CBCL Attent Prob = Child Behavior Checklist (Achenbach and Edelbrock 1983) Attention Problems; Conners Hyper Index = Conners Rating Scales (Conners 1990) Hyperactivity Index.

being more active (Rovet and Alvarez 1996b). These patterns were found to be transient, reflecting the contribution of hormone levels at the time of testing; when the children were reevaluated 2 years later at age 9, the relationships still existed but involved different children, depending on their hormone levels on the day of testing (Rovet and Alvarez 1996a).

In a separate retrospective analysis of the data from the children with CH at their 8-year follow-up visit, Miguel Alvarez and I observed (using several parent-completed behavior problem questionnaires) that the children with CH scored higher than control subjects on scales of conduct and attentional problems. In addition, they were reported as being more organized and more persistent than normal and as having very positive dispositions (J. Rovet and M. Alvarez, "The Relation of Thyroid Function to Attention and Behavior in Eight-Year-Old Children With Congenital Hypothyroidism" [unpublished manuscript], 1994). Regression analyses revealed that scores on scales of conduct problems were positively associated with the starting dosage of levothyroxine (L-T_4); scores on indices of hyperactivity, with T_4 levels at 3 months of age; and a difficult temperament, with low levels of TSH at the time of testing. We also found that the children who received very high starting dosages of L-T_4 were more likely to have behavior problems at age 8 (Rovet and Ehrlich 1995). Because this research was based on relatively crude indices of attention and behavior, we are now studying the effects of neonatal and concurrent TH levels on specific attentional processing subcomponents and on the patients' activity levels.

Implications for Treatment and Management

This chapter has shown the importance of the earliest possible replacement intervention in this population and the need for optimal dosage levels. Dosage should be adjusted to achieve euthyroidism as soon as possible but not to create undue behavioral sequelae. Although it may not yet be possible to reduce the effects of TH insufficiency during pregnancy in CH, the need to shorten the postnatal window should be paramount. This requires close, continuous, and scrupulous monitoring of these children throughout infancy and, ideally, childhood. It is imperative to ensure that TH levels reach the normal range as soon as possible and are continuously maintained in this range, while also preventing hyperthyroxinemia from doses that are too high. Although the extreme behavior problems seen in a small subgroup of patients with juvenile acquired hypothyroidism following thyroxine therapy are extremely rare in this population (see Rovet and Daneman, Chapter 6 in this volume), we have seen children with poor behavioral responses to dose changes that are transient. Although we have not found compliance to be a major issue in our sample, adolescents may be more prone to forgetting to take their medication.

The findings from our studies and those of most others reflect relatively conservative estimates of performance deficits in this population. This is because the children who were observed in these prospective studies received the most optimal care and management at the time because they were seen in tertiary pediatric health care centers. (One exception is Heyerdahl, who studied children across all of Norway and who has reported deficits associated with both early disease and later treatment.) However, the children with CH *not in these studies* may not have all received the same level of care and may be more severely affected. Throughout most of Canada and the United States, most children with CH are followed up mostly by primary care physicians, who are variably informed as to the proper protocols for treatment and management, especially beyond the neonatal period. Although some jurisdictions do provide treatment guidelines, this is often the exception. Indeed, there is very little public information about longer-term management and outcome in these children. A recent survey indicates that unlike other screened metabolic disorders, physicians seldom refer these patients to specialists, under the belief that hypothyroidism is easy to treat and their experience with adult patients applies to children (B. Therrell, Texas Department of Health, personal communication, August 1996). However, the issues are quite different for child than for adult populations. The practice of referral to primary physicians increases the likelihood of poorer management, including the possibility of not dealing adequately with issues such as transient hypothyroidism and hearing, learning, and attentional problems.

Because guidelines for treatment and management of older children with CH are not widely available, there is concern that health maintenance organizations (HMOs) may not allow for sufficient visits to monitor TH levels closely for dosage changes. Furthermore, there is concern that HMOs may restrict the type of thyroid medication the child is to receive. In Canada, cutbacks in federal funding, which have led to reduced provincial budgets for health care, may also restrict the level of care these children receive. In our hospital, for example, children with CH are now followed up by pediatric endocrinologists only to age 3, in contrast to previous years when they were followed up throughout childhood. Even though the majority of children are healthy and no longer in need of specialized care, this may be too early for dealing with problems in speech, hearing, and learning. Many parents whose children are treated by primary health care providers have expressed to us serious concern about the quality of care and timing of dose changes.

Other problems arise from the highly variable (and often nonexistent) information that is provided to parents and parent support groups. The few available pamphlets often present an unrealistic view of long-term outcome. For example, undue emphasis on "normal intelligence" could result in failure to recognize learning problems. Furthermore, unlike other pediatric diseases, there are few avenues for parent support and networking with regard to CH, presumably because it is not considered a serious enough or highly demanding disease. Exceptions include the highly successful annual 1-day programs in Michigan and Illinois, where information on dealing with children with CH is shared among families and with health care specialists.

Conclusions

Although early-treated congenital hypothyroidism following newborn screening is generally associated with significantly reduced morbidity, persisting selective impairments may still occur in these children. They may have language delays, minor motor problems, visuospatial deficits, and attentional problems. About 20% of children may also have hearing impairments. Whereas some problems reflect the severity, duration, and timing of early hypothyroidism, problems with attention appear to result from inappropriate levels of circulating hormone at the time of testing. Continuous regular monitoring is imperative. Better guidelines for physicians and better information for parents are also urgently needed. Although behavior problems are rare in this pediatric population, these children may be at slightly increased risk of ADHD, although this issue has never been definitively determined.

References

Achenbach TM, Edelbrock C: Manual for the Child Behavior Checklist and Revised Child Behavior Profile. Burlington, VT, University of Vermont, 1983

Alves C, Eidson M, Engle H, et al: Changes in brain maturation detected by magnetic resonance imaging in congenital hypothyroidism. J Pediatr 115:600–603, 1989

American Academy of Pediatrics: Newborn screening for congenital hypothyroidism: recommended guidelines. Pediatrics 91:1203–1209, 1993

Aronson R, Rovet JF, Ehrlich RM, et al: Physical development in congenital hypothyroidism detected by screening of neonates. J Pediatr 116:33–37, 1990

Bachrach LK, Burrow GN: Thyroid function in pregnancy. Fetal-maternal relationships. Pediatric and Adolescent Endocrinology 14:1–18, 1985

Bellman SC, Davies A, Fuggle PW, et al: Mild impairment of neuro-otological function in early treated congenital hypothyroidism. Arch Dis Child 74:215–218, 1996

Benda C: Mongolism and Cretinism: A Study of the Clinical Manifestations and the General Pathology of Pituitary and Thyroid Deficiency. London, Heinemann, 1941

Bikker H, den Hartog MT, Baas F, et al: A 20-base pair duplication in the human thyroid peroxidase gene results in a total iodide organification defect and congenital hypothyroidism. J Clin Endocrinol Metab 79:248–252, 1994

Bikker H, Vulsma T, Baas F, et al: Identification of five novel inactivating mutations in the human thyroid peroxidase gene by denaturing gradient gel electrophoresis. Human Mutation 6:9–16, 1995

Bode HH, Vanjonack WJ, Crawford JD: Mitigation of cretinism by breast-feeding. Pediatrics 62:13–16, 1978

Boyages SC, Halpern JP: Endemic cretinism: toward a unifying hypothesis. Thyroid 3:59, 1993

Boyages SC, Halpern JP, Maberly GF, et al: A comparative study of neurological and myxedematous endemic cretinism in western China. J Clin Endocrinol Metab 67:1262–1271, 1988

Bradley D, Young W, Weinberger C: Differential expression of alpha and beta thyroid hormone receptor genes in rat brain and pituitary. Neurobiology 86:7250–7254, 1989

Bradley DJ, Towle HC, Young WS: Spatial and temporal expression of alpha- and beta-thyroid hormone receptor mRNAs, including the beta 2-subtype, in the developing mammalian nervous system. J Neurosci 12:2288–2302, 1992

Bradley DJ, Towle HC, Young S: Alpha and beta thyroid hormone receptor (TR) gene expression during auditory neurogenesis: evidence for TR isoform-specific transcriptional regulation in vivo. Proc Natl Acad Sci U S A 91:439–443, 1994

Brown AL, Fernhoff PM, Milner J, et al: Racial differences in the incidence of congenital hypothyroidism. J Pediatr 99:934–936, 1981

Brucker-Davis F, Skarulis MC, Pikus A, et al: Prevalence and mechanisms of hearing loss in patients with resistance to thyroid hormone. J Clin Endocrinol Metab 81:2768–2772, 1996

Bruininks R: Bruininks-Oseretsky Test of Neuromotor Proficiency. Circle Pines, MN, American Guidance Service, 1978

Bucher H, Prader A, Illig R: Head circumference, height, bone age and weight in 103 children with congenital hypothyroidism before and during thyroid hormone replacement. Helv Paediatr Acta 40:305–316, 1985

Burrow GN, Fisher DA, Larsen PR: Maternal and fetal thyroid function. N Engl J Med 331:1072–1078, 1994

Campos SP, Sandberg DE, Barrick C, et al: Outcome of lower L-thyroxine dose for treatment of congenital hypothyroidism. Clin Pediatr 34:514–520, 1995

Cheron RG, Kaplan MM, Larsen PR, et al: Neonatal thyroid function after propylthiouracil therapy for maternal Graves' disease. N Engl J Med 304:525–528, 1991

Conners CK: The Conners Rating Scales. Toronto, Canada, Multi-Health Systems, 1990

Corey DP, Breakefield XO: Transcription factors in inner ear development. Proc Natl Acad Sci U S A 91:433–436, 1994

Crome L, Stern J: Pathology of mental retardation. Edinburgh, Churchill Livingstone, 1972

Davy T, Daneman D, Walfish PG, et al: Congenital hypothyroidism: the effect of stopping treatment at 3 years. American Journal of Diseases of Children 139:1028–1030, 1985

Debruyne F, Vanderschueren-Lodeweyckz M, Bastijns P: Hearing in congenital hypothyroidism. Audiology 22:404–409, 1983

DeGroot LJ, Larsen PR, Henneman G: The Thyroid and Its Diseases, 6th Edition. New York, Churchill Livingstone, 1996

Delange F, De Vijlder J, Morreale de Escobar G, et al: Significance of early diagnostic data in congenital hypothyroidism, in Research in Congenital Hypothyroidism. Edited by Delange F, Fisher DA, Glinoer D. New York, Plenum, 1989, pp 225–236

DeLong GR, Stanbury JB, Fierror-Benitz R: Neurological signs in congenital iodine-deficiency disorder (endemic cretinism). Dev Med Child Neurol 27:217–324, 1985

Deol MS: The role of thyroxine in the differentiation of the organ of Corti. Acta Otolaryngol 81:429–435, 1976

Derksen-Lubsen G, Verkerk PH: Neuropsychologic development in early treated congenital hypothyroidism: analysis of literature data. Pediatr Res 39:561–566, 1996

Desjardins M, Glorrieux J, Morissette J: The temperament of hypothyroid children, in Advances in Neonatal Screening. Edited by Therrell BL. Amsterdam, Elsevier Science, 1987, pp 105–106

Dubuis JM, Glorieux J, Richer F, et al: Outcome of severe congenital hypothyroidism: closing the developmental gap with early high dose levothyroxine treatment. J Clin Endocrinol Metab 81:222–227, 1996

Ehrlich RM: Thyroxine dose for congenital hypothyroidism. Clin Pediatr 34:522–523, 1995

Eisenstein Z, Weiss M, Katz Y, et al: Intellectual capacity of subjects exposed to methimazole or propylthiouracil in utero. Eur J Pediatr 151:558–559, 1992

Ekins R, Sinha A, Ballabio M, et al: Role of maternal carrier proteins in the supply of thyroid hormones to the fetal-placental unit: evidence of a fetal-placental requirement for thyroxine, in Research in Congenital Hypothyroidism. Edited by Delange F, Fisher DA, Glinoer D. New York, Plenum, 1989, pp 42–60

Emerson C: Thyroid disease during and after pregnancy, in Werner and Ingbar's The Thyroid, 6th Edition. Edited by Braverman LE, Utiger RD. Philadelphia, PA, JB Lippincott, 1991, pp 1263–1279

Farsetti A, Mitsuhashi T, Desvergne B, et al: Molecular basis of thyroid hormone regulation of myelin basic protein gene expression in rodent brain. J Biol Chem 266:23226–23232, 1991

Farsetti A, Desvergne B, Hallenbeck P, et al: Characterization of myelin basic protein thyroid hormone response element and its function in the context of native and heterologous promotor. J Biol Chem 267:15784–15788, 1992

Fellous A, Lennon A, Francon J, et al: Thyroid hormones and neurotubule assembly in vitro during brain development. Eur J Biochem 101:365–376, 1979

Fisher DA: Management of congenital hypothyroidism. J Clin Endocrinol Metab 72:523–529, 1991

Forrest D: Deafness and goiter: molecular genetic considerations (editorial). J Clin Endocrinol Metab 81:2764–2767, 1996

François M, Bonfils P, Leger J, et al: Role of congenital hypothyroidism in hearing loss in children. J Pediatr 123:444–446, 1994

Frank JE, Faix JE, Hermos RJ, et al: Thyroid function in very low birth weight infants: effects on neonatal hypothyroidism screening. J Pediatr 128:548–554, 1996

Fraser GR: Association of congenital deafness with goiter (Pendred's syndrome): a study of 207 families. Ann Hum Genet 28:201–249, 1965

Fuggle PW, Grant DB, Smith I, et al: Intelligence, motor skills and behaviour at 5 years in early treated congenital hypothyroidism. Eur J Pediatr 150:570–574, 1991

Germak J, Foley TP: Longitudinal assessment of L-thyroxine therapy for congenital hypothyroidism. J Pediatr 117:211–219, 1990

Glinoer D, De Nayer P, Bourdoux P, et al: Regulation of maternal thyroid during pregnancy. J Clin Endocrinol Metab 71:276–287, 1990

Gottesman RL, Cerullo FM: Einstein Assessment of School-Related Skills. Cleveland, OH, Modern Curriculum Press, 1988

Gottschalk B, Richman R, Lewandowski L: Subtle speech and motor deficits of children with congenital hypothyroidism treated early. Dev Med Child Neurol 36:216–220, 1994

Gould E, Butcher LL: Developing cholinergic basal forebrain neurons are sensitive to thyroid hormone. J Neurosci 9:3347–3358, 1989

Gupta RK, Bhatia V, Poptani H, et al: Brain metabolite changes on in vivo proton magnetic resonance spectroscopy in children with congenital hypothyroidism. J Pediatr 126:389–392, 1995

Hack M, Taylor G, Klein N, et al: School-age outcomes in children with birth weights under 750 g. N Engl J Med 331:753–759, 1994

Hahn HB, Brown LO, Hillis A, et al: Breast feeding and neonatal screening for congenital hypothyroidism. Texas Med 82:46–47, 1986

Hannigan JH, Martier SS, Naber JM: Independent associations among maternal alcohol consumption and infant thyroxine levels and pregnancy outcome. Alcohol Clin Exp Res 19:135–141, 1995

Hashimoto Y, Furukawa S, Omae F, et al: Correlative regulation of nerve growth factor level and choline acetyltransferase activity by thyroxine in particular regions of infant rat brain. J Neurochem 63:326–332, 1994

Hauser P, Zametkin AJ, Martinez P, et al: Attention-deficit hyperactivity disorder in people with generalized resistance to thyroid hormone. N Engl J Med 328:997–1001, 1993

Hébert R, Laurea E, Vanasse M, et al: Auditory brainstem response audiometry in congenitally hypothyroid children under early replacement therapy. Pediatr Res 20:570–573, 1986

Hernandez JT, Hoffman L, Weavil S, et al: The effect of drug exposure on thyroid hormone levels of newborns. Biochemical Medicine and Metabolic Biology 48:255–262, 1992

Heyerdahl S, Kase BF, Lie SO: Intellectual development in children with congenital hypothyroidism in relation to recommended thyroxine treatment. J Pediatr 118:850–857, 1991

Hollowell JG, Therrell BL, Hannon WH: Newborn Screening for Congenital Hypothyroidism. New York, Oxford University Press (in press)

Hulse JA, Grant DB, Jackson D, et al: Growth, development, and reassessment of hypothyroid infants diagnosed by screening. BMJ 284:1435–1437, 1982

Jastak S, Wilkinson GS: Wide Range Achievement Test—Revised. Wilmington, DE, Jastak Associates, 1984

Juarez de Ku LM, Meserve LA: Perinatal intake of polychlorinated biphenyl (PCB), in Toxin-Induced Models of Neurological Disorders. Edited by Woodruff ML, Nonneman AJ. New York, Plenum, 1994, pp 281–299

Juarez de Ku LM, Sharma-Stokkermans M, Meserve LA: Thyroxine normalizes polychlorinated biphenyl (PCB) dose-related depression of choline acetyltransferase (ChAT) activity in hippocampus and basal forebrain of 150 day-old rats. Toxicology 94:19–30, 1994

Klawans HL, Goetz C, Weiner WJ: Dopamine receptor site sensitivity in hypothyroid and hyperthyroid guinea pigs, in Advances in Neurology, Vol 5. Edited by McDowell FH, Barbeau A. New York, Raven, 1974, pp 846–847

Kooistra LL, Laane C, Vulsma T, et al: Motor and cognitive development in children with congenital hypothyroidism: a long-term evaluation of the effects of neonatal treatment. J Pediatr 124:903–909, 1994.

Kooistra L, van der Meere JJ, Vulsma T, et al: Sustained attention problems in children with early treated congenital hypothyroidism. Acta Paediatr 85:425–429, 1996

Koopman-Esseboom C, Morse DC, Weisglas-Kuperus N, et al: Effects of dioxins and polychlorinated biphenyls on thyroid hormone status of pregnant women and their infants. Pediatr Res 36:468–473, 1994

Kosslyn SM, Flynn RA, Amsterdam JB, et al: Components of high-level vision: a cognitive neuroscience analysis and accounts of neurological syndromes. Cognition 34:203–277, 1990

LaFranchi SH, Hanna CE, Krainz PL, et al: Screening for congenital hypothyroidism with specimen collection at two time periods: results of the Northwest Regional Sreening Program. Pediatrics 76:734–740, 1985

Larsen PR: Ontogenesis of thyroid function, thyroid hormone, and brain development, in The Thyroid and Its Diseases, 6th Edition. Edited by DeGroot LJ, Larsen PR, Henneman G. New York, Churchill Livingstone, 1996, pp 541–567

Lauder J, Krebs H: Do neurotransmitters, neurohumors, and hormones specify critical periods, in Developmental Neuropsychobiology. Edited by Greenough W, Juraska J. New York, Academic Press, 1986, pp 119–174

Legrand J: Effects of thyroid hormones on central nervous system development, in Neurobehavioral Teratology. Edited by Yanat J. Amsterdam, Elsevier, 1984, pp 331–363

Leneman M, Rovet J: "What" happens to the "how" and "where" visual pathways in congenital hypothyroidism. Poster presented at the Hospital for Sick Children Summer Student Symposium, Toronto, July 1995

Levine GD, Therrell BL: Second testing for hypothyroidism. Pediatrics 86:375–376, 1978

Li M, Boyages SC: Detection of widespread beta$_2$ thyroid hormone receptor mRNA in rat brain using cRNA in situ hybridisation histochemistry. Thyroid 5 (suppl 1):S80, 1995

Lucas A, Rennie J, Baker BA, et al: Low plasma triiodothyronine concentrations and outcome in preterm infants. Arch Dis Child 63:1201–1206, 1988

Lucas A, Morley R, Fewtrell MS: Low triiodothyronine concentration in preterm infants and subsequent intelligence quotient (IQ) at 8-year follow-up. BMJ 312:1132–1133, 1996

MacSweeney D, Timms P, Johnson A: Thyro-endocrine pathology, obstetric morbidity and schizophrenia: survey of a hundred families with a schizophrenic proband. Psychol Med 8:151–155, 1978

Madeira MD, Paula-Barbarosa MM: Reorganization of mossy fiber synapses in male and female hypothyroid rats: a stereological study. J Comp Neurol 337:334–352, 1993

Man EB, Brown JF, Serunian SA: Maternal hypothyroxinemia: psychoneurological deficits of progeny. Ann Clin Lab Sci 21:227–239, 1991

Meijer WJ, Verloove-Vanhorick SP, Brand R, et al: Transient hypothyroxinaemia associated with developmental delay in very preterm infants. Arch Dis Child 67:944–947, 1992

Morreale de Escobar G, Obregon MJ, Escobar del Rey F: Transfer of thyroid hormones from the mother to the fetus, in Research in Congenital Hypothyroidism. Edited by Delange F, Fisher DA, Glinoer D. New York, Plenum, 1989, pp 15–30

Moschini L, Costa P, Marinelli E, et al: Longitudinal assessment of children with congenital hypothyroidism detected by neonatal screening. Helv Paediatr Acta 41:415–424, 1986

Munoz A, Rodriguez-Peña A, Perez-Castillo A, et al: Effects of neonatal hypothyroidism on rat brain gene expression. Mol Endocrinol 5:273–280, 1991

New England Congenital Hypothyroidism Collaborative: Neonatal hypothyroidism screening: status of patients at 6 years of age. J Pediatr 107:915–918, 1985

New England Congenital Hypothyroidism Collaborative: Correlation of cognitive test scores and adequacy of treatment in adolescents with congenital hypothyroidism. J Pediatr 124:383–387, 1994

Nicholson JL, Altman J: Thyroid and developing cerebellum. Brain Res 44:13–23, 1972

Nunez J: Differential expression of microtubule components during brain development. Dev Neurosci 8:125–141, 1986

Pendred V: Deaf-mutism and goitre. Lancet 2:532, 1896

Petric K, Rovet J: Math processing in congenital hypothyroidism. Poster presented at the Hospital for Sick Children Summer Student Symposium, Toronto, July 1994

Pluim HJ, de Vijlder JJ, Olie K, et al: Effects of pre- and postnatal exposure to chlorinated dioxins and furans on human neonatal thyroid hormone concentrations. Environ Health Perspect 101:504–508, 1993

Pop VJ, de Vries E, Anneloes L, et al: Maternal thyroid peroxidase antibodies during pregnancy: a marker of impaired child development? J Clin Endocrinol Metab 80:3561–3566, 1995

Porterfield SP, Hendrich CE: The role of thyroid hormones in prenatal and neonatal neurological development—current perspectives. Endocr Rev 14:94–106, 1993

Porterfield SP, Stein SA: Thyroid hormones and neurological development: update 1994. Endocr Rev 3:357–363, 1994

Potter B, Mano M, Belling G, et al: Retarded fetal brain development resulting from severe dietary iodine deficiency in sheep. Neuropathol Appl Neurobiol 8:303–313, 1982

Puymirat J: Effects of dysthyroidism on central catecholaminergic neurons. Neurochem Int 17:969–977, 1985

Puymirat J, Barret A, Picart R, et al: Triiodothyronine enhances the morphological maturation of dopaminergic neurons from fetal mouse hypothalamus cultured in serum-free medium. Neuroscience 10:801–810, 1983

Rastogi RB, Singhal RL: Influence of neonatal and adult hyperthyroidism on behavior and biosynthetic capacity for norepinephrine, dopamine, and 5-hydroxytryptamine in rat brain. J Pharmacol Exp Ther 198:609–618, 1976

Refetoff S, DeWind LT, DeGroot LJ: Familial syndrome combining deaf-mutism, stippled epiphyses, goiter and abnormally high PBI: possible target organ refractoriness to thyroid hormone. J Clin Endocrinol 27:279–294, 1967

Reuss ML, Paneth N, Pinto-Martin JA, et al: The relation of transient hypothyroxinemia in preterm infants to neurologic development at two years of age. N Engl J Med 334:821–827, 1996

Rivkees SA, Hardin DS: Cretinism after weekly dosing with levo-thyroxine for treatment of congenital hypothyroidism. J Pediatr 125:147–149, 1994

Rochiccioli R, Roe B, Alexander F, et al: Resultants du developmente psychomoteur des hypothyroidies dépistées à la naissance. Archives Françaises de Pediatrie 40:537–541, 1983

Rodriguez-Peña A, Ibarrola N, Iniguez MA, et al: Neonatal hypothyroidism affects the timely expression of myelin-associated glycoprotein in the rat brain. J Clin Invest 91:812–818, 1993

Rosman N, Malone M, Helfenstein M, et al: The effect of thyroid deficiency on myelination of the brain. Neurology 22:99–106, 1972

Rovet J: Hypothyroidism: intellectual and neuropsychological functioning, in Psychoneuroendocrinology: Brain, Behavior, and Hormonal Interactions. Edited by Holmes C. New York, Springer-Verlag, 1990, pp 273–322

Rovet J: Neuromotor deficiencies in six year old hypothyroid children identified by newborn screening, in Proceedings of 8th National Neonatal Screening Symposium and XXI Birth Defects Symposium. Edited by Pass K. Washington, DC, Association of State and Territorial Public Health Laboratory Directors, 1991a, pp 378–381

Rovet J: Does newborn screening increase the risk of the vulnerable child syndrome? in Proceedings of 8th National Neonatal Screening Symposium and XXI Birth Defects Symposium. Edited by Pass K. Washington, DC, Association of State and Territorial Public Health Laboratory Directors, 1991b, pp 211–218

Rovet J: Congenital hypothyroidism, in Syndrome of Nonverbal Learning Disabilities: Neurodevelopmental Manifestations. Edited by Rourke BP. New York, Guilford, 1995, pp 255–281

Rovet J: Congenital hypothyroidism: new data on outcome. Paper presented at a conference in honour of the retirement of Robert Ehrlich. Toronto, February 1996a

Rovet J: Math processing in Turner Syndrome, in Turner Syndrome Across the Lifespan. Edited by Rovet J. Toronto, Klein Graphics, 1996b, pp 44–51

Rovet J, Alvarez M: Thyroid hormone and attention in children with congenital hypothyroidism. J Pediatr Endocrinol Metab 9:63–66, 1996a

Rovet J, Alvarez M: Thyroid hormone and attention in school-age children with congenital hypothyroidism. J Child Psychol Psychiatry 37:579–585, 1996b

Rovet JF, Ehrlich RM: Long-term effects of L-thyroxine therapy for congenital hypothyroidism. J Pediatr 126:380–386, 1995

Rovet J, Ehrlich R, Sorbara D: Intellectual outcome in children with fetal hypothyroidism. J Pediatr 110:700–704, 1987

Rovet J, Ehrlich R, Sorbara D: Effect of thyroid hormone level on temperament in infants with congenital hypothyroidism detected by screening of neonates. J Pediatr 114:63–68, 1989

Rovet JF, Ehrlich RM, Sorbara DL: Neurodevelopment in infants and preschool children with congenital hypothyroidism: etiological and treatment factors affecting outcome. J Pediatr Psychol 17:187–213, 1992

Rovet JF, Ehrlich RM, Donner E: Long-term neurodevelopmental correlates of treatment adequacy in screened hypothyroid children. Pediatr Res 33:S91, 1993

Rovet J, Ehrlich R, Altmann D: Psychoeducational outcome in children with early treated congenital hypothyroidism. Poster presented at the International Thyroid Congress, Toronto, September 1995

Rovet J, Walker W, Bliss B, et al: Long term sequelae of hearing impairment in congenital hypothyroidism. J Pediatr 128:776–783, 1996

Sack J, Frucht H, Amado O, et al: Breast milk thyroxine and how cow's milk may mitigate and delay the clinical picture of neonatal hypothyroidism. Acta Paediatr Scand Suppl 277:54–56, 1979

Savard P, Merand Y, DiPaolo T, et al: Effects of thyroid state on serotonin, 5-hydroxyindoleacetic acid and substance P contents in discrete brain nuclei of adult rats. Neuroscience 10:1399–1404, 1983

Shapiro S: Metabolic and maturational effects of thyroxine in the infant rat. Endocrinology 78:527–532, 1966

Silva JE, Larsen PR: Comparison of iodothyronine 5′-deiodinase and other thyroid-hormone-dependent enzyme activities in the cerebral cortex and hypothyroid neonatal rat. J Clin Invest 70:1110–1123, 1982

Simons WF, Fuggle PW, Grant DB, et al: Intellectual development at 10 years in early treated congenital hypothyroidism. Arch Dis Child 71:232–234, 1994

Strait KA, Schwartz HL, Perez-Castillo A, et al: Relationship of c-erbA mRNA content to tissue triiodothyronine nuclear binding capacity and function in developing and adult rats. J Biol Chem 265:10514–10521, 1990

Thorpe-Beeston JG, Nicolaides KH, Felton CV, et al: Maturation of the secretion of thyroid hormone and thyroid-stimulating hormone in the fetus. N Engl J Med 324:532–536, 1991

Tillotson S, Fuggle P, Smith I, et al: Relation between biochemical severity and intelligence in early treated congenital hypothyroidism: a threshold effect. Br Med J 309:440–445, 1994

Ullmann RK, Sleator EK, Sprague RL: ADD-H Comprehensive Teachers Rating Scale. Champaign, IL, MetriTech, 1991

Uziel A, Gabrion J, Ohresser M, et al: Effects of hypothyroidism on the structural development of the organ of corti in the rat. Acta Otolaryngol 92:469–480, 1981

van Wassenaer AG, Kok JH, Endert E, et al: Thyroxine administration to infants of less than 30 weeks' gestational age does not increase plasma triiodothyronine concentrations. Acta Endocrinol 129:129–146, 1993

van Wassenaer AG, Kok JH, de Vijlder JJM, et al: Effects of thyroxine supplementation on neurologic development in infants born at less than 30 weeks' gestation. N Engl J Med 336:21–26, 1997

Vandershueren-Lodewecykx M, deBruyn F, Dooms L, et al: Sensorineural hearing loss in sporadic congenital hypothyroidism. Arch Dis Child 58:419–422, 1983

Veenboer GJ, de Vijlder JJ: Molecular basis of the thyroglobulin synthesis defect in Dutch goats. Endocrinology 132:377–381, 1993

Virgili M, Saverino O, Vaccari M, et al: Temporal, regional and cellular selectivity of neonatal alteration of the thyroid state on neurochemical maturation in the rat. Exp Brain Res 83:556–561, 1991

Vulsma T, Kok JH: Prematurity-associated neurologic and developmental abnormalities and neonatal thyroid function. N Engl J Med 334:857–858, 1996

Vulsma T, Gons MH, de Vijlder JJM: Maternal-fetal transfer of thyroxine in congenital hypothyroidism due to a total organification defect or thyroid agenesis. N Engl J Med 321:13–16, 1989

Wechsler D: The Wechsler Intelligence Scale for Children—Revised. New York, Psychological Corporation, 1974

Withers BT, Reuter SH, Janeke JB: The effects of hypothyroidism on the ears of cats and squirrel monkeys: a pilot study. Laryngoscope 82:779–784, 1972

Chapter 5

Resistance to Thyroid Hormone: Implications for Child Psychiatric Research

Peter Hauser, M.D.

Thyroid hormone and the thyroid hormone receptor are essential for normal behavioral and brain development in many species; in humans, absence of thyroid hormone causes mental retardation (Dussault and Ruel 1987; Porterfield 1994). The importance of thyroid hormone in human neurodevelopment has been demonstrated in subjects with various thyroid dysfunctions. Studies have included children with congenital (Rovet et al. 1993a) (see Rovet, Chapter 4 in this volume) and acquired (Rovet et al. 1993b) (see Rovet and Daneman, Chapter 6 in this volume) hypothyroidism who were treated with thyroid hormone, as well as children and adults with hyperthyroidism (Alvarez et al. 1983; Trzepacz et al.

I wish to thank the numerous investigators who have contributed to the studies of resistance to thyroid hormone subjects at the National Institutes of Health (NIH) and who are referenced in this chapter. In addition I wish to thank Paul Jordan, Joe Lazar, Mary Beth Schultheis, and Edythe Wiggs, who have worked with me on more recent studies of resistance to thyroid hormone subjects and who have not been previously included as coauthors of published studies. Also, many thanks to Dr. Bruce Weintraub, who allowed these studies to take place at NIH. Thanks also to Jirina Hauser for her unwavering support, and to Dr. Michael Davey for a wonderful dinner at the Yamhill Winery in Oregon. I wish also to thank the American Thyroid Association and Audrey McMahon for their support and appreciation of my research. Finally, I wish to thank the various physicians who referred patients to NIH and the families with resistance to thyroid hormone, without whose cooperation the work could not have been done.

1988) (see Bhatara and McMillin, Chapter 7 in this volume) and resistance to thyroid hormone (Brucker-Davis et al. 1995; Hauser et al. 1993a, 1993b; Mixson et al. 1992).

Among thyroid diseases, untreated congenital hypothyroidism (CH) has the most devastating effect, causing a profound and irreversible mental retardation. The economic cost associated with the care of such individuals has prompted government-mandated routine screening of all newborns for low thyroid hormone concentrations (see Pass, Chapter 3 in this volume). Despite newborn screening and adequate thyroid replacement therapy, children with CH may still have residual deficits in language, visuoperception, cognition, and memory abilities and difficult temperament in infancy (see Rovet, Chapter 4 in this volume). These deficits may reflect delays in early neuromotor development and may be due in part to thyroid hormone insufficiency during critical periods of neuronal maturation among other processes. The type of deficit has been demonstrated to involve the cause, severity, timing, or duration of neonatal thyroid hormone insufficiency. However, it has been only in the last 10–15 years that researchers have focused on the behavioral and intellectual effects of other thyroid diseases, such as resistance to thyroid hormone (RTH). RTH is an autosomal dominant disease caused by mutations in the human thyroid hormone receptor β (hTRβ) gene on chromosome 3 (Parilla et al. 1991; Usala et al. 1988). Like CH, it is also associated with lowered IQs (but not mental retardation) and school problems and, in addition, attention-deficit/hyperactivity disorder (ADHD) and language disorders (Brucker-Davis et al. 1995; Hauser et al. 1993a, 1993b; Magner et al. 1986; Mixson et al. 1992; Refetoff et al. 1993).

This chapter first briefly reviews animal and human studies that demonstrate the importance of thyroid hormone and the thyroid hormone receptor in normal behavioral and brain development. The syndrome of resistance to thyroid hormone and the genetic studies that characterize the underlying pathophysiological mechanism of RTH are also reviewed. The chapter then focuses on behavioral and brain imaging studies in subjects with RTH, a disease that disrupts thyroid hormone action and regulation during fetal life as well as in infancy and early childhood. Because the majority of children with RTH develop ADHD, the chapter concludes by suggesting that RTH is relevant to child psychiatric research as a genetic model for ADHD and by suggesting hypotheses for future research.

Thyroid Hormone and Normal Neurodevelopment

The effects of thyroid hormone on early central nervous system (CNS) growth and development and later cognitive functioning are well characterized. A variety of CNS developmental events are influenced by thyroid hormone, including gene expression, growth factors, and cell proliferation, and studies in animals show both organizational and activational effects (Hendrich and Porterfield 1992; Mellström et al. 1991; Munoz et al. 1991; Pipaon et al. 1992). Perhaps the more important and pervasive CNS effect of thyroid hormones is on postproliferation events, which include cerebral and cerebellar neurogenesis and migration, neuronal differentiation, process formation, synaptogenesis, gliogenesis, and myelinogenesis (Lauder 1989). The regulatory control of certain genes, such as the NGFI-A gene, an immediate-early response gene implicated in brain cell proliferation, is directly regulated by triiodothyronine (T_3) in the brain of the neonatal, but not the adult, rat (Pipaon et al. 1992). Also, manipulations of thyroid hormone status can have profound and persistent effects on catecholamine neurotransmitter systems in both the neonatal and the adult rat brain (Dupont et al. 1981; Rastogi and Singhal 1979). These studies are particularly relevant to research on ADHD, as alterations of catecholamine neurotransmitter systems have been implicated in the pathogenesis of ADHD (Shenker 1993).

Although thyroid hormones are necessary for normal CNS function throughout life, they are essential for normal development and maturation of the CNS during a critical developmental period (in utero to 2 years in humans and up to postnatal day 21 in mice). This critical period of neuronal network creation appears to require tightly controlled amounts of thyroid hormone, and thyroid deficiency or excess during this period is associated with permanent neurodevelopmental and behavioral effects (Bernal and Nunez 1995; Porterfield 1994).

It is important to note that the mechanism of thyroid hormone action is initiated by its binding to the thyroid hormone receptor (TR). Two isoforms of the TR (formerly known as the c-erb A) gene, α and β, have been characterized and mapped to human chromosomes 17q11.2–21 and 3p21–25, respectively (Dayton et al. 1984; Gareau et al. 1988). The TR is in the same nuclear hormone receptor superfamily as the glucocorticoid, estrogen, vitamin D, and retinoic acid receptors. These nuclear receptors share a common structure in that they have a ligand-binding domain in the carboxy-terminal region of the receptor protein and a DNA-binding domain in the amino-terminal region of the receptor protein (Evans 1988). The human TRα (hTRα) and the human TRβ (hTRβ) genes each encode for two alternatively spliced isoforms, α1, α2 proteins and β1, β2 proteins (Hodin et al. 1989; Koenig et al. 1988; Mitsuhashi et al. 1988; Nakai et al. 1988). All of the hTR isoforms have a DNA-binding domain in their amino-terminal region that is similar to the DNA-binding domain of the other steroid hormone receptors. The α1, β1, and β2 isoforms have a specific T_3-binding domain in the carboxyl-end of the protein that is not found in the α2 isoform (Mitsuhashi et al. 1988). The binding and activation of hTRα1 and hTRβ proteins by T_3 can modulate the expression of specific thyroid-responsive genes by binding to specific base pair sequences in the regulatory region of these genes known as thyroid hormone response elements (TREs) (see Meier, Chapter 2 in this volume). Furthermore, TRs can heterodimerize with several other nuclear receptors, such as the retinoic acid receptor (RAR) and the 9-*cis* retinoic acid receptor (RXR) (Chin 1992) (see Meier, Chapter 2 in this volume). The TR-RXR heterodimer has been shown to be the most stable and transcriptionally active form. However, TR-TR homodimers may be involved in transcriptional activation and repression with certain TREs. In the liganded state, TR-TR homodimers dissociate from TREs, allowing the TR-RXR heterodimer to be active.

In the rat brain, the differential expression of TRα and TRβ messenger RNAs (mRNAs) has been demonstrated in which TRα was widely distributed throughout the entire brain, whereas the pattern of TRβ was restricted to the neocortex, hippocampus, and anterior pituitary (Bradley et al. 1989). A subsequent study by Bradley and coworkers (1994) found that TRβ expression is restricted to the portion of the inner ear that becomes the cochlea, whereas TRα is also found in inner-ear structures responsible for balance. Also, another study reported a 40-fold increase in rat brain TRβ mRNA between the 19-day-old gestational fetus and the 10-day-old neonate, a period that coincides with T_3-regulated developmental changes of the brain (Strait et al. 1990). In the human fetus, the concentration of TR is low at 10 weeks of gestation, but it increases 10-fold by the 16th week, coincidentally with neuroblast proliferation (Bernal and Pekonen 1984).

Although several T_3-dependent genes have been identified in the rat brain, only the expression of myelin basic protein mRNA has been shown to be mediated by the interaction of the activated thyroid receptor with a TRE in the promoter region of this gene in rat brain (Farsetti et al. 1991). TREs have not yet been identified in the regulatory region of human genes critical for normal brain development.

Resistance to Thyroid Hormone: Definition and Genetic Studies

Resistance to thyroid hormone, first described in 1967 (Refetoff et al. 1967), is one of several hormone resistance syndromes (others include androgen, glucocorticoid, and vitamin D resistance syndromes). Numerous studies have defined the clinical and biochemical parameters of the various hormone resistance syndromes since the description of pseudohypoparathyroidism and the introduction of the concept of hormone resistance more than 50 years ago (Albright et al. 1942). However, it was not until recent advances in molecular genetic technology that the underlying pathophysiological mechanism for the hormone resistance syndromes could be studied directly on a molecular genetic level. Mutations have been identified in the genes that encode for the particular hormone receptor proteins. Furthermore, in vitro studies have shown that these mutations result in functional impairment of the receptor protein. Therefore, the mutations do not represent neutral polymorphisms.

The thyroid gland produces triiodothyronine (T_3) and thyroxine (T_4). The production of these hormones is regulated by negative feedback at the level of the hypothalamus, which produces thyrotropin-releasing hormone (TRH), and at the level of the pituitary, which produces thyrotropin, or thyroid-stimulating hormone (TSH) (see Lash, Chapter 1 in this volume). Hypothyroid states are characterized by low T_3 and T_4 and high TSH concentrations, whereas hyperthyroid states are characterized by high T_3 and T_4 and low TSH levels. RTH, in contrast, is characterized by elevations in T_3 and T_4 concentrations that are accompanied by inappropriately nonsuppressed levels of TSH and reduced responsiveness of pituitary and peripheral tissues to the actions of thyroid hormone (Refetoff et al. 1993). The clinical features of some subjects with RTH are those commonly associated with hypothyroidism, including short stature, delayed bone maturation, and goiter. However, the majority of subjects with RTH are clinically euthyroid, because the elevated thyroid hormone concentrations reflect a compensatory physiological response of the thyroid-pituitary axis to tissue resistance (Brucker-Davis et al. 1995). Clinical, physiological, and biochemical studies of subjects with RTH suggest that there is great variability in the degree of refractoriness to thyroid hormone action among individuals and in various target tissues, including bone, brain, liver, heart, and pituitary (Magner et al. 1986). Even though particular kindreds exhibit discernible patterns of tissue resistance, the degree of resistance in a given tissue can vary among affected subjects within a particular kindred (Magner et al. 1986; Smallridge et al. 1989).

The underlying pathophysiological mechanism for RTH was postulated as an abnormality of the thyroid hormone receptor (Refetoff et al. 1972). However, it was not until c-erb A was identified as the T_3 receptor that the association of RTH to a defective thyroid hormone receptor could be directly studied on a molecular genetic level (Sap et al. 1986; Weinberger et al. 1986). Initial restriction fragment length polymorphism (RFLP) studies demonstrated linkage of the RTH phenotype to the human thyroid receptor β (hTRβ) gene on chromosome 3 (Usala et al. 1988). Subsequent genetic studies of RTH have found distinct mutations in two "hot spots": one in exon 9 and one in exon 10 of the hTRβ gene (Mixson et al. 1992; Parilla et al. 1991; Usala et al. 1990). These two exons code for the hormone-binding domain of the thyroid receptor. The vast majority of the more than 100 different mutations reported have involved only one of the two TRβ alleles of the affected members, confirming the previous familial studies that suggested that RTH is inherited predominantly in an autosomal dominant fashion (Magner et al. 1986; Refetoff et al. 1993). Although a single base insertion (Parilla et al. 1991), a deletion of a single codon (Usala et al. 1991), and major deletion of the DNA and hormone-binding domains of the hTRβ gene (Takeda et al. 1991) have also been identified, most known mutations are single base substitutions that cause a single nonconservative amino acid substitution in the TRβ protein.

In vitro functional studies of several different naturally occurring mutant thyroid receptors have shown a decreased or absent T_3-binding affinity compared to the normal receptor (Cheng et al. 1993; Meier et al. 1992; Parilla et al. 1991). However, no differences were observed in binding to various TREs. A recent study of four different mutant thyroid hormone receptors from families that were included in our behavioral study showed that, in transfected cell cultures, T_3-binding affinity and transcriptional activity were directly correlated (Meier et al. 1992). All four mutant thyroid receptors not only reduced but inhibited the ability of the wild type hTRβ to activate a positive TRE. This dominant negative effect could be reversed by high concentrations of T_3 in two mutant thyroid receptors with partial T_3-binding affinity, but not in the two mutant thyroid receptors with undetectable T_3 binding. It has been postulated that the most likely mechanism for the dominant negative effect is competition between wild type and mutant TRs for binding to various positive and negative TREs on T_3-responsive genes such as myelin basic protein (Farsetti et al. 1991). In the liganded state, TR homodimers dissociate from TREs, allowing the TR-RXR heterodimer to act. However, in order for mutant thyroid receptors to dissociate from TREs, they require greater T_3 concentrations in proportion to their T_3-binding affinities.

It is interesting to note that clinical studies parallel in vitro studies at least in most subjects with RTH. As mentioned above, although clinical features commonly associated with hypothyroidism are found in some subjects with RTH, the majority are clinically euthyroid, because the elevated thyroid hormone concentrations reflect a compensatory physiological response of the thyroid-pituitary axis to tissue resistance (Brucker-Davis et al. 1995).

Resistance to Thyroid Hormone: Behavioral Studies

Studies of neonates with RTH indicate that thyroid hormone concentrations characteristic of this autosomal dominant disease are present at birth (Weiss et al. 1990). Therefore, RTH represents a unique genetic model to study prospectively the neurodevelopmental manifestations of a disruption of thyroid hormone regulation. Initial familial studies described poor school performance, learning disabilities, and symptoms of hyperactivity as among the more commonly reported somatic and neuropsychiatric presentations of RTH (Hopwood et al. 1986; Magner et al. 1986; Pagliara et al. 1983; Usala et al. 1990). However, it was not until our study of 104 affected and unaffected family members that a systematic behavioral study, using structured psychiatric interviews, was undertaken in a large sample of subjects with RTH (Hauser et al. 1993a). We reported a strong and specific association between mutations in the TRβ gene that causes RTH and ADHD. Fifty percent of RTH-affected adults (compared with 7% of unaffected adult family members) and 70% of RTH-affected children (compared with 20% of unaffected child family members) met criteria for the diagnosis of ADHD (Table 5–1). In contrast, the two groups did not differ in the frequency of other psychiatric diagnoses.

Children with RTH had a 10-fold higher likelihood of the diagnosis of ADHD than their unaffected siblings. Also, when the data of adults and children were combined, 76% of males with RTH and 50% of females with RTH had a diagnosis of ADHD (Hauser et al. 1993a). The distribution of ADHD symptoms for the subjects with

Table 5–1. Psychiatric diagnoses of family members with and without resistance to thyroid hormone

	ADULTS		
Diagnosis	RTH + n = 22 (%)	RTH − n = 30 (%)	*
ADHD	11/22 (50)	2/30 (7)	$P \leq .0007$
Major depression	6/22 (27)	6/30 (20)	ns
Anxiety disorders			
Generalized anxiety disorder	2/22 (9)	0/22 (0)	ns
Panic disorder	1/22 (5)	1/30 (3)	ns
Psychoactive substance use disorders	3/22 (14)	3/30 (10)	ns
Antisocial personality disorder	2/22 (9)	1/30 (3)	ns

	CHILDREN		
Diagnosis	RTH + n = 27 (%)	RTH − n = 25 (%)	*
Disruptive behavior disorders	23/27 (85)	7/25 (28)	$P \leq .0001$
ADHD	19/27 (70)	5/25 (20)	$P \leq .0003$
Oppositional defiant disorder	10/27 (37)	5/25 (20)	ns
Conduct disorder	4/27 (15)	1/25 (4)	ns
Mood disorders			
Dysthymic disorder	4/27 (15)	3/25 (12)	ns
Major depression	1/27 (4)	1/25 (4)	ns
Anxiety disorders	4/27 (15)	6/25 (24)	ns
Avoidant personality disorder	0/27 (0)	2/25 (8)	ns
Enuresis	4/27 (15)	1/25 (4)	ns

Note. ADHD = attention-deficit/hyperactivity disorder; RTH = syndrome of resistance to thyroid hormone.
*Statistical analysis with Fisher exact test; ns = not significant.

RTH and their unaffected family members is shown in Figure 5–1.

Our study generated considerable interest in thyroid hormone as it affects attentional processes. Several studies have examined children with ADHD for RTH (Elia et al. 1994; Spencer et al. 1993; Weiss et al. 1993). Although one study found an increased incidence of nonspecific thyroid hormone abnormalities in 3% of their sample (Weiss et al. 1993), none of these studies have demonstrated that children with ADHD also have RTH. However, these studies were limited methodologically, as the sample sizes were relatively small and the subjects were selected from specialized ADHD clinics. Also, attentional processes were not directly quantified.

ADHD research has focused on descriptive studies of the behavioral manifestations of the disorder as well as the effects of treatment with stimulant medications. The symptoms of hyperactivity were emphasized in early descriptive studies of ADHD. In the 1970s researchers demonstrated that, rather than hyperactivity, the symptoms of inattention and poor impulse control were the primary features of ADHD (Barkley 1990). As a result, specific criteria for diagnostic subtypes of ADHD with and without hyperactivity were established in DSM-III (American Psychiatric Association 1980). In DSM-III-R (American Psychiatric Association 1987) ADHD was considered to be one disorder. However, DSM-IV (American Psychiatric Association 1994) reintroduced the distinct subtypes of inattentive and hyperactive-impulsive, with the latter including symptoms of impulsivity. This classification was the result of field studies demonstrating that symptoms of inattention are associated only with academic impairment, whereas symptoms of hyperactivity and impulsivity are associated with a more global impairment (McBurnett 1993). However, as yet no studies have demonstrated a physiological basis for this distinction.

There is little direct evidence that persons with ADHD have neuroanatomic abnormalities or abnormalities of neurotransmitter function. Until recently, there has been a paucity of studies examining neuroendocrine function in ADHD, and the studies have been largely confined to the effects of treatment with sympathomimetic medications (Reeve et al. 1991). The diagnostic validity of

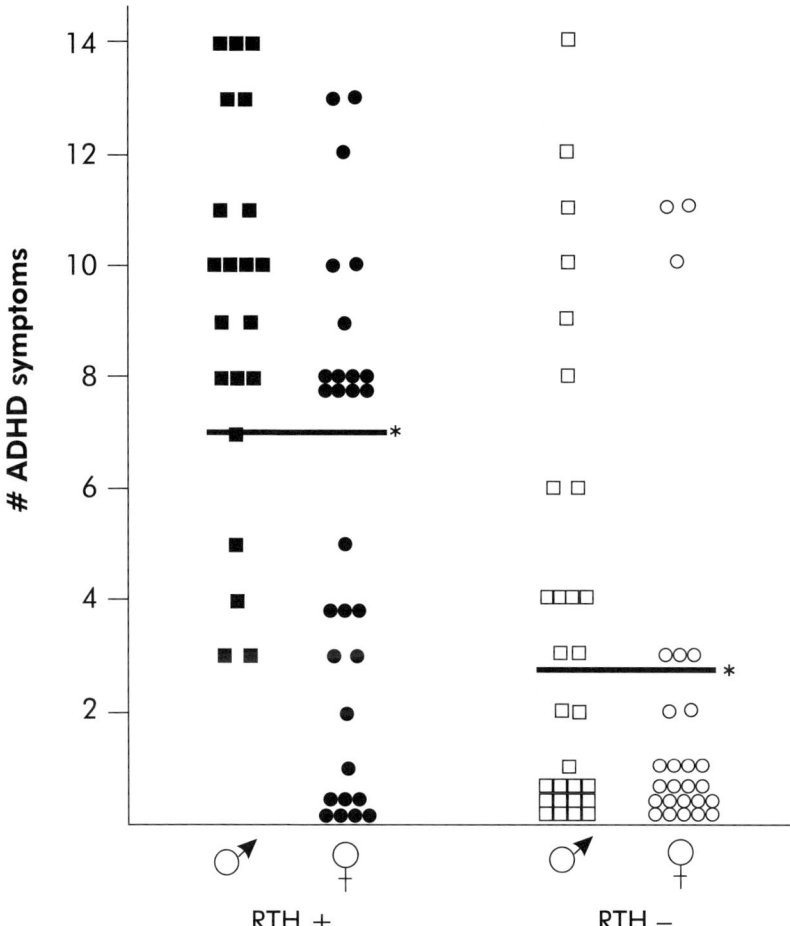

Figure 5–1. Distribution of symptoms of attention-deficit/hyperactivity disorder (ADHD) among subjects with and without resistance to thyroid hormone (RTH). The horizontal lines indicate the mean number of symptoms. The group with resistance to thyroid hormone had a mean of 7.0 symptoms, compared with a mean of 2.8 for the group of unaffected family members ($P < .001$).
Source.   Reprinted from Hauser P, et al.: "Attention-Deficit Hyperactivity Disorder in People With Generalized Resistance to Thyroid Hormone." *New England Journal of Medicine* 328: 997–1001, 1993a. Used with permission.

dividing ADHD into two distinct subtypes, one with and one without hyperactivity, is controversial, since no physiological differences between these two subtypes have been demonstrated. Therefore, my group examined the relationship between thyroid hormones and symptoms of hyperactivity in subjects with RTH and their unaffected family members and hypothesized that there would be significant positive correlations between concentrations of thyroid hormones and symptoms of hyperactivity, but no correlations between concentrations of thyroid hormones and symptoms of inattention. Clinical data were collected on 152 subjects: 75 subjects with RTH and 77 family members without RTH. Each subject was assessed using structured psychiatric interviews based on DSM-III-R criteria. Total T_3 (TT_3), total T_4 (TT_4), and TSH concentrations were measured in each subject. The total number of ADHD symptoms were assigned to either inattention or hyperactivity subgroups using DSM-III-R criteria. The total numbers of ADHD symptoms were then reassigned to inattention or hyperactivity/impulsivity subgroups using DSM-IV criteria. Pearson r correlation coefficients were calculated separately for the RTH and unaffected family member groups to determine the relationships between TSH, TT_3, and TT_4 concentrations and the DSM-III-R and DSM-IV symptom categories of ADHD in both groups (Table 5–2).

TSH concentrations were not significantly correlated with any of the symptom categories in either group. However, in the RTH group both TT_3 and TT_4 concentrations were significantly and positively correlated with total symptoms of ADHD (DSM-III-R) as well as symptoms of inattention (DSM-III-R) and symptoms of hyperactivity (DSM-III-R). When DSM-IV criteria were used, in which symptoms of impulsivity were reassigned from the inattention to the hyperactivity category, only the positive correlation between TT_3 and TT_4 concentrations and symptoms of hyperactivity/impulsivity (DSM-IV) remained significant. In the group of unaffected family members, the relationship between TT_3 concentrations and symptoms of hyperactivity/impulsivity (DSM-IV) was the only significant correlation. These data therefore support the hypothesis that thyroid hormones may provide a physiological basis for the dichotomy between symptoms of inattention and symp-

Table 5–2. Pearson r correlation coefficients for T_3 and T_4 concentrations and symptoms of inattention or hyperactivity

	r for T_3	r for T_4
Subjects with RTH		
Total ADHD symptoms (DSM-III-R)	.406*	.320**
Symptoms of inattention (DSM-III-R)	.322**	.267**
Symptoms of hyperactivity (DSM-III-R)	.492*	.363*
Symptoms of inattention (DSM-IV)	.129	.099
Symptoms of hyperactivity/impulsivity (DSM-IV)	.505*	.417*
Unaffected family members		
Total ADHD symptoms (DSM-III-R)	.221	.048
Symptoms of inattention (DSM-III-R)	.207	.021
Symptoms of hyperactivity (DSM-III-R)	.203	.107
Symptoms of inattention (DSM-IV)	.156	-.031
Symptoms of hyperactivity/impulsivity (DSM-IV)	.276**	.070

Note. ADHD = attention-deficit/hyperactivity disorder; RTH = syndrome of resistance to thyroid hormone; T_3 = triiodothyronine; T_4 = thyroxine.
*$P < .01$ for $n > 70$ and $R > .325$.
**$P < .05$ for $n > 70$ and $R > .250$.

toms of hyperactivity, particularly when DSM-IV criteria are applied.

It is unlikely that RTH is the cause of ADHD in all but a few children. This provokes the question of whether RTH is a reasonable genetic model for studying ADHD. There is no firm evidence that ADHD is a homogeneous phenomenon. The lack of clear biological or genetic markers for ADHD has precluded prospective studies of infants who are later diagnosed with ADHD. Although family studies suggest that relatives of children with ADHD who do not have RTH have much higher risks for ADHD, antisocial personality disorders, and depression than do family members of non-ADHD children (Biederman et al. 1986, 1991), the mechanism of genetic transmission of ADHD remains undetermined. RTH is a well-defined genetic disease that has ADHD as an associated behavioral consequence in the vast majority of cases and therefore is useful as a genetic model for ADHD. Even if there are only a few children with ADHD secondary to RTH, the symptoms observed in these individuals are indistinguishable from those of individuals with ADHD acquired through other mechanisms.

Because studies of neonates with RTH indicate that the thyroid hormone and TSH concentrations characteristic of RTH are present at birth (Weiss et al. 1990), development of a newborn screening method for RTH will allow early identification of these infants. These RTH infants represent a unique sample for prospectively studying the impact of ADHD symptoms on children's emotional and social development. In my group's preliminary study, which was recently published (Mizejewski et al. 1995), it seemed feasible to identify newborns presumed positive for RTH by using dried bloodspots (see Pass, Chapter 3 in this volume).

Several other studies have suggested that RTH may be an important genetic model that will allow researchers to elucidate the underlying pathophysiological mechanisms of ADHD and learning disabilities as well as biological determinants of intelligence. Untreated CH is associated with profound and irreversible mental retardation (Dussault and Ruel 1987). Although RTH is associated with lowered IQs, mental retardation is uncommon. In my group's psychometric study, we evaluated intelligence in 59 subjects with RTH and 50 unaffected family members using the age-appropriate Wechsler Intelligence Scale and Wide Range Achievement Test—Revised (Brucker-Davis et al. 1995; Hauser et al. 1993b). An analysis of variance considering the diagnosis of ADHD, the diagnosis of RTH, and gender was done and showed a main effect for the RTH diagnosis only. The mean IQ scores of subjects with RTH were significantly lower than those of unaffected family members for verbal, performance, and full-scale IQ as well as for reading and arithmetic achievement tests. However, only 3 of 59 subjects (5%) with resistance had a full-scale IQ score under 70, the upper limit for a diagnosis of mild mental retardation. Furthermore, a comparison of 16 RTH subjects with their unaffected siblings closest in age showed that the mean IQs and achievement test scores of the resistance group were more than 10 points lower in all categories (Table 5–3). There was no effect of the ADHD diagnosis on IQ or achievement test scores.

The identified mutations that cause RTH are clustered predominantly in either exon 9 or exon 10 of the hTRβ gene (Parilla et al. 1991). Although subjects with mutations in either of these two "hot spots" are similarly affected with ADHD, language disorders—including delayed language development, dysarthria, and stuttering—have been reported to be significantly more common in subjects with mutations in exon 9 than in exon 10 (Brucker-Davis et al. 1995; Mixson et al. 1992). This difference is interesting to consider, given that a significant percentage of children diagnosed with ADHD are codiagnosed with a specific developmental disorder or learning disability (Shaywitz and Shaywitz 1991). TR affinity for thyroid hormone is variably decreased by both exon 9 and exon 10 mutations, which could be the causative mechanism for the symptoms of ADHD in subjects with RTH. However, exon 9 mutations may additionally alter the thyroid receptor protein such that it no longer interacts with certain auxiliary proteins. This lack of interaction may subsequently change the activity of certain target genes during critical periods of brain development for the substrates of language in subjects with exon 9 mutations.

Table 5–3. Mean IQ and achievement test scores: matched sibling pairs

Test	RTH + ($n = 16$)	RTH − ($n = 16$)	
Verbal IQ[a]	87.1 ± 3.9	102.0 ± 3.6	$P < .002$
Performance IQ	96.9 ± 3.3	107.0 ± 3.5	$P < .02$
Full-scale IQ	91.0 ± 3.3	105.0 ± 3.6	$P < .001$
Reading achievement	78.4 ± 4.8	94.8 ± 4.9	$P < .01$
Arithmetic achievement	76.8 ± 3.9	90.7 ± 5.5	$P < .05$

Note. RTH = syndrome of resistance to thyroid hormone.
[a]IQ and achievement scores are means ± standard error.

Resistance to Thyroid Hormone: Functional and Structural Imaging Studies

Functional Imaging Studies—Positron Emission Tomography

The neurobiological correlates of ADHD have been studied by using positron-emission tomography (PET) and magnetic resonance imaging (MRI) technology. Functional studies, using PET, have been performed in adult subjects who met the diagnostic criteria for ADHD as children. These studies have demonstrated decreases in both global and regional cerebral glucose metabolism, with the greatest decreases occurring in the prefrontal and premotor cortices (Zametkin et al. 1990). Although stimulant medications have been shown to improve the symptoms of ADHD in adults and children (DuPaul and Barkley 1990; Shenker 1993; Wender et al. 1985), administration of these medications (on either a short-term or a long-term basis) has not convincingly demonstrated normalization of cerebral metabolism concomitant with clinical improvement (Matochik et al. 1993, 1994). Therefore, the underlying pathophysiological mechanisms for the cerebral metabolic changes found in adult subjects with ADHD remain elusive.

My group's recent PET study of subjects with RTH suggests an important role for the hTRβ gene in attentional processes (Matochik et al. 1996). PET scans were obtained of 13 adults with RTH (none of whom were receiving thyroid hormone treatment) and 13 control subjects matched as closely as possible for age and sex. Subjects were injected with 18-fluorodeoxyglucose while performing a continuous auditory discrimination task. The task involved the subject pressing a hand-held button when the lowest-volume tone of three different tones was presented through earphones. Each tone was presented 220 times, for a total of 220 targets and 440 distractors. Adults with RTH were greatly impaired in performance of the auditory discrimination task as measured by correct identifications of the target tone (Table 5–4). The mean score of the RTH subjects was 132 out of a possible 220, which was significantly lower than the mean score of 180 for the control group ($P < .0007$, one-tailed t test). In addition, the RTH

Table 5–4. Scores on continuous auditory task by group

	RTH +	RTH –	
Hits[a]	132.4 ± 32.5	179.9 ± 3.6	$P < .0007$
False alarms[a]	38.6 ± 56.8	7.4 ± 7.9	$P < .04$
Accuracy[b]	2.2 ± 1.7	3.6 ± 1.2	$P < .02$

Note. RTH = syndrome of resistance to thyroid hormone.
[a]Scores of hits and false alarms are means ± standard deviation.
[b]Accuracy = log of hits/false alarms + 1.

group had significantly more false alarms and significantly lower performance accuracy than control subjects.

Eight regions known to be associated with sustained attention were sampled and cerebral metabolism measured. Compared with controls, RTH subjects had significantly higher metabolism in the anterior cingulate gyrus and in two areas of the right parietal lobe (Figure 5–2). However, the normalized data (regional absolute value divided by the global value of all slices obtained) showed significant differences only in the anterior cingulate gyrus (RTH group: 1.13 ± 0.07, control group: 1.03 ± 0.05; $P = .0007$).

Studies have shown that metabolism in the anterior cingulate gyrus increases during single word processing tasks and during the Stroop attentional conflict paradigm, suggesting that the anterior cingulate gyrus mediates voluntary control of attention and response selection (Pardo et al. 1991; Petersen et al. 1988). It has been hypothesized that the anterior attentional system initially controls the performance of a particular task and that control is transferred to regions of the right hemisphere that are involved in the performance of a particular task with increasing familiarity of the task (Posner and Petersen 1990). In subjects with RTH, the initial response to an attentional task may be the same as in control subjects (activation of the anterior cingulate gyrus), but subjects with RTH are unable to transfer control to a vigilance subsystem that requires less conscious effort (which may be reflected in a decreased cerebral metabolism). Two studies that demonstrated decreased cerebral blood flow in the anterior cingulate gyrus after subjects practiced a task (and once the task became more automated) sup-

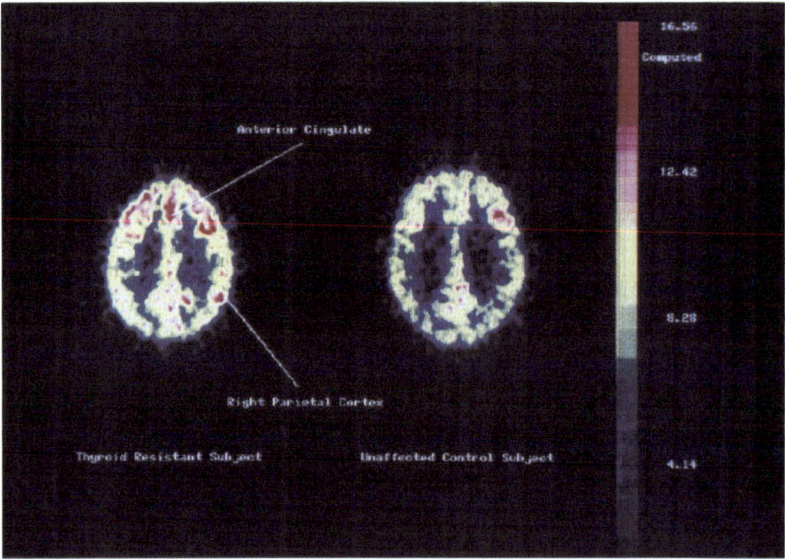

Figure 5–2. Brain images from a subject with resistance to thyroid hormone *(left)* and an unaffected control subject *(right)* through the transaxial plane where the anterior cingulate gyrus was sampled. The occipital lobe is at the bottom of the images. According to the pseudocolor scale to the right of the images, *red* and *yellow* indicate areas of relatively higher glucose metabolism, whereas *green* and *blue* indicate areas of lower metabolism.
Source. Reprinted from Matochik J, et al.: "Abnormalities in Sustained Attention and Anterior Cingulate Metabolism in Subjects With Resistance to Thyroid Hormone." *Brain Research* 723:23–28, 1996. Used with permission.

port this hypothesis (Jenkins et al. 1994; Raichle et al. 1994). The increased metabolism of the anterior cingulate gyrus in patients with RTH may reflect a cerebral metabolic inefficiency in performing a sustained-attention task.

Structural Imaging Studies—Magnetic Resonance Imaging

Although PET studies have implicated frontal brain regions in the pathogenesis of ADHD, these studies have been undertaken in adults and adolescents who had childhood ADHD. The ethical considerations of exposing children to ionizing radiation as well as the discomfort of arterial and intravenous procedures has precluded PET studies of children with ADHD. Therefore, PET studies have provided somewhat limited information because children with ADHD, who have active and more severe symptomatology than adults, have not been studied. However, MRI has allowed structural studies of the developing brain in children both with and without ADHD without the risk of radiation or physical discomfort.

Initial MRI studies of children with and without ADHD revealed that children with ADHD had a narrower right frontal cortex and a reversal of the usual left-greater-than-right asymmetry of the caudate nucleus (Hynd et al. 1991, 1993). In addition, an MRI study of the corpus callosum area found that, compared with subjects without ADHD, children with ADHD had smaller genu (anterior region of the corpus callosum) and splenium (posterior region of the corpus callosum) area measurements (Hynd et al. 1991). Subsequent studies of volumes of the caudate nucleus (the initial Hynd study was an area measurement of the head of the caudate nucleus) found, in contrast to the Hynd study, a normal right-greater-than-left asymmetry of the caudate nucleus in subjects without ADHD (Castellanos et al. 1994, 1996). This caudate nucleus asymmetry was absent in children with ADHD. These studies had large sample sizes and used volumetric measures.

In contrast to the initial corpus callosum study (Hynd et al. 1991), more recent studies have shown a lack of consensus with regard to differences between subjects with and without ADHD (Giedd et al. 1994; Semrud-Clikeman et al. 1994). Both of these recent studies examined only male children. One study found that subjects with ADHD as a group had smaller rostrum and rostral body—but not genu—regions of the corpus callosum (Giedd et al. 1994), whereas the second study (Semrud-Clikeman et al. 1994) found the splenium to be smaller in subjects with ADHD. In summary, the MRI studies of subjects with ADHD support the hypothesis of dysfunction in prefrontal and striatal pathways, but the underlying pathophysiological mechanisms for these changes are not known.

The unknown etiology of the demonstrated structural brain changes found in subjects with ADHD provides justification for the use of MRI technology to study subjects with RTH, because they are a group who have a well-defined genetic disease with a strong and specific association to ADHD (Hauser et al. 1993a). Animal studies have shown that manipulations of thyroid hormone status can have profound and persistent effects on catecholamine neurotransmitter systems in both the neonatal and the adult rat brain (Dupont et al. 1981; Rastogi and Singhal 1979). Furthermore, the regulation of myelin basic protein mRNA expression in rat brain is mediated by the interaction of the activated thyroid hormone receptor with a thyroid response element in the promoter region of this gene (Farsetti et al. 1991). Also, expression of the NGFI-A gene, an immediate-early response gene implicated in the control of brain cell proliferation and aspects of brain development, is directly regulated by T_3 in the brain of the neonatal, but not the adult, rat (Pipaon et al. 1992). Mutant thyroid hormone receptors could disrupt the normal regulation of these genes during fetal life and adversely affect brain and behavioral development. In particular, normal myelinogenesis could be disrupted during fetal and early neonatal life. Because the corpus callosum is the largest delineated white matter tract in the brain and is composed primarily of myelin, it is feasible that this brain structure could be preferentially affected in subjects with RTH. The gross manifestation of this effect could be a smaller corpus callosum.

In a preliminary study, the MRI scans of 23 subjects with RTH, 21 unaffected relatives, and 16 control subjects were measured. My colleagues and I selected only adults for our preliminary study in order to reduce variability secondary to age and the effects of puberty. The demographic data are summarized in Table 5–5.

The images were prepared for measurement using the volume rendering and image editing computer software program ANALYZE, version 6.1 (Biomedical Imaging Resource, Mayo Foundation, Rochester, MN). This software allows automated measurement of regions of interest. The midsagittal slice from each subject was selected and coded. The method used to make measurements of the corpus callosum and cerebrum is described in

Table 5–5. Corpus callosum study: demographic data

	RTH + (n = 23)	RTH − (n = 21)	Control (n = 16)
Age[a]	36.1 ± 9.3	34.7 ± 8.3	35.9 ± 8.8
Sex (M/F)	8/15	11/10	4/12
ADHD[b] (#/total)	11/23	0/21	0/16

Note. ADHD = attention-deficit/hyperactivity disorder; RTH = syndrome of resistance to thyroid hormone.
[a]Ages are means ± standard deviation.
[b]Significantly more RTH + with ADHD; $P < .0001$.

Figure 5–3. In addition, we modified the scheme used by Giedd et al. (1994) to divide the corpus callosum into six subregions (Figure 5–3): cc1 (genu), cc2, cc3, cc4, cc5, and cc6 (splenium).

To establish interrater reliability, the corpus callosum and cerebrum were measured on 14 randomly selected subjects by two raters blind with respect to subject diagnosis and sex. The average interclass correlation for interrater reliability was .95 for the corpus callosum and .94 for the cerebrum.

Each measurement was treated as a dependent variable in a two-way sex by diagnosis analysis of variance (ANOVA). Two-way ANOVA of the cerebral area revealed a significant sex effect ($F = 18.69$, $P < .0001$), with areas being larger in males, and a significant diagnosis effect ($F = 5.86$, $P < .01$). There was no sex by diagnosis interaction. The total corpus callosum, cc1, cc2, cc3, cc4, and cc5 areas did not differ between the sexes or among diagnostic groups. The two-way ANOVA of the cc6 area revealed a significant sex effect ($F = 8.19$, $P < .01$), with areas again being larger in males, and a significant diagnosis effect ($F = 7.87$, $P < .001$). There was no sex by diagnosis interaction. Selected mean area measurements of the subjects with RTH, their unaffected relatives, and control subjects are shown in Table 5–6.

The finding of a smaller splenium in subjects with RTH is in agreement with the study by Semrud-Clikeman et al. (1994), which showed a smaller splenium in children with ADHD compared with control children without ADHD. However, the group of unaf-

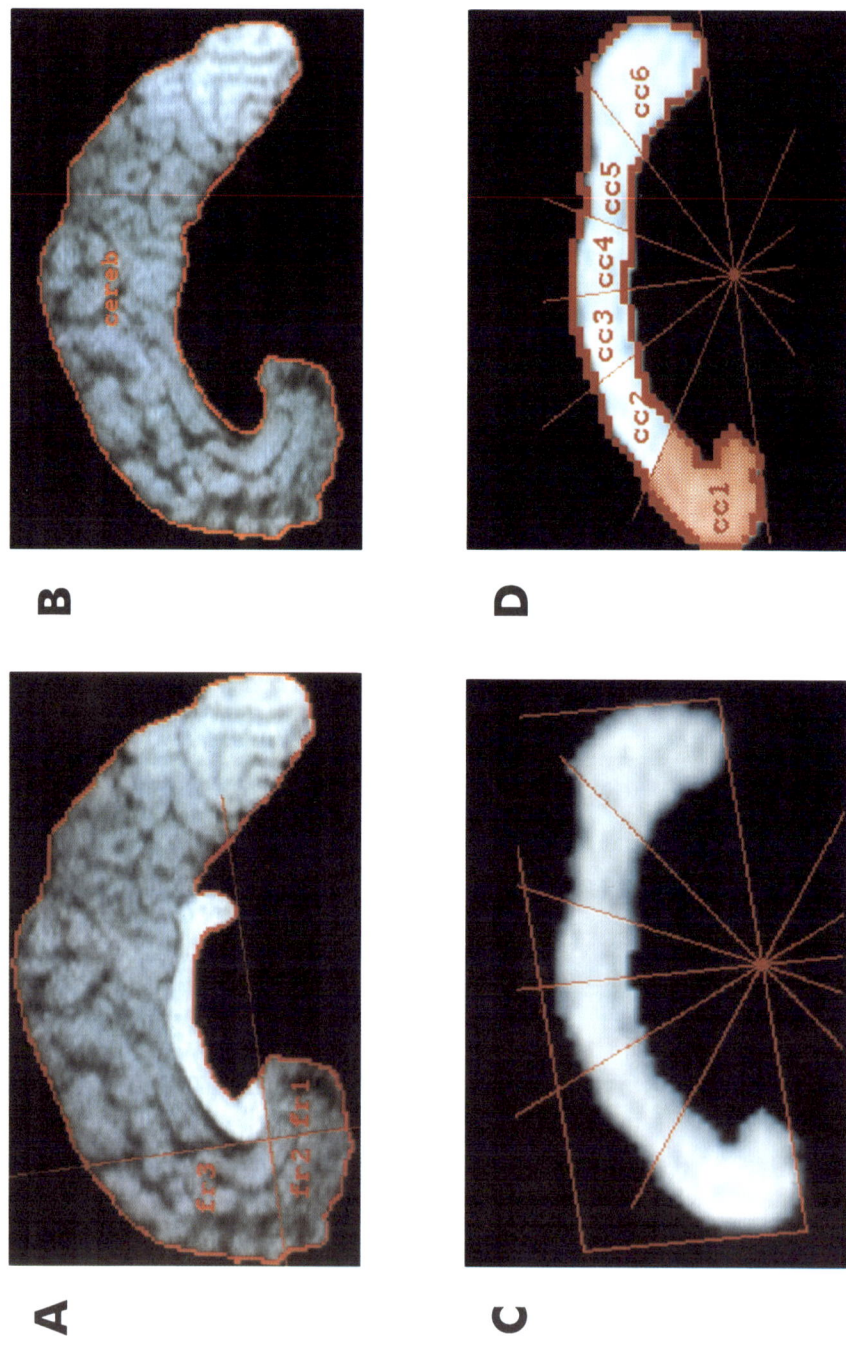

Figure 5–3. Methodology for measuring the areas of the corpus callosum, cerebrum, and six subregions of the corpus callosum. **A.** The cerebrum inclusive of the corpus callosum (CC) is manually traced and a horizontal reference line is drawn from the base of the splenium to the base of the genu. A vertical line is then drawn perpendicular to the horizontal reference line so that it touches the anteriormost aspect of the genu. Automated area measurements are made by selecting the region of interest. **B.** The boundary between the cerebrum and the CC is traced and closed. The automated area measurement is made by selecting the cerebrum (cereb). **C.** The boundary between the cerebrum and the CC is traced and closed. The automated area measurement is made by selecting the CC. A second vertical line is drawn perpendicular to the horizontal reference line so that it touches the posteriormost aspect of the splenium. The length of the horizontal reference line between the perpendicular vertical lines is measured and the midpoint calculated. **D.** A radial divider is placed so that its center is at the midpoint of the horizontal reference line (see C). The CC is thus divided into six subregions: cc1 to cc6. The automated area measurement of each subregion is made by selecting the subregion of interest.

Table 5–6. Corpus callosum study: selected area measurements

	RTH + (n = 23)	RTH – (n = 21)	Control (n = 16)
Cerebrum	72.30 ± 6.80	75.10 ± 7.60	79.10 ± 9.40[a]
CC	6.50 ± 1.00	7.10 ± 0.90	7.30 ± 0.90
cc1	1.66 ± 0.32	1.83 ± 0.34	1.79 ± 0.26
cc6	1.48 ± 0.31	1.65 ± 0.22	1.86 ± 0.25[a]

Note. Values are means in square centimeters ± standard deviation.
RTH = syndrome of resistance to thyroid hormone; CC = corpus callosum; cc1 = first subregion of the corpus callosum; cc6 = sixth subregion of the corpus callosum.
[a]Two-way analyses of variance (ANOVAs) showed a significant sex effect and a significant diagnostic effect but no sex by diagnosis interaction.

fected family members also had smaller splenia than control subjects without ADHD, which suggests that abnormalities in the morphology of the corpus callosum are not necessarily the result of mutations in the hTRβ gene and the ensuing disruption of thyroid hormone regulation during critical periods of brain development. We are currently in the process of increasing our sample size and measuring the scans of children with RTH and their unaffected siblings.

Because there is a significantly higher incidence of language disorders in subjects with RTH than in unaffected family members (Brucker-Davis et al. 1995), we were also interested in assessing our patients for the presence of cerebral anomalies in areas adjacent to the Sylvian fissure that are involved in language function. A classification system has been developed to assess qualitative differences in the perisylvian language regions of the human brain as it is visualized by MRI (Steinmetz et al. 1990). This classification system involves the identification of extra or missing gyri in the parietal operculum of the perisylvian regions in the left and right hemispheres. Sylvian fissure anomalies and multiple Heschl's gyri have been demonstrated in subjects with a family history of reading disability not associated with RTH (Leonard et al. 1993). We obtained MRI scans of 43 subjects with RTH and 32 unaffected family members (Hauser et al. 1993b; Leonard et al. 1995). The scans were assessed by a rater blind to the subject's diagnosis and sex for the presence of Sylvian fissure anomalies and multiple Heschl's gyri (Figure 5–4).

Male subjects with RTH had a significantly increased frequency of cerebral anomalies compared with their unaffected relatives, but female subjects did not. Seventy percent of male subjects with RTH had a left Sylvian fissure anomaly. Our results suggest that abnormal thyroid hormone action in the male fetus early during brain development may be associated with grossly observable cerebral anomalies of the left hemisphere.

Summary

Although studies of families suggest that relatives of children with ADHD have a much higher risk of this disorder (Biederman et al. 1991), the mechanism of genetic transmission of ADHD remains undetermined. Most studies of ADHD lack the prospective developmental approach required for an understanding of the early manifestations of the disorder. Although retrospective accounts of infant hyperactive behavior have been reported by caretakers of children later diagnosed with ADHD, prospective studies of children at risk for developing the disorder are methodologically problematic because biological or genetic markers for ADHD have not been identified. RTH is a well-defined genetic disease, and studies of neonates with RTH indicate that the thyroid hormone and TSH concentrations characteristic of RTH are present at birth (Weiss et al. 1990). This allows early identification of infants with RTH using already existing newborn screening programs. Because the frequency of ADHD in children with RTH is so high—as many as 70% of children with RTH develop ADHD—RTH serves as a genetic model of ADHD and allows the prospective study of behavior, attentional processes, and language and motor development in newborns with RTH. Infant and early childhood predictors of ADHD can be determined, and the validity of these predictors can then be tested in the general population.

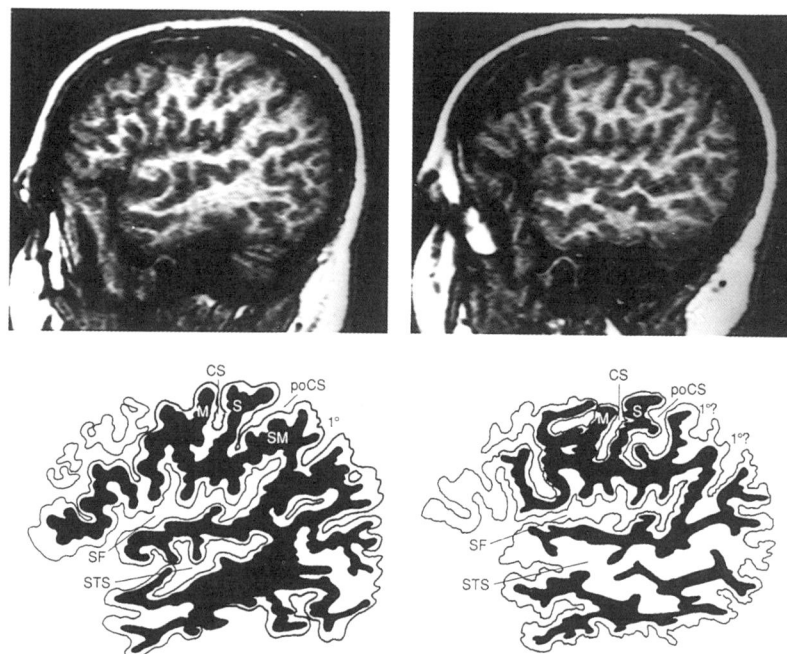

Figure 5–4. Examples of magnetic resonance images and drawings of type 1 and type 3 Sylvian fissures using the Steinmetz classification method (Steinmetz et al. 1990). *(Left)* Unaffected relative: type 1 is the most common and is distinguished by a well-developed posterior ascending ramus that ascends into the supramarginal gyrus (SM). *(Right)* Subject with resistance to thyroid hormone (RTH): type 3 is distinguished by more than one primary fissure of Jensen, resulting in an extra gyrus in the parietal operculum. The posterior ramus ascends between the two "primary" fissures. 1° = primary sulcus; CS = central sulcus; M = motor; poCS = postcentral sulcus; S = sensory; SF = sylvian fissure; SM = supramarginal gyrus; STS = superior temporal sulcus.
Source. Reprinted from Leonard CM, et al.: "Magnetic Resonance Imaging of Cerebral Anomalies in Subjects With Resistance to Thyroid Hormone." *American Journal of Medical Genetics* 60:238–243, 1995. Used with permission.

Another way to use RTH as a genetic model of ADHD is to examine the interaction of various genetic and nongenetic factors with a known genetic abnormality that confers risk for ADHD. In my group's behavioral study, we found that 70% of children with RTH had a diagnosis of ADHD. However, 30% did not have ADHD, suggesting that certain nongenetic factors may protect against the development of ADHD. For example, because RTH is an autosomal dominant disease, identification of newborns with RTH will reveal other family members with RTH. In familial cases of RTH, one parent will also have the disorder, and each child therefore has a 50% chance of having RTH. The effects of maternal compared with paternal inheritance can be studied on the expression of the clinical phenotype. In particular, the consequences of a maternal RTH physiology on the fetal environment and subsequent brain and behavioral development can be studied in both RTH-affected and unaffected offspring. Also, the psychosocial effects of a parent with RTH and ADHD compared with a parent with RTH and no behavioral disorder can be determined. Furthermore, the interaction of certain socioeconomic and psychosocial factors with the consequences of RTH can be studied. By studying the interaction of various nongenetic factors with a known genetic abnormality (a mutant thyroid hormone receptor that causes RTH), we can identify protective and risk factors that may explain the variability and severity of the ADHD phenotype.

The study of single-gene disorders such as RTH can be extended to functional and structural imaging research. Imaging research of ADHD has generally used control subjects without psychiatric illness who are unrelated to the ADHD subjects. This may serve to accentuate differences between groups. In RTH, we are able to identify which family members have a mutation in the thyroid hormone receptor gene and can therefore conduct studies on the basis of genotype rather than phenotype. Furthermore, unaffected family members serve as a comparison group who have genetic and environmental backgrounds similar to those of affected family members with the exception of the mutant gene of interest (in the case of RTH, mutations in the thyroid hormone receptor gene). This allows us to determine whether particular functional or structural abnormalities are specifically associated with a behavioral disorder caused by a single-gene mutation or the consequence of some other genetic or nongenetic factors. Imaging studies of single-gene disorders will allow for greater homogeneity of the patient sample. Also, such studies promise to elucidate the etiology of functional and structural abnormalities that have already been demonstrated in ADHD subjects.

Another important comparison group is made up of subjects with congenital hypothyroidism (CH). Although outcome in children with CH is markedly improved by newborn screening and subsequent early treatment, residual cognitive deficits may still occur that reflect delays in early neuromotor and language development and poorer visuospatial and memory abilities. CH and RTH represent two complementary models for studying attentional processes. In CH, the thyroid receptor is intact but there is an absence of the ligand—thyroid hormone—that activates the receptor during critical periods of brain development. In RTH, there is an excess of thyroid hormone, but it cannot be optimally utilized because the mutant thyroid hormone receptor protein has a decreased affinity for thyroid hormone.

The CH model allows us to study the effects of fetal and early postnatal thyroid hormone absence on behavioral, brain, and cognitive development. Also, because infants and children with treated CH have considerable variation in their circulating thyroid hormone concentrations, the effects of these variations on attentional processes and cognitive and behavioral development can be studied. The RTH model allows us to study the effects of a defective thyroid hormone receptor and the resultant inability to adequately utilize circulating thyroid hormone. This defective thyroid hormone receptor would exert its effect during fetal life as well as in infancy and early childhood. Inclusion of a CH comparison group will allow us to determine whether the defective thyroid hormone receptor is the specific causative factor of ADHD in subjects with RTH.

In both groups, attentional processes and IQ scores are adversely affected, and speech and language development can be delayed. However, there have been no systematic behavioral studies of psychiatric disorders (specifically ADHD) in children with congenital hypothyroidism using structured psychiatric interviews. Such systematic studies are absolutely necessary in order to test the hypothesis that ADHD is overrepresented in this group of children. Furthermore, structural and functional brain imaging studies are justified in children with CH. MRI scans can be obtained in children with little or no discomfort. Although functional imaging studies would entail a greater inconvenience to subjects, such studies could be performed on a limited number of people during their late teens. These studies should be compared with those that have already been completed in subjects with RTH and ADHD. Such comparisons would help to elucidate the role of thyroid hormone and the thyroid receptor in brain development.

In conclusion, by contrasting the neurodevelopmental effects of moderate impairment of thyroid function such as is found in resistance to thyroid hormone with those of congenital hypothyroidism, investigators will generate new hypotheses to test in a research setting. By comparing similarities and differences in measures of attentional processes and language and motor development between infants with CH and those with RTH, we may increase our understanding of the role of thyroid hormone and its receptor in the physiological mechanisms of behavioral, brain, and cognitive development. Such studies may provide new insights into the basic pathogenesis of ADHD as well as of language and other learning disorders.

References

Albright F, Burnett CH, Smith PH, et al: Pseudohypoparathyroidism—an example of Seabright-Bantam syndrome. J Clin Endocrinol Metab 30:922–932, 1942

Alvarez M, Gomez A, Alavez E, et al: Attention disturbance in Graves' disease. Psychoneuroendocrinology 8:451–454, 1983

American Psychiatric Association: Diagnostic and Statistical Manual of Mental Disorders, 3rd Edition. Washington, DC, American Psychiatric Association, 1980

American Psychiatric Association: Diagnostic and Statistical Manual of Mental Disorders, 3rd Edition, Revised. Washington, DC, American Psychiatric Association, 1987

American Psychiatric Association: Diagnostic and Statistical Manual of Mental Disorders, 4th Edition. Washington, DC, American Psychiatric Association, 1994

Barkley RA: A critique of current diagnosis criteria for attention deficit hyperactivity disorder: clinical and research implications. J Dev Behav Pediatr 11:343–352, 1990

Bernal J, Nunez J: Thyroid hormones and brain development. Eur J Endocrinol 133:390–398, 1995

Bernal J, Pekonen F: Ontogenesis of the nuclear 3,5,3'-triiodothyronine receptor in the human fetal brain. Endocrinology 114:677–679, 1984

Biederman J, Munir K, Knee D, et al: A family study of patients with attention deficit disorder and normal controls. J Psychiatr Res 20:263–274, 1986

Biederman J, Faraone S, Keenan K, et al: Family genetic and psychosocial risk factors in DSM-III attention deficit disorder. J Am Acad Child Adolesc Psychiatry 29:526–533, 1991

Bradley DJ, Young WS III, Weinberger C: Differential expression of alpha and beta thyroid hormone receptor genes in rat brain and pituitary. Proc Natl Acad Sci U S A 86:7250–7254, 1989

Bradley DJ, Towle HC, Young WS III: Alpha and beta thyroid hormone receptor (TR) gene expression during auditory neurogenesis: evidence for TR isoform-specific transcriptional regulation in vivo. Proc Natl Acad Sci U S A 91:439–443, 1994

Brucker-Davis F, Skarulis MC, Grace MB, et al: Genetic and clinical features of 42 kindreds with resistance to thyroid hormone: the National Institutes of Health Prospective Study. Ann Intern Med 123:572–583, 1995

Castellanos FX, Giedd JN, Eckburg P, et al: Quantitative morphology of the caudate nucleus in attention deficit hyperactivity disorder. Am J Psychiatry 151:1791–1796, 1994

Castellanos FX, Giedd JN, Marsh WL, et al: Quantitative brain magnetic resonance imaging in attention deficit hyperactivity disorder. Arch Gen Psychiatry 53:607–616, 1996

Cheng S, Ransom SC, McPhie P, et al: Analysis of the binding of 3,3',5-triiodo-L-thyronine and its analogues to mutant human α_1 thyroid hormone receptors: a model of the hormone binding site. Biochemistry 33:4319–4326, 1993

Chin WW: Current concepts of thyroid hormone action: progress notes for the clinician. Thyroid Today 15:1–9, 1992

Dayton AI, Selden JR, Laws G, et al: A human c-erbA oncogene homologue is closely proximal to the chromosome 17 breakpoint in acute promyelocytic leukemia. Proc Natl Acad Sci U S A 81:4495–4499, 1984

DuPaul GJ, Barkley RA: Medication therapy, in Attention-Deficit Hyperactivity Disorder: A Handbook for Diagnosis and Treatment. Edited by Barkley RA. New York, Guilford, 1990, pp 573–612

Dupont A, Dussault JH, Rouleau D, et al: Effect of neonatal thyroid deficiency on the catecholamine, substance P, and thyrotropin-release hormone contents of discrete rat brain nuclei. Endocrinology 108: 2039–2047, 1981

Dussault JH, Ruel J: Thyroid hormones and brain development. Annu Rev Physiol 49:321–334, 1987

Elia J, Gulotta C, Rose SR, et al: Thyroid function and attention-deficit hyperactivity disorder. J Am Acad Child Adolesc Psychiatry 33:169–172, 1994

Evans RM: The steroid and thyroid hormone receptor superfamily. Science 240:889–895, 1988

Farsetti A, Mitsuhashi T, Desvergne B, et al: Molecular basis of thyroid hormone regulation of myelin basic protein gene expression in rodent brain. J Biol Chem 266:23226–23232, 1991

Gareau J, Houle B, Leduc F, et al: A frequent HindIII RFLP on chromosome 3p21–25 detected by a genomic c-erbAβ sequence. Nucleic Acids Res 16:1223, 1988

Giedd JN, Castellanos FX, Casey BJ, et al: Quantitative morphology of the corpus callosum in attention deficit hyperactivity disorder. Am J Psychiatry 151:665–669, 1994

Hauser P, Zametkin AJ, Martinez P, et al: Attention-deficit hyperactivity disorder in people with generalized resistance to thyroid hormone. N Engl J Med 328:997–1001, 1993a

Hauser P, Wiggs E, Leonard CM, et al: Neurobiologic correlates of generalized resistance to thyroid hormone (abstract 274A). Paper presented at the American Federation of Clinical Research Annual Meeting, Washington, DC, May 1993b

Hendrich CE, Porterfield SP: Serum growth hormone levels in hypothyroid and GH-treated thyroidectomized rats and their progenies. Proc Soc Exp Biol Med 201:296–302, 1992

Hodin RA, Lazar MA, Wintman BI, et al: Identification of a thyroid hormone receptor that is pituitary-specific. Science 244:76–79, 1989

Hopwood NJ, Sauder SE, Shapiro B, et al: Familial partial peripheral and pituitary resistance to thyroid hormone: a frequently missed diagnosis? Pediatrics 78:1114–1122, 1986

Hynd GW, Semrud-Clikeman M, Lorys AR, et al: Corpus callosum morphology in attention-deficit hyperactivity disorder: morphometric analysis of MRI. Journal of Learning Disabilities 24:141–146, 1991

Hynd GW, Hern KL, Novey ES, et al: Attention deficit hyperactivity disorder and asymmetry of the caudate nucleus. J Child Neurol 8:339–347, 1993

Jenkins IH, Brooks DJ, Nixon PD, et al: Motor sequence learning; a study with positron emission tomography. J Neurosci 14:3775–3790, 1994

Koenig RJ, Warne RL, Brent GA, et al: Isolation of a cDNA clone encoding a biologically active thyroid hormone receptor. Proc Natl Acad Sci U S A 85:5031–5035, 1988

Lauder JM: Thyroid influences on the developing cerebellum and hippocampus of the rat, in Iodine and the Brain. Edited by Delong GR, Robbins J, Condliffe PG. New York, Plenum, 1989, pp 79–90

Leonard CM, Voeller KKS, Lombardino LJ, et al: Anomalous cerebral structure in dyslexia revealed with MR imaging. Arch Neurol 50: 461–469, 1993

Leonard CM, Martinez P, Weintraub BD, et al: Magnetic resonance imaging of cerebral anomalies in subjects with resistance to thyroid hormone. Am J Med Genet 60:238–243, 1995

Magner JA, Petrick P, Menezes-Ferreira MM, et al: Familial generalized resistance to thyroid hormones: report of three kindreds and correlation of patterns of affected tissues with the binding of [^{125}I]triiodothyronine to fibroblast nuclei. J Endocrinol Invest 9:459–470, 1986

Matochik JA, Nordahl TE, Gross M, et al: Effects of acute stimulant medication on cerebral metabolism in adults with hyperactivity. Neuropsychopharmacology 8:377–386, 1993

Matochik JA, Liebenauer LL, King AC, et al: Cerebral glucose metabolism in adults with attention deficit hyperactivity disorder after chronic stimulant treatment. Am J Psychiatry 151:658–664, 1994

Matochik J, Zametkin A, Cohen RM, et al: Abnormalities in sustained attention and anterior cingulate metabolism in subjects with resistance to thyroid hormone. Brain Res 723:23–28, 1996

• McBurnett K, Lahey B, Pfiffner L: Diagnosis of attention deficit disorders in DSM-IV: scientific basis and implications for education. Except Child 60:108–117, 1993

Meier CA, Dickstein BM, Ashizawa K, et al: Variable transcriptional activity and ligand binding of mutant beta$_1$ T$_3$ receptors from four families with generalized resistance to thyroid hormone. Mol Endocrinol 6:248–258, 1992

Mellström B, Naranjo JR, Santos A, et al: Independent expression of the α and β c-erb A genes in developing rat brain. Mol Endocrinol 5:1339–1350, 1991

Mitsuhashi T, Tennyson GE, Nikodem VM: Alternative splicing generates messages encoding rat c-erbA proteins that do not bind thyroid hormones. Proc Natl Acad Sci U S A 85:5804–5805, 1988

Mixson AJ, Parrilla R, Ransom S, et al: Correlations of language abnormalities in the β-thyroid receptor in 13 kindreds with generalized resistance to thyroid hormone: identification of four novel mutations. J Clin Endocrinol Metab 75:1039–1045, 1992

Mizejewski GJ, Morris JE, Hauser P, et al: A strategy for newborn screening for resistance to thyroid hormone: relevance to attention deficit hyperactivity disorder. Screening 4:61–70, 1995

Munoz A, Rodriguez-Peña A, Perez-Castillo A, et al: Effects of neonatal hypothyroidism on rat brain gene expression. Mol Endocrinol 5:273–280, 1991

Nakai A, Sakurai A, Bell GI, et al: Characterization of a third human thyroid hormone receptor coexpressed with other thyroid hormone receptors in several tissues. Mol Endocrinol 2:1087–1092, 1988

Pagliara AS, Caplan RH, Gunderson CB, et al: Peripheral resistance to thyroid hormone in a family: heterogeneity of clinical presentation. J Pediatr 103:228–232, 1983

Pardo JV, Fox PT, Raichle ME: Localization of a human system for sustained attention by positron emission tomography. Nature 349:61–64, 1991

Parilla R, Mixson AJ, McPherson J, et al: Characterization of seven novel mutations of the c-erbAβ gene in unrelated kindreds with generalized thyroid hormone resistance: evidence for two "hot spot" regions of the ligand binding domain. J Clin Invest 88:2123–2130, 1991

Petersen SE, Fox PT, Posner MI, et al: Positron emission tomographic studies of the cortical anatomy of single-word processing. Nature 331:585–589, 1988

Pipaon C, Santos A, Perez-Castillo A: Thyroid hormone up-regulates NGFI-A gene expression in rat brain during development. J Biol Chem 267:21–23, 1992

Porterfield SP: Vulnerability of the developing brain to thyroid abnormalities: environmental insults to the thyroid system. Environ Health Perspect 102 (suppl 2):125–130, 1994

Posner MI, Petersen SE: The attention system of the human brain. Annu Rev Neurosci 13:25–42, 1990

Raichle ME, Fiez JA, Videen TO, et al: Practice-related changes in human brain functional anatomy during nonmotor learning. Cereb Cortex 4:8–26, 1994

Rastogi RB, Singhal RL: Effect of neonatal hypothyroidism and delayed L-triiodothyronine treatment on behavioral activity and norepinephrine and dopamine biosynthetic systems in discrete regions of rat brain. Psychopharmacology 62:287–293, 1979

Reeve E, Garfinkel B: Neuroendocrine and growth regulation: the role of sympathomimetic medication, in Ritalin: Theory and Patient Management. Edited by Greenhill LL, Osman BB. New York, Mary Ann Liebert, 1991, pp 289–300

Refetoff S, Dewind LT, DeGroot LJ: Familial syndrome combining deaf-mutism, stippled epiphyses, goiter and abnormally high pbi: possible target organ refractoriness to thyroid hormone. J Clin Endocrinol Metab 27:279–294, 1967

Refetoff S, DeGroot LJ, Bernard B, et al: Studies of a sibship with apparent hereditary resistance to the intracellular action of thyroid hormone. Metabolism 21:723–756, 1972

Refetoff S, Weiss RE, Usala SJ: The syndromes of resistance to thyroid hormone. Endocr Rev 14:348–399, 1993

Rovet JF, Ehrlich RM, Donner E: Long-term neurodevelopmental correlates of treatment adequacy in screened hypothyroid children. Pediatr Res 33:91, 1993a

Rovet JF, Daneman D, Bailey JD: Psychologic and psychoeducational consequences of thyroxine therapy for juvenile acquired hypothyroidism. J Pediatr 122:543–549, 1993b

Sap J, Munoz A, Damm K, et al: The c-erb-A protein is a high-affinity receptor for thyroid hormone. Nature 324:635–640, 1986

Semrud-Clikeman M, Filipek PA, Biederman J, et al: Attention deficit hyperactivity disorder: magnetic resonance imaging morphometric analysis of the corpus callosum. J Am Acad Child Adolesc Psychiatry 33:875–881, 1994

Shaywitz BA, Shaywitz SE: Comorbidity: a critical issue in attention deficit disorder. J Child Neurol 6 (suppl):S13–S20, 1991

Shenker A: The mechanism of action of drugs used to treat attention-deficit hyperactivity disorder: focus on catecholamine receptor pharmacology. Adv Pediatr 39:337–382, 1993

Smallridge RC, Parker RA, Wiggs EA, et al: Thyroid hormone resistance in a large kindred: physiologic, biochemical, pharmacologic, and neuropsychologic studies. Am J Med 86:289–296, 1989

Spencer T, Biederman J, Wilens T, et al: Attention deficit hyperactivity disorder and thyroid abnormalities. Poster presented at the American Academy of Child and Adolescent Psychiatry Annual Meeting, San Antonio, TX, October 1993

Steinmetz H, Ebeling U, Huang Y, et al: Sulcus topography of the parietal opercular region: an anatomic and MRI study. Brain Lang 48:515–533, 1990

Strait KA, Schwartz HL, Perez-Castillo A, et al: Relationship of c-erbA mRNA content to tissue triiodothyronine nuclear binding capacity and function in developing and adult rats. J Biol Chem 265:10514–10521, 1990

Takeda K, Balzano S, Sakuri A, et al: Screening of nineteen unrelated families with generalized resistance to thyroid hormone for known point mutations in the thyroid hormone receptor β gene and the detection of a new mutation. J Clin Invest 87:496–502, 1991

Trzepacz P, McCue M, Klein I, et al: A psychiatric and neuropsychological study of patients with untreated Graves' disease. Gen Hosp Psychiatry 10:49–55, 1988

Usala SJ, Bale AE, Gesundheit N, et al: Tight linkage between the syndrome of generalized thyroid hormone resistance and the human c-erbA β gene. Mol Endocrinol 2:1217–1220, 1988

Usala SJ, Tennyson GE, Bale AE, et al: A base mutation of the c-erbA thyroid hormone receptor in a kindred with generalized thyroid hormone resistance: molecular heterogeneity in two other kindreds. J Clin Invest 85:93–100, 1990

Usala SJ, Menke JB, Cugini CD, et al: A mutation in codon 315 of C-erbAβ in a kindred with generalized hormone resistance and dyslexia (abstract). Clinical Research 39:293A, 1991

Weinberger C, Thompson CC, Ong ES, et al: The c-erb-A gene encodes a thyroid hormone receptor. Nature 324:641–646, 1986

Weiss RE, Balzano S, Scherberg NH, et al: Neonatal detection of generalized resistance to thyroid hormone. JAMA 264:2245–2250, 1990

Weiss RE, Stein MA, Trommer B, et al: Attention-deficit hyperactivity disorder and thyroid function. J Pediatr 123:539–545, 1993

Wender PH, Reimherr FW, Wood DR: A controlled study of methylphenidate in the treatment of attention deficit disorder, residual type, in adults. Am J Psychiatry 142:547–552, 1985

Zametkin AJ, Nordahl TE, Gross M, et al: Cerebral glucose metabolism in adults with hyperactivity of childhood onset. N Engl J Med 323:1361–1366, 1990

Chapter 6

Behavioral and Cognitive Abnormalities Associated With Juvenile Acquired Hypothyroidism

Joanne Rovet, Ph.D., and Denis Daneman, M.D.

Juvenile acquired hypothyroidism (JAH) is a form of primary hypothyroidism that develops during childhood or adolescence following a period of previously normal thyroid function. Although the peak age is late childhood, onset can occur as early as infancy. Like congenital hypothyroidism (CH), JAH is characterized by low levels of thyroid hormone and elevated thyrotropin. However unlike CH, JAH is distinguished by the presence of high thyroid antibody titers. JAH involves a number of characteristic physical features, including short stature and slow growth, dry skin, coarse hair, and occasionally goiter. There are no remarkable behavioral features of JAH other than lassitude and sometimes poor school performance. A few children presenting with de novo psychiatric disorders, including attention-deficit disorder, have been found to be hypothyroid (Bhatara et al. 1993).

It is not uncommon, after the initiation of treatment for JAH, for behavioral problems to arise in some children. Problems range

---

This work was originally conducted in collaboration with Dr. John Bailey, whose concern for these children and clinical acumen spearheaded these investigations. We also appreciate Donna Sorbara, Jeannine Pinnsonneault, Lindsay Ireland, and Dr. Susan Bradley for their contributions to this study. This research was made possible by grants from the Ontario Ministry of Health and the Ontario Mental Health Foundation.

from frank psychopathology to attention and learning difficulties. This chapter reviews aspects of JAH and associated behavioral manifestations. Several case studies are described as well as findings from a prospective follow-up study of children with newly diagnosed JAH. The implications of our findings for treatment and management of this disease are also discussed.

Disease Characteristics

JAH is reported to be the single most frequent thyroid disorder of childhood and adolescence (Fisher 1993). The female:male sex ratio is between 6:1 and 11:1 (Fisher 1993), and there is a strong family history of thyroid disease (Badenboop et al. 1990) in as many as 30% of children with JAH (LaFranchi 1992). Typically, JAH is a single-gland disorder involving just the thyroid. However, it can co-occur with other endocrine deficiency syndromes, particularly insulin-dependent diabetes mellitus. JAH is also common among children with chromosome abnormalities, specifically Down, Turner, and Klinefelter syndromes (LaFranchi 1992).

The most frequent cause of JAH is chronic lymphocytic autoimmune thyroiditis, or Hashimoto's thyroiditis (HT), although JAH may also be caused by ingestion of excess iodine, drugs with antithyroid activity, or naturally occurring environmental goitrogens, such as cabbage and groundwater bacteria (Fisher 1993). In a survey of more than 5,000 11- to 18-year-olds in the southwestern United States, JAH due to HT alone was estimated at 1.3%, whereas in Kentucky, where groundwater bacteria rates are high, the prevalence rate for hypothyroidism of any form was estimated at 5% (LaFranchi 1992).

The exact immunological pathogenesis of HT is not known, although several mechanisms have been posited. These include a virus or bacterium that contains a protein similar to thyroid hormone (molecular mimicry) and origin within the thyroid epithelial cells themselves (Dayan and Daniels 1996). HT occurs in genetically predisposed individuals from a failure of immune surveillance that results in inflammatory destruction of the thyroid gland

(LaFranchi 1992). A wide spectrum of antibodies may be produced in HT, including antithyroglobulin antibody, antimicrosomal (antiperoxidase) antibody, thyroid growth–blocking antibody, thyroid growth–stimulating antibody, TSH-binding inhibitory immunoglobulin, and TSH receptor stimulating immunoglobulin. The type, timing, and predominance of antibodies may determine the clinical presentation (LaFranchi 1992).

The peak age at onset of JAH is 10–11 years, but the condition may occur at any age (LaFranchi 1979) and is most commonly found in adolescent girls (LaFranchi 1992). Although JAH rarely occurs before the age of 3 years, Foley et al. (1994) described four infants with JAH whose clinical and biochemical presentation resembled late-diagnosed CH except that they had high thyroid antibody titers.

The onset of JAH is usually insidious. In the majority of children, severe JAH is diagnosed only after an extended fall-off in linear growth. Clinical features of JAH include dry skin, coarse hair, and puffiness (Ingbar and Woeber 1974); a goiter may or may not be present (Dayan and Daniels 1996). Affected infants may also have an enlarged tongue. There may be a disproportionate appearance of body segments, with an increased upper to lower body ratio, and dentition and skeletal maturity may be delayed. For the majority of adolescents with JAH, puberty is typically delayed; however, there has been an association with precocious puberty in several cases (Van Wyk and Grumbach 1960). Mild lassitude, fatigue, cold intolerance, bradycardia, and poor school performance are common behavioral symptoms (Ingbar and Woeber 1974).

The differential diagnosis of JAH is based on laboratory tests showing a decreased concentration of circulating thyroid hormones (thyroxine [T_4], free T_4, and triiodothyronine [T_3]) and an elevated serum thyroid-stimulating hormone (TSH) concentration. The presence of thyroid antibodies confirms a diagnosis of Hashimoto's thyroiditis. Bone age is often used as a marker for dating the onset of JAH (LaFranchi 1979). Computed tomography and magnetic resonance imaging of the brain may reveal an enlarged sella turcica due to pituitary thyrotroph hypertrophy (LaFranchi et al. 1986). An empty sella may also appear.

Treatment is levothyroxine (L-T_4) replacement given orally in a single daily dose, determined by the child's size. The recommended daily dose levels by age are 8–10 μg/kg at 3–6 months of age, 6–8 μg/kg from 6 to 12 months (LaFranchi 1992), 6 μg/kg from 1 to 5 years, 4 μg/kg from 6 to 10 years, and 2–3 μg/kg from 11 to 20 years (Fisher 1993). According to Fisher (1993), the optimal maintenance dosage of L-T_4 should normalize serum TSH and maintain serum T_4 in the middle or upper range of normal for age. A prudent approach based on our studies described below is to provide low dosages initially, with gradual increases until the minimal dosage needed to suppress TSH to the normal range is achieved (Rovet et al. 1993). Many patients require smaller dosages of L-T_4 than are currently recommended (Fisher 1990; Rezvani and DiGeorge 1977); excessive dosages should be avoided, because they may lead to accelerated skeletal maturation and compromised final adult height (LaFranchi 1992). Excessive dosage may also cause hyperthyroid symptoms and signs. Regular clinical and biochemical evaluations should be performed to guide changes in L-T_4 dosage until an optimal level has been achieved.

Behavioral Manifestations

The severe mental deficiency typically associated with late-treated congenital hypothyroidism is seldom if ever seen in JAH. However, school achievement has been reported to be poorer than normal (LaFranchi 1992), and lower intelligence may occur if JAH presents in infancy and treatment is delayed. For example, among the four very young patients described by Foley et al. (1994), the two with JAH of 5–6 months' duration were significantly delayed in their development, whereas the one with onset prior to 6 months of age, but only of 2 months' duration, was mildly retarded (the one child who was diagnosed immediately after onset at 1.1 year was normal). These observations suggest that timing is critical—the earlier the onset, the worse the prognosis. In children who develop hypothyroidism after the age of 3, mental retardation is not usually observed. In fact, children with JAH have anecdotally been described as very good, if not overachieving, students, which may be attributed to their overly pliant behavior and decreased activity levels in the hypothyroid state.

Before treatment, behavior problems are rarely seen in children with JAH, although one teenager who presented with psychosis was subsequently found to be hypothyroid, and he improved markedly following L-T_4 therapy (Bhatara et al. 1993). The relationship between attention-deficit/hyperactivity disorder (ADHD) and varying forms of dysthyroidism has become a topic of recent interest and debate (Alessi et al. 1993; Ciaranello 1993; Elia 1995) and is being studied by several groups (Eberle 1995; Elia et al. 1994; Hauser et al. 1993; Rovet and Alvarez 1996; Spencer et al. 1995; Weiss et al. 1993). In a small proportion of children with ADHD (Weiss et al. 1993), clinical and subclinical hypothyroidism have been observed. What has emerged from this literature is the question whether children with ADHD, especially those with a fall-off in growth, should be screened for thyroid dysfunction (Bhatara et al. 1994; Ciaranello 1993). A recent report from our laboratory has shown no evidence of hypothyroidism in children with ADHD, although free and total T_4 levels are consistently at the lower end of the normal range, as are TSH levels (Bass et al. 1996). This suggests possible hyporegulation of the pituitary.

In contrast to the relative paucity of behavior problems among children with JAH before they begin receiving thyroxine therapy, there are numerous reports of adults and children demonstrating adverse behavioral reactions once replacement therapy is initiated (Josephson and Mackenzie 1980). In adults, both cognitive and affective disturbances have been described (Josephson and Mackenzie 1980), and one case has been reported in which a patient receiving L-T_4 therapy committed a murder that was attributed to myxedema madness (Easson 1980). In children, neurological complications have included headaches, visual impairment with papilledema, and pseudotumor cerebri (Huseman and Torbelson 1984; McVie 1984; Rohn 1985; Van Dop et al. 1983; Van Wyk and Grumbach 1960), whereas learning and behavior problems have been reported to coincide with improvements in physical symptoms (DeGroot et al. 1984). We have seen dramatic behavioral reactions in a small proportion of pediatric patients with JAH in response to thyroxine therapy. These include inability to learn, attention problems, conduct problems, aggression, and psychosis (Rovet et al. 1993).

Although there have been a few anecdotal reports, there have been few if any empirical studies of intellectual and behavioral outcome in children with JAH. Our experience with three adolescents who demonstrated significant and marked behavior abnormalities after starting therapy for JAH (see below) prompted us to conduct a controlled study of JAH in childhood (also described below). Our findings suggest that severe behavior problems are rare in this population; however, there is a definite need for further study.

Case Studies

Case 1

A 13.5-year-old girl was diagnosed with JAH after a 3-year period of slow growth, inactivity, fatigue, lack of pubertal development, and changes in skin color. On examination, she had low T_4 levels and an elevated TSH concentration. She was started on a regimen of 150 µg L-T_4. Before the initiation of replacement therapy, she was described in her school reports as an above-average student with superior math abilities and advanced artistic talents, and she was exceptionally neat, well organized, and persevering.

Two months after starting treatment, she was noted to be more active and less tired and she demonstrated a dramatic improvement and maturation of her physical appearance. However, she was doing quite poorly at school. Six months following the initiation of therapy, her eighth-grade teacher noted, "In class she became listless and inattentive. The quality of her work deteriorated substantially. Her writing became messy. Her grade average dropped from 75% to approximately 55% during one term." One year after diagnosis, her dosage of levothyroxine was reduced from 150 µg to 100 µg, but she was still unable to concentrate and was performing exceedingly poorly at school. She obtained only 3 of 8 credits in her first year of high school.

When assessed psychologically in our unit 1.5 years after diagnosis and initiation of treatment, she had a full-scale IQ score of 98 with equivalent levels of verbal and performance IQ. On tests of memory, attention, and visuomotor ability, she scored in the average range and showed no specific deficits. Her handwriting was very messy and her figure drawings were sketchy and of poor quality. On achievement testing, she scored 2.6 grades below expectation in reading and 4.0 grades below in arithmetic. Retesting 1 year later while she was receiving 75 μg thyroxine revealed improved perceptual abilities, whereas verbal skills remained as before; she had made minimal achievement gains and was falling progressively behind.

A psychiatric consultation indicated "features of organic brain syndrome as a result of thyroxine's causing a fairly marked deterioration in concentration and attention skills." Her high school performance continued to deteriorate, and she had to switch from an academic program to a more technical placement, necessitating changing high schools. Her family was supportive but devastated by these changes.

Case 2

A 12-year-old boy was diagnosed with JAH after a 2-year history of slow growth. He was treated with 100 μg of levothyroxine daily. He had previously been an honor student and indicated no signs of hyperactivity or major behavior problems.

Twelve days after starting treatment, he was admitted to a local hospital with acute psychosis. A computed tomographic scan was normal, but an electroencephalogram (EEG) revealed a petit mal variant with myoclonic jerks. His dosage of L-T_4 was reduced for 3 days and then returned to 100 μg, and he was given primidone 25 μg twice daily. Recovery from psychosis occurred within 1 week and his EEG improved. Five months later, when first seen in our hospital, he was clinically euthyroid but was reported to have significant difficulties with concentration, organization, and behavior. He was also hyperactive and failing most subjects at school.

He received a psychological evaluation in our unit 1.5 years after diagnosis. The results showed a full-scale IQ of 116, with his performance IQ (PIQ) significantly higher than his verbal IQ (VIQ). On tests of figure copying, drawing, and achievement, he indicated above-average ability, but he showed a deficit in short-term recall. He was also impulsive and hyperactive.

Because of a low T_4 concentration and elevated TSH on one occasion, his daily dosage of L-T_4 was increased to 125 µg. However, as this was also associated with increased hyperactivity and forgetfulness, his dosage was immediately reduced to 100 µg. Unfortunately, his inattention, memory problems, and inability to complete school assignments continued, and he was now reportedly speaking "double time" and failing most subjects at school. He was also frequently suspended for conduct problems. EEG testing at this time was normal. Subsequent psychological testing indicated a significant decline in arithmetic, slower response times, and a behavior profile of a clinically hyperactive child.

A psychiatric consultation revealed "a vulnerable youngster, whose basic behavioral difficulties have probably been aggravated by thyroxine." Although he was not seen again by us, a later consultation with his mother indicated her grave concerns about his behavior and deteriorating school performance.

Case 3

A 16-year-old boy was diagnosed with JAH after the development of obesity and lethargy and a 3-year period of growth failure. Although he was initially treated with 150 µg of L-T_4, his dosage was reduced because of deterioration in math, poor concentration, frequent upsets, agitation, conduct problems, and excessive talkativeness, as well as an attempted sexual assault on an older neighbor.

Our psychological evaluation revealed a cooperative and quiet boy, lacking in affect and not overly impulsive. His full-scale IQ was 95, and he showed an advantage in VIQ over PIQ. Although he demonstrated exceptional abstract reasoning ability, his short-term memory (auditory and visual), visual discrimination, visuomotor, and arithmetic abilities were quite poor. His behavior problems included somatic complaints, communication difficulties, and delinquent behavior. School problems and difficulties with attention persisted, even when his dosage was reduced to 75 µg daily.

A psychiatric consultation suggested that with thyroxine therapy it was difficult for him to control preexisting concerns regarding his parents' recent separation and lack of paternal involvement, along with frustration, increased sexual tension, and normally poor impulse control. There was no further follow-up

Summary

Each of the three patients described above had severe behavioral or learning difficulties that started soon after initiation of L-T_4 replacement therapy for severe JAH. All showed marked declines in school performance. Psychological assessment revealed IQs in the normal to high normal range with no obvious pattern of impairment. One teenager had equivalent verbal and nonverbal abilities, one was better in the verbal domain, and one was better in the nonverbal. They all had significant problems in attention and impulse control, which were relieved slightly if at all when dosage levels were lowered. Unfortunately, each child became mildly clinically hypothyroid. In at least one case (case 2), significant behavior problems have persisted.

A Prospective Study of Newly Diagnosed Juvenile Acquired Hypothyroidism

Given our experience with the three teenagers described above, we designed and conducted a prospective study of an unselected series of children and adolescents with newly diagnosed JAH. The goals of this study were to evaluate intelligence, behavior, and achievement before and after the first 2 years of therapy and to determine the prevalence of behavior and learning problems. We also sought to document the incidence of adverse reactions and whether adverse reactions correlated with persisting behavior problems.

The study involved assessing all newly diagnosed children who presented with severe hypothyroidism between June 1983 and October 1987 at the Endocrine Clinic of Toronto's Hospital for Sick Children (HSC) (see Rovet et al. 1993 for details). All were diagnosed with JAH on the basis of elevated TSH concentration

(> 20 mU/L), low total T_4 level (> 50 nmol/L), thyroid antibodies, and the presence of clinical symptoms. The patients were tested immediately after the diagnosis was made and before the initiation of treatment with L-T_4. They were given a brief battery (1.5 hours) of psychometric tests that included an age-appropriate Wechsler intelligence test (Wechsler Preschool and Primary Scale of Intelligence [WPPSI; Wechsler 1967] or Wechsler Intelligence Scale for Children, Revised [WISC-R; Wechsler 1974]), a test of visuomotor integration (Beery and Buktenica 1989), a test of impulsivity using a modification of the Matching Familiar Figures Test (Rovet 1980), and the Wide Range Achievement Test—Revised (Jastak and Wilkinson 1984). Parents completed Achenbach's Child Behavior Checklist (Achenbach and Edelbrock 1983). This battery was restricted in scope and duration to allow an assessment without notice on the day the diagnosis was made. Initiation of treatment followed this first assessment.

Subjects were reassessed on three subsequent occasions: 3 months, 1 year, and 2 years after diagnosis. At 3 months, only the Wechsler subtests that could be reliably repeated within a short period were given (i.e., arithmetic, vocabulary, digit span, picture completion). The entire battery was readministered at 1 and 2 years. Thyroid function tests (T_4 and TSH) were also conducted on each day of testing. We reviewed medical charts for indications of headaches, visual disturbance, papilledema, pseudotumor cerebri, signs and symptoms of hypothyroidism or hyperthyroidism, and behavioral changes.

We succeeded in studying the majority of newly presenting patients with severe JAH, which included 17 girls and 6 boys ranging in age from 4.9 to 16.5 years (mean ± SD = 11.1 ± 3.2 years). Premorbidly, only one child (4.5%) was found to be retarded, whereas two (9%) had borderline intelligence. Figure 6–1, which distributes IQ scores by age, shows that the three children who were functioning below normal were diagnosed after age 10, whereas the youngest two children, both diagnosed at age 5, had normal IQs. Unlike the case for CH, age at onset does not seem to be critical for JAH.

Table 6–1, which presents the mean scores from all testing ses-

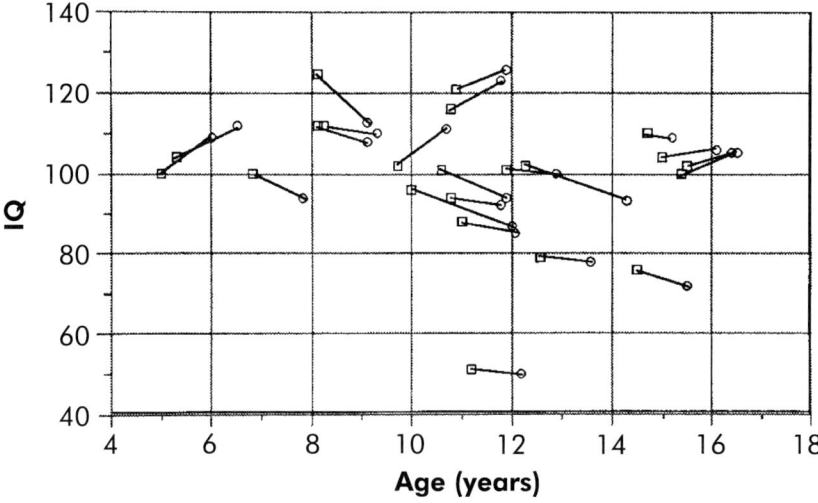

Figure 6–1. Individual pretreatment and posttreatment IQ levels in juvenile acquired hypothyroidism. The majority of posttreatment assessments are at 12 months postdiagnosis.

sions, shows that before the initiation of therapy, the intelligence of the subjects was in the normal range (although about one-third of a standard deviation below normal). As indicated by lower VIQ than PIQ scores and by lower scores on several verbal subtests (information, arithmetic, vocabulary, digit span), subjects' verbal abilities were lower than their nonverbal abilities, whereas all nonverbal subtests were in the normal range. Their visuomotor skills were average. Achievement test results were slightly below average, particularly for arithmetic, which was at the 38th percentile. The subjects did not indicate any problems with attention, as measured by the Freedom from Distractibility (FFD) composite score of the Wechsler tests (Kaufman 1975), impulsivity testing (data not provided), and parent questionnaires.

After initiation of treatment, four children (17%) developed de novo behavior problems, such as temper tantrums, moodiness, aggression, and irritability (Table 6–2). A comparable number (not

Table 6–1. Test results for subjects with juvenile acquired hypothyroidism over a 2-year period

Test	Pretreatment	3 months	12 months	24 months
WISC/WPPSI (%)				
VIQ	91.9		90.3	89.1
PIQ	100.1		105.8	101.4
Full-scale IQ	95.6		96.8	94.6
Information	8.8		8.5	7.7
Similarities	10.4		10.0	9.0
Arithmetic*	7.1	7.1	7.8	5.9
Vocabulary	9.3	9.6	9.1	7.5
Digit span	9.4	8.8	9.7	9.6
Picture completion	10.1	10.7	11.0	10.9
Block design	10.5		10.0	9.3
Coding**	10.5	10.2	10.7	8.2
Beery (%)**	55.0	49.1	44.0	44.2
WRAT-R (%)				
Reading	42.1	27.9	43.3	37.3
Spelling	44.7	38.4	38.8	41.7
Arithmetic	37.6	29.9	29.9	29.7

Note. At 3 months, only the Wechsler subtests that could be reliably repeated within a short period were given (Arithmetic, Vocabulary, Digit Span, Picture Completion). Beery = Developmental Test of Visual Motor Integration (Beery and Buktenica 1989); PIQ = performance IQ; VIQ = verbal IQ; WISC = Wechsler Intelligence Scale for Children—Revised (Wechsler 1974); WPPSI = Wechsler Preschool and Primary Scale of Intelligence (Wechsler 1967); WRAT-R = Wide Range Achievement Test—Revised (Jastak and Wilkinson 1984). Based on repeated measures analyses of variance (ANOVA), $^*P < .01$; $^{**}P < .05$.

necessarily the same children) had problems concentrating. In contrast, 22% were described as showing significantly improved behavior, demonstrated by increased energy levels and a better attitude.

Table 6–2. Incidence of adverse events following treatment of juvenile acquired hypothyroidism

	n (%)
Headaches	5 (22)
Papilledema	3 (13)
Pseudotumor cerebri	3 (13)
Temporary hair loss	2 (9)
Seizures	0 (0)
Lack of concentration	4 (17)
Behavior problems	4 (17)

Across the group, no major changes in intelligence were observed, as shown in Table 6–1. However, as Figure 6–1 shows, six children did decline, whereas a comparable number improved. Repeated measures analyses of variance revealed that performance on arithmetic and coding subtests declined significantly. Although these are subtests that partially make up the FFD composite of attention, the total composite score itself was not significantly affected. A significant decline in visuomotor integration was also observed over the 2-year period. There were no effects on impulsivity, behavior problems, or social competence (data not presented). Individually, none of the children had difficulties of the magnitude of the three cases presented above.

Parents reported on questionnaires that the children declined significantly in writing ($P < .001$), arithmetic ($P < .03$), and spelling ($P < .001$) and that they showed a significant increase in academic problems ($P < .01$). Achievement testing of the children following treatment did not reveal that the group had changed significantly (Table 6–1). However, examination of the grade level scores of individual children revealed that only about one-third showed appropriate progress, whereas one-third showed no gain at 3 months but caught up by 1 year and one-third failed to make the expected gains in reading or arithmetic or both at 1 and 2 years.

To determine whether children with different achievement profiles varied with regard to their original hypothyroidism, we assigned subjects to three groups on the basis of their achievement performance. Group A consisted of eight children who made the expected gains, group B consisted of eight children who showed delayed gains, and group C consisted of six children who made no gains. Figure 6–2 shows the thyroid function test results and dosage levels of the three groups. They differed significantly in their hormone levels at diagnosis, with group C (no gains) being the most severely hypothyroid, as indicated by lower serum T_4 levels ($P < .05$) and higher serum TSH concentrations ($P < .01$). Group B (delayed gains) was intermediate, having T_4 values that were between the other two groups and TSH levels that were significantly lower ($P < .01$) than those of group C. Once receiving treatment, the groups did not differ in T_4 or TSH levels; however, group A (expected gains), which had the mildest hypothyroidism to start, was the slowest to achieve euthyroidism. The dosage levels of group C were higher, although not significantly different, than those of group A. Group C was also slightly older than groups A and B (mean ages of 13.6, 10.4, and 10.5 years, respectively). The groups did not differ in adverse events and none in the no-gains group had headaches, papilledema, or pseudotumor cerebri, which suggests that these events were not associated with poor school learning.

A similar series of comparisons was conducted for the neuropsychological test results of the three groups. After 1 year of therapy, group C declined significantly in full-scale IQ and scored lower on the verbal comprehension factor, block design, and similarities subtests. The groups did not differ significantly on any of the behavioral parameters, including parent-reported attention problems; in fact, parents reported fewer problems in group C (Figure 6–3, right panel). However, on direct testing, group C showed a trend for lower FFD scores ($P = .08$) (see Figure 6–3, left panel), suggestive of poorer attention. Because this was observed at baseline and did not change with therapy, a de novo attention deficit attributed to L-T_4 therapy does not appear to be contributing to the lack of achievement in the no-gains group. However, the small sample sizes and crude measure of attention may have limited our power to detect a real effect.

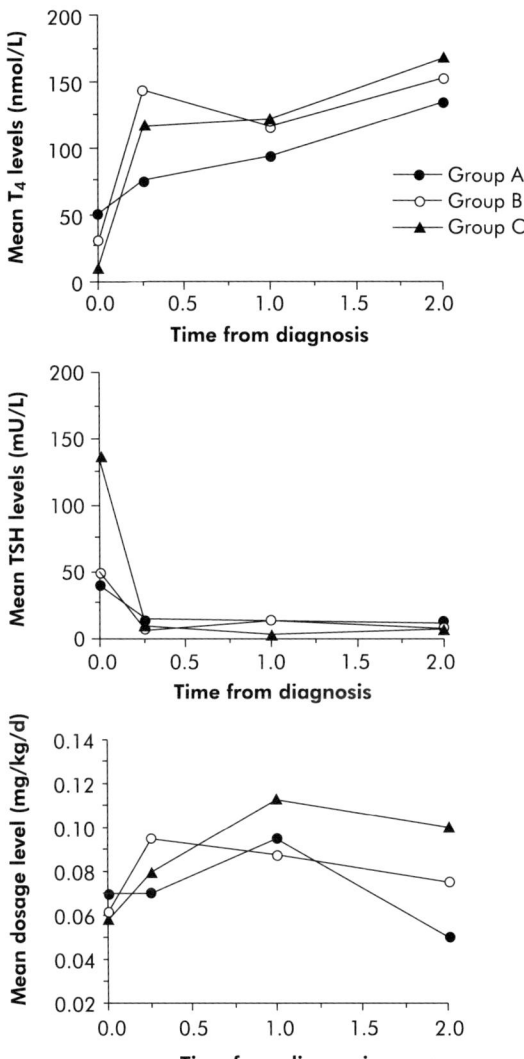

Figure 6–2. Changes in total thyroxine (T_4) concentration *(upper panel)*, thyrotropin concentration *(middle panel)*, and dosage of L-thyroxine *(lower panel)* for three achievement groups: filled circles, group A (expected-gains group); open circles, group B (delayed-gains group); triangles, group C (no-gains group). T_4 was lower ($P < .05$) and TSH was higher at baseline in the no-gains group.

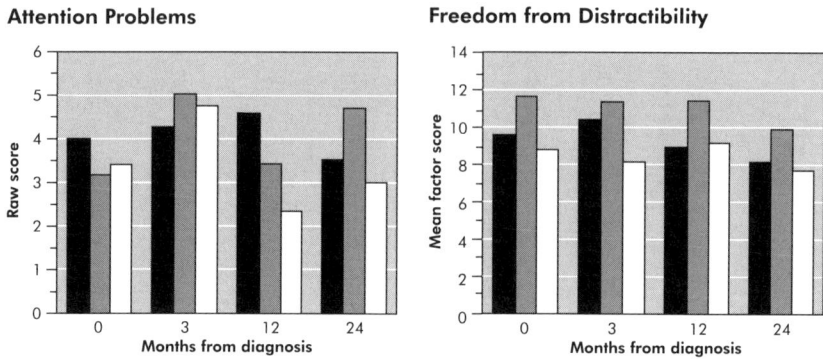

Figure 6–3. Attention measure results. Group A (expected gains) is shown in *dark bars;* group B (delayed gains) in *stippled bars;* group C (no gains) in *white bars*. A high Child Behavior Checklist (Achenbach and Edelbrock 1983) Attention Problems score signifies more attention problems, whereas a lower Wechsler (1974) Freedom from Distractibility score signifies poorer attention.

Correlational analyses were computed on indices of thyroid function and behavior. The results revealed that before the initiation of therapy, there was an association between measures of visual perceptual abilities (which were generally better than verbal) and degree of hypothyroidism. Children who were more severely hypothyroid did poorer on visuospatial tasks. In contrast, reading and arithmetic achievement were positively associated with hypothyroidism prior to therapy: children who were more hypothyroid did better in these areas. Once the children were receiving therapy, their levels of thyroid hormone were correlated with degree of impulsivity, verbal ability, and class placement. In particular, children with higher thyroid hormone levels were less impulsive, more skilled verbally, and less likely to be in a special class. However, children whose thyroid hormone levels were within or above the high normal range scored lower in reading, suggesting the need to maintain thyroid hormone levels well within the normal range.

In summary, the results of this prospective study indicate that the severe behavioral symptomatology seen in the three original cases is rare, whereas moderate symptoms and declines in school achievement occur in about 25% of cases. Children at greatest risk appear to be those with the more severe and long-standing hypothyroidism initially, who achieve euthyroidism quickly, and whose thyroid hormone levels are subsequently high. Attentional skills did not appear to be seriously compromised by implementation of therapy, nor did attention predict decrements in achievement. However, care should be taken in interpreting these data, because the attentional indices we used in this study may not have been adequately sensitive for the effects we observed.

Mechanisms for Poorer Outcome in Juvenile Acquired Hypothyroidism

The three case studies and our prospective study show that some children with JAH are at risk for severe behavioral reactions (including attentional dysfunction) and severe learning problems following administration of L-T_4 therapy, although these reactions are rare. Milder learning problems are evident in as many as 25% of children, who fail to make adequate gains in school following initiation of treatment. Children who are more vulnerable tend to be those with more severe hypothyroidism and who achieve euthyroidism very quickly, as well as those whose thyroid hormone concentrations are subsequently maintained at a high level.

There are several explanations for our findings. First is the possibility that some of the children were actually overachievers in the hypothyroid state because of their lower levels of arousal and activity. The lack of gain on becoming euthyroid may have actually represented a normalization to their true level, because of increased activity and arousability. Our finding of a significant correlation between low thyroid hormone values at diagnosis and higher achievement before, but not after, initiation of treatment lends credibility to this interpretation.

Alternatively, the poor outcome in some children may reflect a neurotransmitter imbalance, which was initiated by thyroid hormone deficiency and stimulated by administration of L-T_4. The different behavioral manifestations we observed in the three patients with extreme reactions may have reflected effects on different neurotransmitter systems (Klawans et al. 1974; Prange 1969; Puymirat 1985; Rastogi and Singhal 1976; Savard et al. 1983). It is known that in hypothyroidism, receptor sensitivity to central nervous system catecholamines is decreased and there is a compensatory rise in catechol concentration (Josephson and Mackenzie 1979). With rapid thyroid hormone normalization using high levels of thyroxine replacement, a hypercatecholaminergic state may be precipitated (Johnston and Singer 1982), which leads to hyperactivity and impaired learning. In support of this interpretation is the anecdotal observation from case 1: following initiation of therapy, the patient showed a dramatic deterioration in her handwriting and artwork reminiscent of the production deficits in children with ADHD. Because it is known that these graphomotor deficits improve in ADHD with methylphenidate therapy (Lerer et al. 1977), a known augmentor of catecholamine activity, it may be that children with JAH in the hypothyroid state resemble methylphenidate-treated hyperactive children and, when given thyroxine, revert to a state similar to untreated hyperactive children. The seizures and severe behavioral disturbance (Johnston and Singer 1982) observed in cases 2 and 3 may reflect similar neurotransmitter imbalances, which may be operating on different neurotransmitter systems.

A third possibility is that the levels of thyroid hormones in blood do not represent those in brain and that for some children the blood thyroid hormone levels may be normal but those at the level of the central nervous system are not. This reflects the fact that there are different deiodinase enzymes for converting T_4 to T_3 in the brain than in the periphery and the fact that the type II 5′-deiodinase found in the brain is sensitive to catecholamine levels (Silva and Landsberg 1993). It is possible that the children who responded more extremely to L-T_4 therapy had different catecholamine levels (possibly owing to their different dysthyroid states), which enhanced deiodination of T_4 to T_3 and so exposed their brains to higher levels of T_3.

Implications for Treatment and Management of Juvenile Acquired Hypothyroidism

Our studies have shown that there may be adverse behavioral sequelae following treatment of some children with JAH. In particular, children with more severe and long-standing hypothyroidism and who achieve euthyroidism quickly appear to be at highest risk, although there may also be milder problems associated with subsequent high thyroid hormone levels. These results suggest the need for caution in treating children with JAH and for regular and close monitoring of these children, both hormonally and behaviorally, especially if their hypothyroidism is severe and long-standing. Although current results from the three cases and the prospective study showed that adolescents were at greater risk, we know of and have more recently seen problems in children as young as age 5. Adverse psychological effects of thyroxine therapy for JAH represent an extremely disconcerting problem for parents, who express loss of their previously normal child, and for physicians, who may see themselves as partly responsible for these problems.

Our results indicate that a prudent but as yet untested approach is to provide a low dosage initially and to gradually increase it until the minimal dosage needed to suppress TSH to the normal range is found. This differs from the treatment of congenital hypothyroidism, in which achieving euthyroidism as quickly as possible is critical to prevent brain damage and permanent neuropsychological impairment (see Lash, Chapter 1, and Rovet, Chapter 4, in this volume). However, for the youngest children with JAH, who are undergoing major brain development, achieving euthyroidism quickly to prevent mental retardation may outweigh the potential for curbing behavior and temperament problems (Rovet et al. 1989).

Although extreme reactions to L-T_4 therapy may be rare among children with JAH, the question remains as to what should be done for these patients. A 9-year-old boy we saw recently with JAH, who following L-T_4 therapy acquired ADHD and learning problems reminiscent of case 1, was successfully treated with methylphenidate. Not only was he once again able to focus and sustain his attention, but he showed markedly improved behavior and school performance and was able to return to the gifted program he was originally in. We are also aware of another child presenting with a similar history for whom β-blockade with propranolol proved successful in controlling the behavioral disturbance. These anecdotal observations suggest the need for continued study of these children, including studies of stimulant/ blockade on attentional performance.

Conclusions

JAH represents a unique condition with iatrogenic behavioral effects of treatment with L-thyroxine in a small proportion of patients. Further research should focus on the impact of different $L-T_4$ replacement regimens and on the use of other medications (e.g., methylphenidate or β-blockade) if indicated.

References

Achenbach TM, Edelbrock C: Manual for the Child Behavior Checklist and Revised Child Behavior Profile. Burlington, VT, University of Vermont, 1983

Alessi N, Hottois MD, Coates JK: The gene for ADHD? Not yet. J Am Acad Child Adolesc Psychiatry 32:1073–1074, 1993

Badenboop K, Schwarz G, Walfish PG, et al: Susceptibility to thyroid autoimmune disease: molecular analysis of HLA-D region genes identifies new markers for goitrous Hashimoto's thyroiditis. J Clin Endocrinol Metab 71:1131–1137, 1990

Bass A, Rovet J, Lobaugh N, et al: Thyroid hormone (TH) and attention in children with attention deficit hyperactivity disorder (ADHD) (abstract). Thyroid 6:S58, 1996

Beery K, Buktenica N: Developmental Test of Visual Motor Integration. Chicago, IL, Follett, 1989

Bhatara V, Bandettini F, McMillin MJ: Psychosis associated with untreated hypothyroidism: a review of neuropsychiatric findings in children and adolescents with thyroid disorders. Journal of Child and Adolescent Psychopharmacology 3:199–212, 1993

Bhatara VS, Kummer M, McMillin JM, et al: ADHD and the thyroid (abstract). J Am Acad Child Adolesc Psychiatry 33:1057, 1994

Ciaranello RD: Attention deficit-hyperactivity disorder and resistance to thyroid hormone—a new idea? (editorial: comment). N Engl J Med 328:1038–1039, 1993

Dayan CM, Daniels GH: Chronic autoimmune thyroiditis. N Engl J Med 335:99–107, 1996

DeGroot LJ, Larsen PR, Refetoff S, et al: The Thyroid and Its Diseases, 5th Edition. New York, Wiley, 1984, p 627

Easson WM: Myxedema psychosis: insanity defense in homicide. J Clin Psychiatry 41:316–318, 1980

Eberle AJ: Hyperactivity and Graves' disease (letter). J Am Acad Child Adolesc Psychiatry 34:973, 1995

Elia J: Hyperactivity and Graves' disease (reply to letter). J Am Acad Child Adolesc Psychiatry 34:973–974, 1995

Elia J, Gulotta C, Rose SR, et al: Thyroid function and attention-deficit hyperactivity disorder. J Am Acad Child Adolesc Psychiatry 33:169–172, 1994

Fisher DA: The thyroid, in Clinical Pediatric Endocrinology. Edited by Kaplan SA. Philadelphia, PA, WB Saunders, 1990, pp 87–126

Fisher DA: Acquired juvenile hypothyroidism, in Werner and Ingbar's The Thyroid, 7th Edition. Edited by Braverman LE, Utiger RD. Philadelphia, PA, JB Lippincott, 1993, pp 1228–1236

Foley TP, Abbassi V, Copeland KC, et al: Hypothyroidism caused by chronic autoimmune thyroiditis in very young infants. N Engl J Med 330:466–468, 1994

Hauser P, Zametkin AJ, Martinez P, et al: Attention-deficit hyperactivity disorder in people with generalized resistance to thyroid hormone. N Engl J Med 328:997–1001, 1993

Huseman CA, Torbelson RD: Pseudotumor cerebri following treatment of hypothalamic and primary hypothyroidism. American Journal of Diseases of Children 138:927–931, 1984

Ingbar SH, Woeber KA: The thyroid gland, in Textbook of Endocrinology, 5th Edition. Edited by Williams RH. Philadelphia, PA, WB Saunders, 1974, pp 95–232

Jastak S, Wilkinson GS: Wide Range Achievement Test—Revised. Wilmington, DE, Jastak Associates, 1984

Johnston MV, Singer HS: Brain neurotransmitters and neuromodulators in pediatrics. Pediatrics 70:57–68, 1982

Josephson AM, Mackenzie TB: Appearance of manic psychosis following rapid normalization of thyroid status. Am J Psychiatry 136:846–847, 1979

Josephson AM, Mackenzie TB: Thyroid-induced mania in hypothyroid patients. Br J Psychiatry 41:316–318, 1980

Kaufman A: Factor analysis of the WISC-R at 11 age levels between 6.5 and 16.5 years. J Consult Clin Psychol 43:135–147, 1975

Klawans HL, Goetz C, Weiner WJ: Dopamine receptor site sensitivity in hypothyroid and hyperthyroid guinea pigs, in Advances in Neurology, Vol 5. Edited by McDowell FH, Barbeau A. New York, Raven, 1974, pp 846–847

LaFranchi SH: Hypothyroidism. Pediatr Clin North Am 26:35–51, 1979

LaFranchi S: Thyroiditis and acquired hypothyroidism. Pediatr Ann 21:32–39, 1992

LaFranchi SH, Hanna CE, Krainz PL: Primary hypothyroidism, empty sella, and hypopituitarism. J Pediatr 108:571–573, 1986

Lerer RJ, Lerer MP, Artner J: The effects of methylphenidate on the handwriting of children with minimal brain dysfunction. J Pediatr 91:127–132, 1977

McVie R: Abnormal TSH regulation, pseudotumor cerebri, and empty sella after replacement therapy in juvenile hypothyroidism. J Pediatr 105:768–770, 1984

Prange AJ: Enhancement of imipramine antidepressant activity by thyroid hormone. Am J Psychiatry 126:457–469, 1969

Puymirat J: Effects of dysthyroidism on central catecholaminergic neurons. Neurochem Int 17:969–977, 1985

Rastogi RB, Singhal RL: Influence of neonatal and adult hyperthyroidism on behavior and biosynthetic capacity for norepinephrine, dopamine and 5-hydroxytryptamine in rat brain. J Pharmacol Exp Ther 198:609–618, 1976

Rezvani I, DiGeorge AM: Reassessment of the daily dose of oral thyroxine for replacement therapy of hypothyroid children. J Pediatr 91:291–297, 1977

Rohn R: Pseudotumor cerebri following treatment of hypothyroidism. American Journal of Diseases of Children 138:927–931, 1985

Rovet J: A parametric measure of reflection–impulsivity. Journal of Applied Developmental Psychology 1:221–225, 1980

Rovet J, Alvarez M: Thyroid hormone and attention in school-age children with congenital hypothyroidism. J Child Psychol Psychiatry 37: 579–585, 1996

Rovet J, Ehrlich R, Sorbara D: Effect of thyroid hormone level on temperament in infants with congenital hypothyroidism detected by screening of neonates. J Pediatr 114:63–68, 1989

Rovet JF, Daneman D, Bailey JD: Psychologic and psychoeducational consequences of thyroxine therapy for juvenile acquired hypothyroidism. J Pediatr 122:543–549, 1993

Savard P, Merand Y, DiPaolo T, et al: Effects of thyroid state on serotonin, 5-hydroxyindoleacetic acid and substance P contents in discrete brain nuclei of adult rats. Neuroscience 10:1399–1404, 1983

Silva JE, Landsberg L: Catecholamines and the sympathoadrenal system in thyrotoxicosis, in Werner and Ingbar's The Thyroid, 7th Edition. Edited by Braverman LE, Utiger RD. Philadelphia, PA, JB Lippincott, 1993, pp 1228–1236

Spencer T, Biederman J, Wilens T, et al: ADHD and thyroid abnormalities: a research note. J Child Psychol Psychiatry 36:879–885, 1995

Ullmann RK, Sleator EK, Sprague RL: ADD-H Comprehensive Teachers Rating Scale. Champaign, IL, MetriTech, 1991

Van Dop C, Conte FA, Koch TK, et al: Pseudotumor cerebri associated with initiation of levothyroxine therapy for juvenile hypothyroidism. N Engl J Med 308:1076–1080, 1983

Van Wyk JJ, Grumbach MM: Syndrome of precocious menstruation and galactorrhea in juvenile hypothyroidism: an example of hormonal overlap in pituitary feedback. J Pediatr 47:416–435, 1960

Wechsler D: The Wechsler Preschool and Primary Scale of Intelligence. New York, Psychological Corporation, 1967

Wechsler D: The Wechsler Intelligence Scale for Children—Revised. New York, Psychological Corporation, 1974

Weiss RE, Stein MA, Trommer B, et al: Attention-deficit hyperactivity disorder and thyroid function. J Pediatr 123:539–545, 1993

Chapter 7

Behavioral and Cognitive Abnormalities Associated With Pediatric Thyrotoxicosis

Vinod S. Bhatara, M.D., M.S., and
J. Michael McMillin, M.D., F.A.C.P.

Background

History

The phenomenon of conspicuous cognitive-behavioral changes occurring in association with thyrotoxicosis was first described by Caleb Parry (1825) in his original report on hyperthyroidism in 1786 and was later mentioned by Graves (1835). The cognitive-behavioral changes associated with thyrotoxicosis in the classic descriptions were observed in adults, but these effects were later documented in children and adolescents (Barnes and Blizzard 1977; Saxena et al. 1964). Today, despite advances in the biochemical diagnosis of thyroid disorders, correct interpretation of cognitive and behavioral disturbances secondary to pediatric thyrotoxicosis remains important. Subtle cognitive-behavioral changes are among the earliest symptoms of pediatric thyrotoxicosis and often antedate medical diagnosis by 6–12 months (Barnes and Blizzard 1977). The knowledge of behavioral and cognitive phenomena in pediatric thyrotoxicosis is obviously important for early and correct medical diagnosis, and early detection of thyrotoxicosis is vital because symptoms can be potentially reversed with antithyroid therapy.

Prevalence

The prevalence of thyrotoxicosis in the general population is estimated to be between 0.15% and 0.5%, with British studies reporting a higher prevalence than American studies (Furszyfer et al. 1970; Vanderpump and Tunbridge 1996). The higher end of the range represents the British prevalence figures in women, and the lower end, the American figures in men. Only about 5% of all thyrotoxic patients are below 15 years of age (Dallas and Foley 1990; Saxena et al. 1964). Thyrotoxicosis is more common in adolescents than in children, and prevalence progressively increases with age. The disease is much more common in girls than in boys, with a female:male ratio between 3.5:1 and 6:1 (Barnes and Blizzard 1977; Zimmerman and Lteif 1998).

Etiology and Pathophysiology

Differentiating between the terms *thyrotoxicosis* and *hyperthyroidism* is useful in order to understand the relationship between the two conditions (Foley 1992). Although these two terms are often used interchangeably, in a narrower sense thyrotoxicosis is defined as the clinical syndrome characterized by excessive levels of unbound circulating thyroid hormones (Braverman and Utiger 1996). It is usually, but not always, caused by overactivity of the thyroid gland (referred to as hyperthyroidism). Occasionally, excessive circulating thyroid hormone is caused by ingestion of thyroid hormones (thyrotoxicosis of extrathyroid origin). Usually thyrotoxicosis is caused by excessive levels of circulating thyroxine (T_4); triiodothyronine (T_3) toxicosis also occurs, but it is rare (Root 1994). Hyperthyroidism refers strictly to overactivity of the thyroid gland.

Thyrotoxicosis with hyperthyroidism. The vast majority of cases of pediatric thyrotoxicosis are caused by autoimmune hyperthyroidism, known as Graves' disease (LaFranchi and Mandel 1996). Historically, Parry (1825) and Graves (1835) postulated that the psychological state of the patient played a role in the development of hyperthyroidism. However, it is currently accepted that Graves' disease has an autoimmune etiology, and a purely psychogenic etiology is unlikely. Autoimmune thyroid diseases result from a complex interplay between genetic predisposition and environmental factors (McKenzie and Zakarija 1996; McLachlan and Rapoport 1996). A high proportion of patients with Graves' disease have a positive family history for hyperthyroidism, hypothyroidism, or goiter (Barnes and Blizzard 1977). It is now known that thyrotropin (thyroid-stimulating hormone [TSH])-receptor antibodies that stimulate the thyroid gland (termed thyroid-stimulating antibodies [TSAbs]) cause Graves' disease (Davies 1996). However, the trigger that initiates the production of TSAbs remains elusive (Hershman 1995)

Leakage thyrotoxicosis. Thyrotoxicosis can be caused by destruction of the thyroid gland, causing release of preformed thyroid hormone into the circulation. The most common form of leakage thyrotoxicosis is "de Quervain's," or subacute, thyroiditis, which is most likely a postviral inflammation of the thyroid (Lazarus 1996). It has a characteristic triphasic clinical picture of thyroid tenderness associated with the signs and symptoms of thyrotoxicosis as the inflammatory process releases thyroid hormone. This is followed by a hypothyroid phase when all thyroid hormone has been released. Finally, when the thyroid recovers, the patient becomes euthyroid. Surgical manipulation of the thyroid and bacterial infections can also rarely cause leakage thyroiditis (Basgoz and Swartz 1996).

Thyrotoxicosis of extrathyroidal origin. Ingestion of thyroid hormones (intentional or unintentional) is the most frequent cause of thyrotoxicosis of extrathyroidal origin (Greer 1996). In younger children, ingestion of thyroid hormone is usually accidental (Cohen et al. 1989). However, in adolescents, thyroid hormone abuse may be associated with an eating disorder (Braunstein et al. 1986). In rare instances, thyrotoxicosis can also be caused by ingestion of contaminated meat (McMillin 1988). Epidemics of thyrotoxicosis factitia due to ingestion of contaminated meat in the tristate area of South Dakota, Iowa, and Minnesota (Hedberg et al. 1987) led to the U.S. Department of Agriculture's prohibiting the use of neck trim (containing thyroid tissue) in the preparation of edible meat products.

Currently, the term *thyrotoxicosis factitia* is used to describe excessive thyroid hormone administration of diverse causes, including acute or chronic thyroid hormone overdose, prescribed thyroid hormone therapy, and ingestion of food contaminated with thyroid tissue (Cohen et al. 1989). However, historically, the term was used in a narrower sense. It referred to a "psychoneurotic disturbance" in patients who secretly ingest thyroid hormone to obtain attention, lose weight, or receive compensation (Greer 1996).

Iodine-induced thyrotoxicosis. Iodine plays an important role in central nervous system (CNS) development and function as part of thyroid hormone physiology (Pharoah and Connolly 1995). Thyrotoxicosis can occur in iodine-deficient persons with goiter following iodine supplementation or in patients with preexisting thyroid disease who have received large doses of iodine through diet, medication, or radiocontrast dyes (Fradkin and Wolff 1983; Jackson 1925; Roti and Vagenakis 1996; Stewart et al. 1971). For example, a 22-day-old infant developed iodine-induced thyrotoxicosis following mediastinal lavage with povidone iodine (Betadine) (Bryant and Zimmerman 1995). Other potential sources of excess iodine include medications such as amiodarone and clioquinol; vitamin preparations containing iodine; iodine-rich products available from health food stores such as kelp and dulse; radiocontrast materials such as iothalamate; or povidone used to purify water (Liel and Alkan 1996; Roti and Vagenakis 1996).

Neonatal thyrotoxicosis. In neonates, Graves' disease usually results from transplacental passage of TSAbs into the fetal circulation (Dirmkiss and Munro 1975). Although it is usually associated with active maternal Graves' disease, it can also occur in infants of mothers in whom Graves' disease is not present (LaFranchi and Mandel 1996).

General Clinical Features of Thyrotoxic States

Graves' disease. In the pediatric form of Graves' disease, the clinical features are similar to those of adult hyperthyroidism, but there are two important differences (Bhatara et al. 1995; Sills 1994). First, growth and development are uniquely affected in thyrotoxic children and adolescents. Acceleration of linear growth and early epiphyseal maturation are often present in children and adolescents who have onset of thyrotoxicosis before the pubertal growth spurt. However, there is no change in final adult height. Second, the disease is not fulminant as it is in many adults (DiGeorge and LaFranchi 1996). In children, tachycardia may be the only presenting sign (Joseph 1996). Table 7–1 presents general medical and cognitive-behavioral features of pediatric thyrotoxicosis and their estimated frequency on the basis of the existing literature.

Thyrotoxicosis factitia. The clinical features shown in Table 7–1 are also seen in thyrotoxicosis factitia, but autoimmune features such as thyromegaly, infiltrative ophthalmopathy, and dermopathy do not occur (Burch et al. 1996; Greer 1996). A history of thyroid hormone ingestion in the absence of a goiter and hyperthyroidism confirms the diagnosis.

Neonatal thyrotoxicosis. The onset of neonatal thyrotoxicosis is usually prenatal, when it is manifested by tachycardia (LaFranchi and Mandel 1996). However, the disease may not be noticed until several days after birth, because clinical signs and symptoms are nonspecific. These include low birth weight, microcephaly, ventricular enlargement, hyperphagia, poor weight gain despite excessive food intake, irritability, exophthalmos, synostosis, tachypnea, tachycardia, and goiter (Foley 1991). Because of its association with clinical features of multiple systems, neonatal thyrotoxicosis can be mistaken for congenital heart disease or drug withdrawal.

Thyrotoxic storm. The acute syndrome thyrotoxic storm appears to be increasingly rare with earlier recognition and treatment of thyrotoxicosis (Wartofski 1996). Although it may occur in pa-

Table 7–1. Estimated frequency of signs and symptoms of pediatric thyrotoxicosis

General medical features	Frequency	Cognitive-Behavioral features	Frequency
Goiter	6	Drop in schoolwork and attention; decreased performance IQ	5
Tachycardia	4	Hyperactivity	5
Increased pulse pressure	4	Dysphoria (irritability or restlessness)	5
Hypertension	4	Positive behavioral response to antithyroid treatment	5
Exophthalmos	4	Mood swings (cries easily)	3–4
Fine tremor	4	Restless sleep and insomnia	3
Increased appetite	3	Rapid speech	2
Weight loss	3	Psychotic symptoms	1
Thyroid bruit	3	Mania	1
Increased sweating	3	Apathy	1
Heart murmur	3	Tics (coughing, eye blinking)	1
Palpitations	2	Psychological precipitant	1
Heat intolerance	2	Borderline IQ or mental retardation	1
Fatigue	2	Ingestion of thyroid hormone or iodine	1
Headache	1	Aggressiveness	1
Diarrhea	1	Other symptoms (e.g., symptoms of an eating disorder, delirium)	1

Note. 1 = 0%–20%; 2 = 21%–40%; 3 = 41%–60%; 4 = 61%–80%; 5 = 81%–95%; 6 = >95%.

Sources. Barnes and Blizzard 1977; Daneman and Howard 1980; Eberle 1995; Kogut et al. 1965; Money and Drash 1967; Money et al. 1966; Saxena et al. 1964; Vaidya et al. 1974.

tients with masked or apathetic thyrotoxicosis, most patients have rather obvious and exaggerated manifestations of thyrotoxicosis. Because it is often precipitated by infection, it may become difficult to determine whether the hyperpyrexia and tachycardia associated with infection in a thyrotoxic patient predict impending crisis or merely reflect the infectious process. The CNS symptoms are consistent with an acute metabolic encephalopathy and include delirium, lability, restlessness, agitation, confusion, psychosis, and coma (Aiello et al. 1989).

Cognitive-Behavioral Abnormalities in Thyrotoxic Youth

Although there is a paucity of objective data on cognitive and behavioral correlates of thyrotoxicosis in all age groups (Whybrow 1996), there is a relatively larger body of literature on the subject in adults.

Adult Thyrotoxicosis Versus Pediatric Thyrotoxicosis

A comparison of the literature on cognitive-behavioral aspects of thyrotoxicosis in adults with that in children and adolescents reveals two major differences between the groups. First, pediatric thyrotoxicosis (but not adult thyrotoxicosis) has prominent and unique neurodevelopmental effects. Second, actual or perceived differences in the incidence of dysphoria and symptoms of attention-deficit/hyperactivity disorder (ADHD) appear to exist between the two groups. A fidgety or restless adult is labeled anxious, but similar symptoms in children and adolescents are described as symptoms of ADHD.

Background: Cognitive-Behavioral Features in Adult Thyrotoxicosis

Although the true incidence of cognitive-behavioral abnormalities in adult thyrotoxicosis is not known (Whybrow 1996), certain trends emerge from the existing data (Alvarez et al. 1983; Bennett and Cambor 1961; Hermann and Quarton 1965; Jadresic 1990; Kathol and Dalahunt 1983; Kathol et al. 1986; Kleinschmidt and Waxenberg 1956; Lidz and Whitehorn 1949; MacCrimmon et al. 1979; Reus 1993; Rockey and Griep 1980; Stern et al. 1996; Trzepacz et al. 1988; Whybrow et al. 1969). Problems in behavior and cognition are very common in the early presentation of thyrotoxicosis. Although a variety of neurobehavioral and cognitive changes are observed, an anxious or irritable dysphoria seems to be by far the most frequent emotional symptom in thyrotoxic adults (Stern and Prange 1995). A subjective feeling of impaired concentration may be one of the earliest and most persistent symptoms of thyrotoxicosis. By contrast, frank psychiatric symptoms such as psychosis, delirium, and mania are rare (Bursten 1961; Lidz and Whitehorn 1949; Whybrow 1996). Psychosis is usually associated with cognitive clouding, suggesting possible delirium (Whybrow et al. 1969).

Using a survey questionnaire pertaining to neuropsychiatric complaints, Stern and associates (1996) queried patients with Graves' disease about their symptoms. Of the 137 respondents who provided data, a vast majority reported psychiatric symptoms while they were hyperthyroid. Irritability and anxiety were the most frequently endorsed symptoms on the questionnaire; other mood or somatic symptoms were also common. More than half of the respondents experienced anger, crying, insomnia, fatigue, weight loss, sensation of shakiness, and shortness of breath. Most of the patients also reported significant decline in their memory, attention, planning, and productivity during hyperthyroidism. Many patients continued to have residual cognitive impairment even after peripheral euthyroidism had been achieved.

Other studies also support the view that thyrotoxicosis is usually associated with anxiety. Using objective criteria, Kathol and Dalahunt (1983) demonstrated the incidence of generalized anxiety disorder and depression to be three to four times higher in hyperthyroid adults than in the general population. They also found that thyrotoxicosis was more specifically and more frequently associated with anxiety disorders than with depression.

The severity of anxiety symptoms (but not of depressive symptoms) correlated with other symptoms of thyrotoxicosis and thyroxine (T_4) level. Subsequently, Kathol et al. (1986), in a prospective study, found that in 21 of 23 cases of generalized anxiety disorder associated with thyrotoxicosis, anxiety resolved completely after euthyroidism was attained. Rarely, thyrotoxicosis can play a role in the development of disruptive, antisocial, or aggressive behavior. Davis and colleagues (1971) described cases of three adult thyrotoxic men without previous criminal records who committed felonies while their thyroid disorder was poorly controlled. In one case, an unsuccessful attempt was made to defend a man charged with larceny on the grounds that thyrotoxicosis was the cause.

Subtle cognitive abnormalities have also been observed in thyrotoxic adults. Frequently, thyrotoxic adults complain of diminished attention and concentration as well as memory problems (Stern and Prange 1995). Whybrow and colleagues (1969) found thyrotoxic adults to show impaired performance on the Porteus-Maze and Trail Making tests, and task impairment was found to correlate with degree of serum T_4 elevation. MacCrimmon et al. (1979) found that in a sample of 19 thyrotoxic adult women, impaired performance on cognitive tests requiring maximal concentration and memory (but not on simple cognitive tests) was significantly associated with elevated serum T_4 concentration. However, Alvarez and associates (1983) reported no correlation between performance and any thyroid function test results. Collectively these studies suggest that cases of adult thyrotoxicosis may be associated with impairment of visual tracking, visual attention, planning, motor efficiency, and sustained attention; but auditory attention and reaction time are not affected.

Cognitive-Behavioral Features and Syndromes in Pediatric Thyrotoxicosis

The cognitive-behavioral abnormalities associated with pediatric thyrotoxicosis range from subtle changes to frank mental retardation or psychosis. The degree of abnormality is dependent on four factors: 1) time of onset and course of thyrotoxicosis; 2) severity of the disease, especially in utero; 3) developmental phase of the individual; and 4) cause (Porterfield 1994). The abnormalities associated with early or less severe thyrotoxicosis are mild, whereas frank neuropsychiatric problems are seen only in severe thyrotoxicosis. In young children, neurodevelopmental effects of thyroid hormone excess are important. Although thyroid hormone excess can have adverse effects in any age group, it may produce irreversible CNS damage during a critical period extending until 2 or 3 years of age (Porterfield 1994; Rodier 1994; Root 1996). Generally, the nature of cognitive-behavioral abnormalities is independent of the cause of thyrotoxicosis; however, each etiological subtype may have its own unique features. In the following section, thyrotoxicosis is subtyped by these four factors, and several syndromes are elucidated by thyrotoxicosis subtype (Table 7–2).

Early thyrotoxicosis. At onset, thyrotoxicosis is frequently associated with subtle cognitive-behavioral symptoms. An unexplained drop in school performance is one of the most sensitive early symptoms of thyrotoxicosis in children and adolescents (Bhatara et al. 1996). Because school achievement requires coordination of a number of complex tasks, it is in this area that the earliest signs of thyrotoxicosis are often seen. Other early behavioral and cognitive changes include deterioration of handwriting, symptoms of ADHD, behavioral problems, emotional outbursts, difficulty in sleeping, and restlessness (DiGeorge and LaFranchi 1996). New-onset ADHD symptoms after age 7 are not typical of classic ADHD and necessitate a thorough investigation of other medical or psychiatric causes (Elia 1994).

Mild thyrotoxicosis. In the majority of cases, pediatric thyrotoxicosis is mild. It is often associated with a variety of mild to moderate cognitive-behavioral signs and symptoms including those described for early thyrotoxicosis. Typically, thyrotoxic children come to the attention of teachers or caretakers because of deteriorating school performance or lower performance than verbal IQ scores on their psychometric testing (Alvarez et al. 1996; Money et al. 1966). Some common symptoms are hyperactivity, inatten-

Table 7–2. Cognitive-behavioral changes associated with pediatric thyrotoxic syndromes

Thyrotoxic syndrome	Signs and symptoms
Thyrotoxicosis with hyperthyroidism	
Early	Subtle changes in cognition and behavior, an unexplainable drop in school achievement, poor penmanship, impaired attention, and hyperactivity
Mild	Deteriorating school performance, decreased performance IQ, hyperactivity, impaired attention, anxious dysphoria, restlessness, irritability, mood swings, tremors, poor sleep, and fatigue
Severe	Severe cognitive impairment, delirium, delusions, paranoia, hallucinations, agitation, mania or depression, tremors, and fatigue
Thyrotoxic storm	Symptoms of an acute and severe encephalopathy, including delirium, lability, restlessness, agitation, confusion, and coma
"Apathetic"	Psychomotor retardation, depression
Neonatal	Irritability, difficulty in accepting consolation; long-term effects can include hyperactivity and varying degrees of intellectual and developmental impairments associated with craniosynostosis
Thyrotoxicosis without hyperthyroidism	
Iodine-induced	Cognitive and behavioral features are poorly documented but are probably similar to those of other forms of thyrotoxicosis
Thyrotoxicosis factitia	Cognitive and behavioral features are similar to those of other forms of thyrotoxicosis. Manifestations depend on the patient's age, comorbidity (such as an eating disorder), dose of thyroid hormone ingested, delay in diagnosis, and whether thyrotoxicosis is mild or severe

tion, anxious dysphoria, emotional lability, restlessness, irritability, mood swings, tremors, poor sleep, and fatigue. Frank neuropsychiatric abnormalities (such as mania, delusions, or hallucinations) are rare.

Severe thyrotoxicosis. In cases of severe pediatric thyrotoxicosis, cognitive and behavioral abnormalities are fulminant. Such cases of thyrotoxicosis are rare and can manifest as delusions, delirium, hallucinations, agitation, mania, or paranoia. Mania or psychosis usually occurs in susceptible children or adolescents with a personal or family history of bipolar disorder (Weller et al. 1996). Perhaps, as in adults (Whybrow 1996), careful application of DSM-IV (American Psychiatric Association 1994) criteria may reveal some cases of "psychosis" to fulfill the diagnostic criteria of delirium.

Thyrotoxic storm. The cognitive and behavioral features in the acute form of severe thyrotoxicosis known as thyrotoxic storm are also fulminant (Wartofski 1996). Acute encephalopathy due to thyrotoxic storm can manifest as delirium, lability, restlessness, agitation, confusion, or even coma (Aiello et al. 1989).

Apathetic thyrotoxicosis. The term *apathetic thyrotoxicosis* (or *masked thyrotoxicosis)* is used to denote a clinical picture resembling depression; rather than being hyperactive, patients present with psychomotor retardation, confusion, and apathy (Bauer et al. 1987). The apathetic type of pediatric thyrotoxicosis is very rare, but cases have been reported (McKendrik and Newns 1965; Money and Drash 1967).

Neonatal thyrotoxicosis. Thyroid excess during the prenatal or neonatal periods may have both short-term and long-term effects. Typically, thyrotoxic neonates are noted to be irritable at or shortly after birth. They have difficulty in accepting consolation and are hyperactive. Long-term effects of prenatal thyroid excess have been demonstrated by Daneman and Howard (1980). Confirming the findings of earlier and smaller case series (Hollingworth and Mabry 1976; Wilroy and Etteldorf 1971), these researchers found the majority of their patients to show hyperactivity and varying degrees of intellectual impairment (despite early and vigorous antithyroid treatment). To our knowledge, anatomic or neuroimaging studies in these children have not been done and are needed.

Thyrotoxicosis factitia. The manifestations of thyrotoxicosis factitia probably depend on the extent of exposure to exogenous thyroid hormones (dose and duration), developmental status and susceptibility of the individual, and other personality factors. Once the diagnosis is clear, the signs and symptoms can usually be reversed by avoidance of the exogenous source of thyroid hormone. Lehrner and Weir (1984) reviewed nine cases of acute thyroid ingestion in seven very young children (ages 20–39 months). The behavioral symptoms ranged from none to brief irritability and agitation to psychosis. Caudill and Lardinois (1991) reported a case of severe thyrotoxicosis from accidental thyroid hormone ingestion that presented as acute psychosis. Similarly, iatrogenic thyrotoxicosis may be seen in cases of overzealous thyroid replacement therapy in hypothyroidism or in use of thyroid hormone for indications other than hypothyroidism, such as thyroid augmentation of antidepressant treatment (Beyer et al. 1993). Braunstein et al. (1986) reported a case of a 16-year-old girl with thyrotoxicosis factitia due to ingestion of diet pills containing thyroid hormone. The symptoms consisted of fatigue, weight loss, and headaches. In that case, ingestion of thyroid hormone was unintentional, but historically, secretive ingestion of thyroid hormone to obtain attention, lose weight, or receive compensation has been noted (Greer 1996). Bhatara et al. (1995) described the case of a 4-year-old boy who exhibited violent aggressiveness due to thyrotoxicosis factitia caused by ingestion of beef contaminated with bovine thyroid hormone ("hamburger thyrotoxicosis" [McMillin 1988]).

Rarely, iatrogenic thyroid hormone excess caused by thyroid hormone replacement treatment of pediatric hypothyroidism may be associated with delirium, psychosis, or mania (Bhatara et al. 1993). More frequently, initiation of thyroid therapy in hypothyroid children is associated with transient symptoms such as ADHD characteristics, as well as problems with learning, achievement, or behavior (Rovet et al. 1993).

Iodine-induced thyrotoxicosis. Cognitive-behavioral features of iodine-induced thyrotoxicosis are similar to those of other types of thyrotoxicosis, but a background history of iodine deficiency or an eating disorder may be elicited. The following case, involving a 17-year-old girl with a restrictive type of anorexia nervosa who was eating a large amount of kelp, is illustrative. She presented with a suppressed TSH level suggestive of subclinical thyrotoxicosis, apparently induced by iodine-rich kelp (T. Soundy, Human Services Center, Yankton, South Dakota, personal communication, July 1996).

Behavioral and Cognitive Syndromes That May Mimic Pediatric Thyrotoxicosis

Thyrotoxicosis in children and adolescents may mimic subtle behavioral disorders (new-onset ADHD, drop in school grades) or overt cognitive-behavioral disorders (anxiety, mood, cognitive, or psychotic disorders) (Bhatara et al. 1995). A literature review revealed that most descriptions of cognitive and behavioral abnormalities of pediatric thyrotoxicosis were confined to the endocrinological literature (Barnes and Blizzard 1977; Kogut et al. 1965; Saxena et al. 1964; Vaidya et al. 1974), although behavioral scientists have been involved in a few studies (Eberle 1995; Money and Drash 1967). The cognitive and behavioral findings from these studies are summarized in Table 7–3.

The studies summarized in Table 7–3 were primarily methodologically flawed retrospective studies of poorly defined samples that used vague behavioral terms such as "nervousness." Despite their limitations, an overall finding from these studies is that symptoms of ADHD, mild cognitive impairment, and irritable or anxious dysphoria are overrepresented in pediatric thyrotoxicosis and in those who are treated with thyroid replacement therapy for hypothyroidism (Rovet et al. 1993).

Table 7–3. Frequency of cognitive-behavioral abnormalities in pediatric thyrotoxicosis

Study	N	Drop in school performance (%)	Hyperactivity (%)	Irritable or anxious dysphoria (%)	Other abnormalities
Saxena et al. 1964	70	44	44	100	Other common symptoms were fatigue, muscle weakness, increased appetite, and tremors
Kogut et al. 1965	45	No data	27	89	Other common symptoms were increased appetite and tremors
Money et al. 1966	22	No data	No data	No data	Significant verbal-performance IQ discrepancy in favor of verbal IQ
Money and Drash 1967	29	61	61	61	Restless sleep in 52%
Vaidya et al. 1974	75	No data	No data	60	Unspecified emotional disorder in 50%
Barnes and Blizzard 1977	100	40	38	92	4 children became psychotic after thyroid surgery. Other problems included anxiety, suicidal ideas, neuroses, and anorexia nervosa
Daneman and Howard 1980	9	No data	No data	No data	In 5 of the 6 patients with neonatal thyrotoxicosis who underwent intelligence testing, a varying degree of intellectual impairment was found
Eberle 1995	23	95	87	No data	47% had impaired concentration, 53% had mood swings, and 73% slept poorly

Symptoms of Attention-Deficit/Hyperactivity Disorder

Clinicians have long known that cognitive and behavioral symptoms of pediatric thyrotoxicosis are similar to those of ADHD, but the phenomenon is poorly studied. Impaired concentration and inattention are classic and early symptoms of thyrotoxicosis (Alvarez et al. 1996; Bhatara et al. 1996).

Relationship of ADHD symptoms and thyrotoxicosis The literature suggests that thyrotoxicosis may induce, mimic, or exacerbate symptoms of ADHD in susceptible children and adolescents (Bhatara et al. 1995). A recent case report suggests that preexisting ADHD can be aggravated by thyrotoxicosis. Leo and colleagues (1996) described a case of a 15-year-old boy whose ADHD was diagnosed when he was 2 years old. He showed marked and transient exacerbation of ADHD symptoms with clinical and laboratory evidence of subacute thyroiditis. His symptoms responded to propranolol. After definitive treatment of thyrotoxicosis, he no longer required propranolol.

Although the relationship between ADHD and pediatric thyrotoxicosis symptoms remains elusive, this issue is receiving increasing study. Although the phenomenology of attentional processes in primary ADHD and that of ADHD symptoms in thyrotoxicosis have not been directly compared, the work of the Toronto group (Rovet and her associates at the Hospital for Sick Children) has provided preliminary data suggesting that attentional processes are impaired differently in primary ADHD and thyrotoxicosis with ADHD-like symptoms. During hyperthyroidism, nine thyrotoxic children were found to have impairments in the shift and disengage, but not sustain, subcomponents of attention (Alvarez et al. 1996). These impairments were reversible with antithyroid medication and attainment of euthyroidism. In contrast to thyrotoxic children, children with primary ADHD scored lower than control subjects on stimulus processing indices of attention tests, which included the abilities to detect, concentrate, activate, and select information (Bass et al. 1996). The children with ADHD did not differ from control subjects in their ability to focus or to sustain attention over time or in their executive processing skills such as suppress, inhibit, or shift. Thus, it appears that disturbance of attention may be more selective in thyrotoxicosis than in ADHD and that ADHD symptoms in thyrotoxicosis are reversible with antithyroid agents.

The Toronto group also examined the relationship between thyroid hormone level and attention. Using children with congenital hypothyroidism (CH) treated with levothyroxine (L-T_4) as a model to study thyroid hormone–attention relationships, Rovet and Alvarez (1996) subgrouped their subjects by their T_4 and TSH levels at the time of testing. Nearly 10% of children who had high T_4 values with inappropriately elevated TSH (similar to the profile in resistance to thyroid hormone [RTH]) had the poorest performance of all the children on two measures specific to attention (Freedom from Distractibility and Digit Span), whereas their intelligence and achievement were comparable if not superior to that of the other CH groups. T_4 levels were primary predictors of attention. Rovet and Alvarez proposed that high T_4 and high TSH levels at the time of testing may contribute to impairments of attention. They speculated that thyroid hormone may play a role in pathogenesis of a subset of ADHD.

Prevalence of ADHD symptoms in thyrotoxicosis. The endocrinological literature supports the clinical experience that symptoms of ADHD are very common in thyrotoxicosis (Table 7–3). More recent estimates from the child psychiatry literature (Eberle 1995; Elia 1995) also suggest that the frequency of ADHD symptoms is higher than reported earlier by the endocrinological literature. Eberle (1995) found that hyperactivity was present in 87% and poor concentration in 47% of thyrotoxic patients whose charts were reviewed. Elia (1995) also observed that ADHD symptoms were extremely common early symptoms of pediatric thyrotoxicosis and frequently preceded the thyroid diagnosis. Clearly, research data are needed to support these clinical or retrospective observations.

Prevalence of thyrotoxicosis in ADHD. Four studies on the prevalence of thyroid abnormalities in ADHD suggest that cases of thyrotoxicosis in the general population of children with ADHD are rare. In their sample of 277 children with ADHD, Weiss et al. (1993) observed the rates of thyroid abnormalities in ADHD (5.4%) to be higher than in the general population (> 1%). However, most of the abnormalities were of low magnitude, and it was hypothyroidism—not hyperthyroidism or RTH—that accounted for the increased prevalence of thyroid dysfunction. These findings were not in agreement with studies by Spencer et al. (1995) and Elia et al. (1994), who found no significant thyroid abnormalities in their ADHD subjects. In a study involving 37 children (ages 7–12 years) with ADHD, Bass et al. (1996) observed free and total T_4 values to be atypically low but in the euthyroid range, whereas TSH levels were also low, which may suggest a hyposensitivity at the level of the pituitary. Overall, the data from these studies suggest that thyrotoxicosis is not usually seen in the "garden-variety" ADHD.

Mechanism by which ADHD symptoms may be produced. Very little is known about the genesis of cognitive-behavioral anomalies in pediatric thyrotoxicosis, and the exact mechanism by which thyroid hormone modifies behavior remains to be discovered. However, Dratman (1993) pointed out that CNS thyroid hormone metabolism is tightly regulated. Thus, despite an excess of circulating T_3 and T_4 in the peripheral tissues, a variety of protective mechanisms may maintain nearly normal CNS thyroid concentrations. However, these protective physiological mechanisms can fail in thyrotoxicosis, particularly in patients who are genetically vulnerable. In such cases, Dratman (1993) suggested, thyrotoxicosis is associated with serious behavioral disturbances because the CNS is overly sensitive to thyroid excess when it finally occurs.

The specific mechanisms that result in the production of ADHD symptoms in thyrotoxicosis are not known. Alvarez et al. (1996) suggested that anxiety does not play a major role in the pathogenesis of inattention because there was a lack of correlation between anxiety and deficits of attention in their nine thyrotoxic subjects. Moreover, in their experience, thyrotoxic children were not unduly anxious. However, it seems plausible that thyroid toxicity can both mimic and trigger many psychiatric symptoms, including ADHD symptoms, through its CNS effects and effects on biogenic amines. Alvarez et al. (1996) proposed that impairments of attention in thyrotoxicosis are consequences of thyroid-induced activation of the prefrontal cortex (the cerebral substrate underlying the shift and disengage functions of attentional processing). Their hypothesis is consistent with the proposal by Hunt et al. (1991) that CNS hyperarousal (reflecting increased noradrenergic activity) may lead to excessive activity and impair information processing in a subtype of ADHD.

Once inattention and hyperactivity are established, interactions between excessive thyroid hormone and biogenic amines (especially catecholamines) may magnify the symptoms: it is known that thyroid hormones can produce a positive gain in the actions of catecholamines (Silva 1996). Also, the sympathoadrenal system and thyroid hormones may have a synergistic relationship in maintenance of CNS homeostasis (Bauer et al. 1987). The available data, though often conflicting, indicate that thyroid hormone excess could increase sympathetic activity through an increased number of CNS β-adrenergic receptors, enhanced receptor sensitivity to catecholamines, increased catecholamine sensitivity at a postreceptor site, or direct sympathomimetic actions. It is conceivable that high circulating levels of thyroid hormones can produce a hypercatecholaminergic state by 1) direct thyroid hormonal effects on CNS thyroid receptors and 2) upregulation of CNS catechol receptors produced by excessive T_3 and T_4 (Silva 1996). It has been suggested that ADHD symptoms probably result from increased CNS noradrenergic function caused by thyrotoxicosis because β-adrenergic blocking agents decrease symptoms such as anxiety in thyrotoxicosis independently of the levels of thyroid hormones (Stern and Prange 1995). Thus, it is possible that the ADHD symptoms in thyrotoxicosis result from a combination of increased peripheral sympathoadrenal activity and disturbances in CNS brain thyroid economy.

Irritable or Anxious Dysphoria and Emotional Lability

Frequently, thyrotoxicosis is associated with development of irritability, anxiety, or emotional lability. Irritability seems to antedate medical referral in 40%–50% of cases, and occasionally children become aggressive (Eberle 1995; Money and Drash 1967). In Money and Drash's (1967) sample, 2 of their 23 thyrotoxic children were aggressive. Bhatara et al. (1995) described a case of possible thyrotoxicosis-induced violent aggressiveness and fire setting in a 4-year-old boy affected by an epidemic of thyrotoxicosis factitia caused by ingestion of beef contaminated with bovine thyroid tissue. Their patient was not violent during two admissions to a hospital (where he did not eat thyroid-laced meat) and became aggressive on returning home (where contaminated ground beef was served). Bhatara and associates concluded that pediatric thyrotoxicosis may induce or trigger marked behavioral deterioration, including the aggressive type in vulnerable persons.

In some thyrotoxic children, it is not irritability but emotional lability that is the most prominent symptom. Previously well-controlled children have been observed to cry easily, become angry, or have mood swings during hyperthyroidism. Like children with bipolar mood disorder, thyrotoxic children may also sleep poorly. But in contrast to bipolar disorder, the energy level is lower in thyrotoxicosis. Thyrotoxic children, like their adult counterparts, often complain of being tired. The prevalence of bipolar mood disorder in pediatric thyrotoxicosis is not known, but the prevailing view is that those with family histories of the disorder may rarely present with "manic-like" symptoms (Weller et al. 1996; Whybrow 1996).

It is not known how common the symptoms of irritable or anxious dysphoria are in pediatric thyrotoxicosis. Observations published by Alvarez et al. (1996) suggest that anxiety in thyrotoxic children may be less common than in thyrotoxic adults. Contrary to expectations and findings in adults, Alvarez et al. (1996) found both treated and untreated thyrotoxic children to be less anxious than control subjects on the Children's Personality Questionnaire. The level of anxiety was unaffected by the antithyroid treatment and did not correlate with any measures of attention.

At present, there continues to be a paucity of studies on the prevalence of anxious dysphoria in pediatric thyrotoxicosis. Studies similar to the ones by Kathol et al. (1986) in adults, documenting the frequency of generalized anxiety disorder by standardized diagnostic criteria and carefully distinguishing anxiety symptoms from those of ADHD, need to be undertaken. Meanwhile, there is no evidence to support the traditional view that the ADHD and cognitive symptoms associated with pediatric thyrotoxicosis are due to anxiety (Alvarez et al. 1996).

Cognitive Symptoms

Thyrotoxic youth frequently demonstrate mild problems of early achievement. Rarely, mental retardation can be a consequence of fetal or neonatal hypothyroidism (see Neurodevelopmental Problems, below). Perhaps the earliest study that systematically examined cognition in pediatric thyrotoxicosis was conducted by Money and associates (1966), who reported the IQ scores and school performances of 22 juvenile patients with thyrotoxicosis. The distribution of full-scale IQs of the patients closely approximated that of the general population, but verbal IQ (VIQ) scores were significantly higher than performance IQ (PIQ) scores. Although the VIQ-PIQ discrepancy persisted, the full-scale IQs improved after antithyroid treatment. Alvarez et al. (1996) also found PIQ to be lower than VIQ during hyperthyroidism, but VIQ-PIQ differences were not statistically significant. However, the thyrotoxic group had significantly lower scores on Block Design and Object Assembly subtests during hyperthyroidism than after attainment of euthyroidism. The PIQ scores of untreated thyrotoxic children were significantly below those of control subjects, and both VIQ and PIQ scores improved modestly after attainment of euthyroidism. Although the findings of Alvarez et al. are limited by the sample size ($N = 9$), they support the observations of Money et al. (1966) that untreated thyrotoxic children may exhibit visuospatial difficulties.

One of the earliest signs of thyrotoxicosis is a dramatic drop in school performance, occurring in up to 95% of thyrotoxic children and adolescents (Eberle 1995). Because some of the cognitive deficits associated with deteriorating school performance can be reversed with propranolol, it has been suggested that sympathoadrenal abnormalities (such as an upregulation of catechol receptors) may be aggravating thyroid-induced cognitive dysfunction. These neurocognitive difficulties possibly result from a combination of increased peripheral sympathoadrenal activity, thyroid hormone excess in the CNS, disrupted normal homeostasis, and (in younger children) neurodevelopmental effects of thyroid hormone. Some neurocognitive findings in thyrotoxicosis are consistent with prefrontal lobe dysfunction (Bhatara et al., in press; Stern and Prange 1995). For example, disturbances in areas of organization, conceptualization, and mental flexibility might be explained by a prefrontal lobe dysfunction associated with thyrotoxicosis. Data from functional imaging techniques such as positron-emission tomography (PET) and magnetic resonance spectroscopy (MRS) are needed to define the role of prefrontal lobe dysfunction that may link hyperthyroidism with its associated neurocognitive abnormalities. Data from a pilot proton MRS study in adults tentatively suggested a decrease of choline/creatine ratios in the prefrontal cortex during hyperthyroidism in Graves' disease, which appeared to be reversible with antithyroid treatment (Bhatara et al., in press). However, these findings were limited by a small sample size and await confirmation in a definitive study. Electroencephalographic data are available that suggest that multiple nonspecific CNS abnormalities are associated with autoimmune thyrotoxicosis in adults (DeLong 1996).

Neurodevelopmental Problems

Thyroid hormones are vital for normal CNS development (see Chapter 8). Thyroid excess during a critical period (starting in utero and extending until 2–3 years of age) may produce irreversible CNS dysfunctions, with manifestations ranging from subtle cognitive abnormalities to mental retardation (Porterfield 1994; Rodier 1994). Excessive thyroid hormone during the prenatal or neonatal period may disturb or accelerate the orderly patterns of CNS development. Although the normal stages of CNS development and differentiation may be achieved more rapidly, cell division is prematurely arrested (Anand and Nemeroff 1996; Bernal and Nunez 1995). If the developing brain is exposed to excessive thyroid hormones, proliferation ends and differentiation starts prematurely, resulting in reductions in the total number of neuronal cells.

Fetal and neonatal thyrotoxicosis may cause cognitive, behavioral, and psychomotor impairments in both animals and humans later in life (Chiovato et al. 1992; Lauder 1977; Mestman et al. 1995). The factors that may define cognitive and behavioral manifestations for the child with fetal and neonatal thyrotoxicosis are the time of onset and severity of thyrotoxicosis (Porterfield 1994). Adult rats exposed to excessive thyroid hormone during their neonatal period were found to have multiple abnormalities of morphology, behavior, and learning (Patel et al. 1979). The rodents showed neurochemical and morphological changes in hippocampal formation and reductions in brain weight and the number of brain cells (Dussault and Ruel 1987; Pavlides et al. 1991). In humans, long-term effects of thyroid hormone excess before birth has been shown by several case series, which found varying levels of intellectual retardation (Daneman and Howard 1980; Hollingworth and Mabry 1976; Wilroy and Etteldorf 1971). These findings underscore the importance of early diagnosis, particularly during the prenatal and neonatal periods.

Differential Diagnosis and Thyroid Screening

Because problems of attention, cognition, mood, and behavior are very common in its early presentation, pediatric thyrotoxicosis may be misdiagnosed as a primary psychiatric disorder or the diagnosis may be delayed. For example, the mean time between the presumed onset of illness and the first visit was 8.8 months in Barnes and Blizzard's (1977) sample. In such cases, psychiatric syndromes due to thyrotoxicosis and primary psychiatric disorders are difficult to differentiate.

Because clinical features of thyrotoxicosis may mimic the symptoms of a primary psychiatric disorder, it is important to know the features that distinguish a primary psychiatric disorder from a behavioral disorder due to thyrotoxicosis. Physical symptoms of thyrotoxicosis are not present in a primary psychiatric disorder; however, they also may not be detected in early thyrotoxicosis. Early symptoms of thyrotoxicosis tend to be subtle. On the basis of our literature review, we consider the following high-risk situations to be indications for the performance of thyroid function tests (free T_4 and TSH): 1) new onset of ADHD after age 7; 2) sudden and unexplained drop in grades; 3) sudden behavior change, especially in girls; 4) persistent resting tachycardia; 5) presence of goiter or thyroid nodule; 6) strong family history of a thyroid disease or an autoimmune disease; and 7) presence of autoimmune diseases (American Association of Clinical Endocrinologists 1995; Bhatara et al. 1994; Joseph 1996; Ladenson 1996; Surks et al. 1990).

Thyrotoxicosis may be easily confused with a primary anxiety disorder because symptoms such as shakiness, palpitations, sweating, decreased sleep, fatigue, shortness of breath, nervousness, irritability, and diminished concentration are present in both thyrotoxicosis and anxiety. However, in contrast to anxiety disorders, which tend to have waxing and waning intensity, thyrotoxicosis is usually progressive. Moreover, unlike the situation in anxiety, the resting pulse rate in thyrotoxicosis and sinus tachycardia is persistent. Some features unique to thyrotoxicosis that are not seen in anxiety are goiter, exophthalmos, heat intolerance, warm and moist skin, increased appetite, weight loss, hyperactive reflexes, and muscle wasting. Subjective feeling of anxiety or dysphoria is more prominent in anxiety, which is also often associated with fear of dying, dizziness, unreality, chest pain, and faintness. Patients with thyrotoxicosis and patients with anxiety may both have a fine tremor of the fingertips. However, the fingertips of thyrotoxic patients are warm and dry, whereas those of anxious patients are cool and moist.

Early changes in thyrotoxicosis are frequently subtle. The cognitive features of central dysfunction caused by thyrotoxicosis may range from subtle learning problems and inattention to severe cognitive problems. Clinicians working with children need to be aware that learning problems or inattention may be among the earliest manifestations of a thyroid disease, frequently antedating the medical diagnosis (Bhatara et al. 1996). New-onset ADHD symptoms after age 7 are not typical of ADHD and require a thorough investigation of other medical or psychiatric causes (Elia 1994). Because the prevalence of thyrotoxicosis is higher in girls, any clinical features suggestive of thyrotoxicosis in girls—such as persistent resting tachycardia and/or mild goiter—are indications for thyroid function testing (Bhatara et al. 1994; Eberle 1995).

DSM-IV and Thyrotoxicosis

DSM-IV (American Psychiatric Association 1994) has established criteria for the diagnosis of psychiatric syndromes caused by general medical conditions such as thyrotoxicosis. According to DSM-IV, diagnosis of a psychiatric syndrome due to thyrotoxicosis requires the clinical judgment that thyrotoxicosis and the psychiatric syndrome are etiologically related through a physiological mechanism. The presence of a temporal association between the onset and the time course of thyrotoxicosis and that of the psychiatric syndrome is suggestive of an etiological association. Another consideration that may provide evidence of a plausible etiological association between a psychiatric syndrome and a general medical condition is the presence of features that are atypical of the primary mental disorder. Absence of personal or family history of a primary mental disorder may also be supportive of a causal relationship between thyrotoxicosis and behavioral syndromes. However, there are times when the cognitive and behavioral symptoms antedate the signs, symptoms, and hormonal changes of thyrotoxicosis; differential diagnosis of primary psychiatric disorder and thyrotoxicosis is difficult in such cases.

Although DSM-IV does provide diagnostic terms for psychiatric disorders secondary to general medical disorders such as thyrotoxicosis (e.g., mental disorder not otherwise specified due to a thyrotoxicosis), we believe that a more specific and "child-oriented" coding option (e.g., behavior change due to thyrotoxicosis, disruptive type) should be considered for inclusion in the next DSM (Bhatara and McMillin, in press).

Summary and Conclusions

In describing multiple and varied cognitive-behavioral findings in pediatric thyrotoxicosis, two approaches were used in this chapter. First, we subtyped pediatric thyrotoxicosis into four factors (time of onset, severity, age, and etiology) and described behavioral changes in each subtype. Second, we described neuropsychiatric syndromes that are mimicked by pediatric thyrotoxicosis.

Thyrotoxicosis in children may mimic subtle neurobehavioral or cognitive problems (deficits of learning or achievement, new-onset ADHD symptoms, drop in school grades) or overt psychiatric syndromes (anxiety, mood, psychotic, or cognitive disorders). This review of literature on neurobehavioral and cognitive problems has implications not only for clinicians and researchers, but also for teachers. This is because they may be the first ones to observe early symptoms of thyrotoxicosis in their pupils and can prevent misdiagnosis or delay in endocrinologic diagnosis by medical referrals.

The findings of Alvarez et al. (1996) that children with thyrotoxicosis are at risk for disturbance in shift and disengage subcomponents of attentional processes, if confirmed, may also have classroom implications. Teachers need to be aware that disturbance in attention may adversely affect school performance in one or more areas of learning, and thyrotoxic children may find it hard to shift attention. By monitoring the attention of thyrotoxic children very closely, teachers can collaborate with the treating physicians in maintaining attentional processes and the hormone levels in the optimal range for normalizing potential processes. In particular, they can help with shifting tasks and in disengaging and reengaging. This is because the school tasks facing thyrotoxic children are continuously shifting as the new information is presented to them, and the process of shifting requires disengaging from the previous task and shifting focus to the new information. Teachers might also provide explicit clues for the introduction of new tasks and give multiple explanations and forewarnings about impending changes. Similarly, teachers and other school personnel might be educated about possible visuospatial difficulties in thyrotoxic children, so that suitable adjustments can be made at school.

Several research questions that remain unanswered include the prevalence of various cognitive-behavioral abnormalities and syndromes in pediatric thyrotoxicosis, the mechanism by which ADHD symptoms are produced, and whether pediatric thyrotoxicosis differentially affects visuospatial functioning and the right cortical hemisphere. Answering these questions will ultimately improve the lives of children with thyrotoxicosis.

References

Aiello DP, DuPlessis AJ, Pattishall EG III, et al: Thyroid storm presenting with coma and seizures. Clin Pediatr 28:571–573, 1989

Alvarez MA, Gomez A, Alavez E, et al: Attention disturbance in Graves' disease. Psychoneuroendocrinology 8:451–454, 1983

Alvarez MA, Guell R, Chong D, et al: Attentional processing in hyperthyroid children before and after treatment. J Pediatr Endocrinol Metab 9:447–454, 1996

American Association of Clinical Endocrinologists and the American College of Endocrinology: AACE clinical practice guidelines for the evaluation and treatment of hyperthyroidism and hypothyroidism. Endocrine Practice 1:56–62, 1995

American Psychiatric Association: Diagnostic and Statistical Manual of Mental Disorders, 4th Edition. Washington, DC, American Psychiatric Association, 1994

Anand KJS, Nemeroff CB: Developmental psychoneuroendocrinology, in Child and Adolescent Psychiatry: A Comprehensive Textbook, 2nd Edition. Edited by Lewis M. Baltimore, MD, Williams & Wilkins, 1996, pp 64–86

Barnes H, Blizzard RM: Antithyroid drug therapy for toxic diffuse goiter (Graves' disease): thirty year experience in children and adolescents. J Pediatr 91:313–320, 1977

Basgoz N, Swartz MN: Infections of the thyroid gland, in Werner and Ingbar's The Thyroid: A Fundamental and Clinical Text, 7th Edition. Edited by Braverman L, Utiger R. Philadelphia, PA, Lippincott-Raven, 1996, pp 1049–1056

Bass A, Rovet J, Lobaugh N, et al: Thyroid hormone and attention in children with attention-deficit hyperactivity disorder. Poster presented at the 69th annual meeting of the American Thyroid Association, San Diego, CA, November 14–November 17, 1996

Bauer MS, Droba M, Whybrow PC: Disorders of the thyroid and parathyroid, in Handbook of Clinical Psychoneuroendocrinology. Edited by Nemeroff CB, Loosen PT. New York, Guilford, 1987

Bennett A, Cambor C: Clinical study of hyperthyroidism: comparison of male and female characteristics. Arch Gen Psychiatry 4:160–165, 1961

Bernal J, Nunez J: Thyroid hormones and brain development. Eur J Endocrinol 133:390–398, 1995

Beyer J, Burke M, Meglin D, et al: Organic anxiety disorder: iatrogenic hyperthyroidism. Psychosomatics 34:181–184, 1993

Bhatara V, McMillin JM: Disruptive disorders, thyrotoxicosis, and DSM-IV (letter). J Am Acad Child Adolesc Psychiatry (in press)

Bhatara V, Bandettini F, McMillin MJ: Psychosis associated with untreated hypothyroidism: a review of neuropsychiatric findings in children and adolescents with thyroid disorders. J Child Adolesc Psychopharmacol 3:199–212, 1993

Bhatara V, Kummer M, McMillin MJ, et al: Screening for thyroid disease in ADHD. ADHD Reports 2(4):7–9, 1994

Bhatara V, McMillin MJ, Kummer M: Fire setting and aggressive behavior in a 4-year-old boy associated with ingestion of ground beef contaminated with bovine thyroid tissue: a case report and review of neuropsychiatric findings in pediatric thyrotoxicosis. J Child Adolesc Psychopharmacol 5:255–271, 1995

Bhatara V, McMillin JM, Tervo R, et al: Learning disorders and the thyroid (letter). J Am Acad Child Adolesc Psychiatry 35:406, 1996

Bhatara V, Tripathi R, Sankar R, et al: Frontal lobe proton magnetic resonance spectroscopy in Graves' disease: a pilot study. Psychoneuroendocrinol (in press)

Braunstein GD, Koblin R, Sugawara M, et al: Unintentional thyrotoxicosis factitia due to a diet pill. West J Med 145:388–391, 1986

Braverman LE, Utiger RD: Introduction to thyrotoxicosis, in Werner and Ingbar's The Thyroid: A Fundamental and Clinical Text, 7th Edition. Edited by Braverman L, Utiger R. Philadelphia, PA, Lippincott-Raven, 1996, pp 522–524

Bryant WP, Zimmerman D: Iodine-induced hyperthyroidism in a newborn. Pediatrics 95:434–436, 1995

Burch HB, Gorman CA, Bahn RS, et al: Graves' disease—ophthalmopathy, in Werner and Ingbar's The Thyroid: A Fundamental and Clinical Text, 7th Edition. Edited by Braverman L, Utiger R. Philadelphia, PA, Lippincott-Raven, 1996, pp 592–594

Bursten B: Psychosis associated with thyrotoxicosis. Arch Gen Psychiatry 6:267–269, 1961

Caudill T, Lardinois C: Severe thyrotoxicosis presenting as acute psychosis. West J Med 155:292–293, 1991

Chiovato L, Tonacchera M, Lapi P, et al: Thyroid autoimmunity and neuropsychological development. Acta Med Austriaca 19 (suppl 1): 91–95, 1992

Cohen JH, Ingbar SH, Braverman LE: Thyrotoxicosis due to ingestion of excess thyroid hormone. Endocr Rev 10:113–124, 1989

Dallas J, Foley TP: Hyperthyroidism, in Pediatric Endocrinology: A Clinical Guide. Edited by Lifshitz F. New York, Marcel Dekker, 1990, pp 483–500

Daneman D, Howard NJ: Neonatal thyrotoxicosis: intellectual impairment and craniosynostosis in later years. J Pediatr 97:257–259, 1980

Davies TF: The pathogenesis of Graves' disease, in Werner and Ingbar's The Thyroid: A Fundamental and Clinical Text, 7th Edition. Edited by Braverman L, Utiger R. Philadelphia, PA, Lippincott-Raven, 1996, pp 525–536

Davis PJ, Rappeport JR, Lutz H, et al: Three thyrotoxic criminals. Ann Intern Med 74:743–745, 1971

DeLong GR: The neuromuscular system and brain in thyrotoxicosis, in Werner and Ingbar's The Thyroid: A Fundamental and Clinical Text, 7th Edition. Edited by Braverman L, Utiger R. Philadelphia, PA, Lippincott-Raven, 1996, pp 645–652

DiGeorge AM, LaFranchi S: Hyperthyroidism, in Nelson's Textbook of Pediatrics, 15th Edition. Edited by Nelson WE, Behrman RE, Kleigman RM, Arvin AM. Philadelphia, PA, WB Saunders, 1996, pp 1600–1602

Dirmkiss SM, Munro DS: Placental transmission of thyroid-stimulating immunoglobulins. BMJ 2:665–670, 1975

Dratman MB: Cerebral versus peripheral regulation and utilization of thyroid hormones, in The Thyroid Axis and Psychiatric Illness. Edited by Joffe R, Levitt A. Washington, DC, American Psychiatric Press, 1993, pp 1–94

Dussault JH, Ruel J: Thyroid hormones and brain development. Annu Rev Physiol 49:321–334, 1987

Elia J: Resistance to thyroid hormones. Symposium presented at the 41st Annual Meeting of the American Academy of Child and Adolescent Psychiatry, New York, October 26th, 1994

Elia J: ADHD and the thyroid (reply to letter). J Am Acad Child Adolesc Psychiatry 33:1058, 1994

Elia J, Gulotta C, Rose SR, et al: Thyroid function and attention-deficit hyperactivity disorder. J Am Acad Child Adolesc Psychiatry 33:169–172, 1994

Foley T: Maternally transferred thyroid disease in the infant: recognition and treatment, in Advances in Perinatal Thyroidology. Edited by Bercu B, Shulman D. New York, Plenum, 1991, pp 209–226

Foley T: Thyrotoxicosis in childhood. Pediatr Ann 21:43–49, 1992

Fradkin J, Wolff J: Iodide-induced thyrotoxicosis. Medicine 62:1–20, 1983

Furszyfer J, Kurland LT, McCohaney WM, et al: Graves' disease in Olmstad County, Minnesota, 1935 through 1967. Mayo Clin Proc 45:636–641, 1970

Graves RJ: Newly observed affection of the thyroid gland in the females. London Medical and Surgical Journal 7:516–525, 1835

Greer MA: Thyrotoxicosis of extrathyroid origin, in Werner and Ingbar's The Thyroid: A Fundamental and Clinical Text, 7th Edition. Edited by Braverman L, Utiger R. Philadelphia, PA, Lippincott-Raven, 1996, pp 592–594

Hedberg CW, Janssen RS, Meyers B, et al: An outbreak of thyrotoxicosis caused by the consumption of bovine thyroid gland in ground beef. N Engl J Med 316:993–998, 1987

Hermann H, Quarton L: Psychological changes and psychogenesis in thyroid hormone disorders. Journal of Clinical Endocrinology 25:527–538, 1965

Hershman JM: Does thyroxine therapy prevent Graves' hyperthyroidism? (editorial). J Clin Endocrinol Metab 80:1479–1480, 1995

Hollingworth DR, Mabry CC: Congenital Graves' disease. American Journal of Diseases of Children 130:148–151, 1976

Hunt RD, Mandl L, Lau S, et al: Neurobiological theories of ADHD and Ritalin, in Ritalin: Theory and Patient Management. Edited by Greenhill L, Osman B. New York, Mary Ann Liebert, 1991, pp 267–288

Jackson AS: Iodine hyperthyroidism: an analysis of fifty cases. Boston Medical and Surgical Journal 193:1138, 1925

Jadresic D: Psychiatric aspects of hyperthyroidism. J Psychosom Res 34:603–615, 1990

Joseph JG: Tachycardia in a 7-year-old boy. Emergency and Office Pediatrics 9:17–20, 1996

Kathol R, Dalahunt J: The relationship of anxiety and depression to symptoms of hyperthyroidism using operational criteria. Gen Hosp Psychiatry 8:23–28, 1983

Kathol R, Turner R, Dalahunt J: Depression and anxiety associated with hyperthyroidism: response to antithyroid therapy. Psychosomatics 27:501–505, 1986

Kleinschmidt H, Waxenberg S: Psychophysiology and psychiatric management of thyrotoxicosis: a two year follow up study. Mt Sinai J Med 23:131–153, 1956

Kogut M, Kaplan S, Colipp P, et al: Treatment of hyperthyroidism in children: analysis of forty-five cases. N Engl J Med 272:217–221, 1965

Ladenson PW: Diagnosis of thyrotoxicosis, in Werner and Ingbar's The Thyroid: A Fundamental and Clinical Text, 7th Edition. Edited by Braverman L, Utiger R. Philadelphia, PA, Lippincott-Raven, 1996, pp 708–712

LaFranchi S, Mandel SH: Graves' disease in neonatal period and childhood, in Werner and Ingbar's The Thyroid: A Fundamental and Clinical Text, 7th Edition. Edited by Braverman L, Utiger R. Philadelphia, PA, Lippincott-Raven, 1996, pp 1000–1008

Lauder JM: The effects of early hypo- and hyperthyroidism on the development of rat cerebellar cortex: kinetics of cell proliferation in the external granular layer. Brain Res 126:31–51, 1977

Lazarus JH: Silent thyroiditis and subacute thyroiditis, in Werner and Ingbar's The Thyroid: A Fundamental and Clinical Text, 7th Edition. Edited by Braverman L, Utiger R. Philadelphia, PA, Lippincott-Raven, 1996, pp 577–591

Lehrner LW, Weir MR: Acute ingestion of thyroid hormones. Pediatrics 73:313–317, 1984

Leo RJ, Khin NA, Cohen GN: ADHD and thyroid dysfunction (letter). J Am Acad Child Adolesc Psychiatry 35:1572–1573, 1996

Lidz T, Whitehorn J: Psychiatric problems in the thyroid clinic. JAMA 139:698–701, 1949

Liel Y, Alkan M: "Travelers' thyrotoxicosis": transitory thyrotoxicosis induced by iodinated preparations for water purification. Arch Intern Med 156:807–810, 1996

MacCrimmon DJ, Wallace JE, Goldberg WM, et al: Emotional disturbance and cognitive deficits in hyperthyroidism. Psychosom Med 41:331–340, 1979

McKendrik T, Newns G: Thyrotoxicosis in children: a follow-up study. Arch Dis Child 40:71–76, 1965

McKenzie JM, Zakarija M: Antibodies in autoimmune thyroid disease, in Werner and Ingbar's The Thyroid: A Fundamental and Clinical Text, 7th Edition. Edited by Braverman L, Utiger R. Philadelphia, PA, Lippincott-Raven, 1996, pp 1032–1048

McLachlan SM, Rapoport B: Genetic factors in thyroid disease, In Werner and Ingbar's The Thyroid: A Fundamental and Clinical Text, 7th Edition. Edited by Braverman L, Utiger R. Philadelphia, PA, Lippincott-Raven, 1996, pp 1032–1048

McMillin JM: Hamburger thyrotoxicosis: the endocrinologist as sleuth. Thyroid Today 11(2):1–9, 1988

Mestman J, Goodwin M, Montoro M: Thyroid disorders in pregnancy. Endocrinol Metab Clin North Am 24:41–71, 1995

Money J, Drash P: Juvenile thyrotoxicosis: symptoms and antecedents leading to referral and diagnosis. Journal of Special Education 2:83–91, 1967

Money J, Weinberg R, Lewis V: Intelligence quotient and school performance in twenty-two children with a history of thyrotoxicosis. Bulletin of The Johns Hopkins Hospital 118:275–281, 1966

Parry CH: Collections from the unpublished writings of the late C.H. Parry, Vol 2. London, Underwoods, 1825

Patel A, Lewis P, Bailey P: Effects of thyroxine on postnatal cell acquisition in the rat brain. Brain Res 35:57–72, 1979

Pavlides C, Westlind-Danielsson A, Nyborg H, et al: Neonatal hyperthyroidism disrupts hippocampal LTP and spatial learning. Exp Brain Res 85:559–564, 1991

Pharoah PO, Connolly KJ: Iodine and brain development. Dev Med Child Neurol 38:464–469, 1995

Porterfield SP: Vulnerability of the developing brain to thyroid abnormalities: environmental insults to the thyroid insults. Environ Health Perspect 102 (suppl 2):125–130, 1994

Reus V: Psychiatric aspects of thyroid disease, in The Thyroid Axis and Psychiatric Illness. Edited by Joffe RT, Levitt AJ. Washington, DC, American Psychiatric Press, 1993, pp 171–195

Rockey P, Griep R: Behavioral dysfunction in hyperthyroidism: improvement with treatment. Arch Intern Med 140:1194–1197, 1980

Rodier P: Vulnerable periods and processes during central nervous system development. Environ Health Perspect 102 (suppl 2):121–124, 1994

Root AW: Free triiodothyronine toxicosis in two adolescents. J Pediatr 124:276–278, 1994

Root AW: Editorial review: endocrine and metabolism. Curr Opin Pediatr 8:387–388, 1996

Roti E, Vagenakis AG: Effects of excess iodide: clinical aspects, in Werner and Ingbar's The Thyroid: A Fundamental and Clinical Text, 7th Edition. Edited by Braverman L, Utiger R. Philadelphia, PA, Lippincott-Raven, 1996, pp 316–329

Rovet J, Alvarez M: Thyroid hormone and attention in children with congenital hypothyroidism. J Pediatr Endocrinol Metab 9:63–66, 1996

Rovet J, Daneman DL, Bailey JD: Psychologic and psychoeducational consequences of thyroxine therapy for juvenile acquired hypothyroidism. J Pediatr 122:543–549, 1993

Saxena KM, Crawford JD, Talbot NB: Childhood thyrotoxicosis: a long-term perspective. BMJ 2:1153–1158, 1964

Sills IN: Hyperthyroidism. Pediatr Rev 15:417–420, 1994

Silva JE: Catecholamines and the sympathoadrenal system in thyrotoxicosis, in Werner and Ingbar's The Thyroid: A Fundamental and Clinical Text, 7th Edition. Edited by Braverman L, Utiger R. Philadelphia, PA, Lippincott-Raven, 1996, pp 661–670

Spencer T, Biederman J, Wilens T, et al: ADHD and thyroid abnormalities: a research note. J Child Psychol Psychiatry 36:879–885, 1995

Stern RA, Prange AJ: Neuropsychiatric aspects of endocrine disorders, in Comprehensive Textbook of Psychiatry/VI, 6th Edition, Vol 1. Edited by Kaplan H, Sadock B. Baltimore, MD, Williams & Wilkins, 1995, pp 241–245

Stern RA, Robinson B, Thorner AR, et al: A survey study of neuropsychiatric complaints in patients with Graves' disease. J Neuropsychiatry Clin Neurosci 8:181–185, 1996

Stewart JC, Vidor GI, Buttifield IH, et al: Epidemic thyrotoxicosis in Northern Tasmania: studies of clinical features and iodine nutrition. Aust N Z J Med 1:203–211, 1971

Surks MI, Chopra IJ, Mariash CN, et al: American thyroid association guidelines for use of laboratory tests in thyroid disorders. JAMA 264:1529–1532, 1990

Trzepacz P, McCue M, Klein I, et al: Psychiatric and neuropsychological response to propranolol in Graves' disease. Biol Psychiatry 23:678–683, 1988

Vaidya VA, Bongiovanni A, Parks J, et al: Twenty-two years' experience in the medical management of juvenile thyrotoxicosis. Pediatrics 54:565–570, 1974

Vanderpump MPJ, Tunbridge WMG: The epidemiology of thyroid disease, in Werner and Ingbar's The Thyroid: A Fundamental and Clinical Text, 7th Edition. Edited by Braverman L, Utiger R. Philadelphia, PA, Lippincott-Raven, 1996, pp 474–482

Wartofski L: Thyrotoxic storm, in Werner and Ingbar's The Thyroid: A Fundamental and Clinical Text, 7th Edition. Edited by Braverman L, Utiger R. Philadelphia, PA, Lippincott-Raven, 1996, pp 701–707

Weiss RE, Stein MA, Trommer B, et al: Attention-deficit hyperactivity disorder and thyroid function. J Pediatr 123:539–545, 1993

Weller E, Weller R, Svadjian H: Mood disorders, in Child and Adolescent Psychiatry—A Comprehensive Textbook, 2nd Edition. Edited by Lewis M. Baltimore, MD, Williams & Wilkins, 1996, pp 650–665

Whybrow PC: Behavioral and psychiatric aspects of thyrotoxicosis, in Werner and Ingbar's The Thyroid: A Fundamental and Clinical Text, 7th Edition. Edited by Braverman L, Utiger R. Philadelphia, PA, Lippincott-Raven, 1996, pp 696–700

Whybrow PC, Prange AJ, Treadway CR: Mental changes accompanying thyroid gland dysfunction: a reappraisal using objective psychological measurements. Arch Gen Psychiatry 20:48–63, 1969

Wilroy R, Etteldorf J: Familial hyperthyroidism including two siblings with neonatal Graves' disease. J Pediatr 78:625–632, 1971

Zimmerman D, Lteif A: Thyrotoxicosis in children. Endocrinol Metab Clin North Am 27:109–126, 1998

Chapter 8

Neurodevelopmental Changes Associated With Thyroid-Disrupting Contaminants

Vinod S. Bhatara, M.D., M.S., J. Michael McMillin, M.D., F.A.C.P., and Peter Hauser, M.D.

Over the past decade, endocrine-disrupting agents in the environment have received considerable attention as possible causes of certain disease states. However, the primary focus has been on estrogen disrupters (Fry 1995), and synthetic chemically induced disruptions of the thyroid system have been relatively neglected. Until recently, interest in disruptions of the hypothalamic-pituitary-thyroid axis was essentially confined to natural causes such as iodine deficiency or naturally occurring goitrogens. Today, there is considerable public health concern about the effects of several ubiquitous synthetic compounds (such as dioxins and dioxin-like compounds [DLCs]) on the thyroid and other endocrine systems (Kavlock et al. 1996).

In her classic work, *Silent Spring,* Rachel Carson (1962) warned about the public health hazards from pesticides. Heavy and repetitive use of dichlorodiphenyl trichloroethane (DDT) was linked with decreased survival of various bird species, thinner eggshells, and adverse effects on the reproductive system. The reproductive effects were later attributed to the estrogen-mimicking effects of DDT (Fry 1995). The effects of DDT on the thyroid economy were studied in birds, but not in humans. When pigeons were exposed to low levels of DDT, the birds were found to have thyrotoxicosis. However, at high levels of DDT exposure, the pigeons developed hypothyroidism (Rattner 1984). The 1996 publication of *Our Stolen Future* (Colborn et al. 1996) rekindled public concern about the effects of synthetic endocrine disrupters on health and development (Ginsburg 1996). Several European and North American organizations have urged greater attention to synthetic chemical endocrine disrupters (Baldwin 1996; Brouwer et al. 1995; Kavlock et al. 1996). A consensus appears to be emerging that children are at risk for toxicity from synthetic chemical endocrine disrupters during prenatal and early postnatal developmental stages (Alleva et al. 1998). A national research strategy to fill the gaps in knowledge about endocrine-disrupting chemicals in the environment is being developed (Kavlock et al. 1996).

Definition of a Thyroid Disrupter

In this chapter, a thyroid system disrupter (TD) is defined as an exogenous substance that disturbs thyroid homeostasis through alterations in synthesis, secretion, transport, metabolism, binding action, or elimination of endogenous thyroid hormones (Ginsburg 1996; Kavlock et al. 1996). The term *TD* is used here to denote exogenous causes of thyroid system disruption only; endogenous causes of disturbance in the thyroid homeostasis (e.g., autoimmunity, iodine deficiency, puberty, pregnancy, and the postpartum state) are not covered (Chiovato et al. 1992). This term does include iatrogenic causes of thyroid disruption (such as antithyroid drugs and radioiodine therapy) and xenobiotics disturbing thyroid economy by immunological mechanisms (e.g., autoimmune thyroid disease associated with interferon alfa, other cytokines, or *Yersinia enterocolitica* infection) (Schultz et al. 1989). A discussion of endogenously caused thyroid disruption is beyond the scope of this chapter. However, it should be noted that exogenously and endogenously induced thyroid disruptions can amplify each other's effects.

This definition also recognizes that some compounds (such as dioxins), particularly in low doses, may have thyroid-disrupting effects in developing organisms but not in adults. This vulnerability of embryonic, fetal, and neonatal tissues—and particularly the central nervous system (CNS)—suggests that developing organisms may "see" TDs in a different way (possibly even by different mechanisms) than do adults (Kavlock et al. 1996). Generally, the developing CNS is the system most frequently disrupted by teratogens, perhaps for several reasons (Rodier 1994). The key reason may be that CNS development takes much longer than development of other body systems. The developing CNS is therefore subject to injury over a longer period. Other factors include the poor ability of the CNS to replace missing elements and the absence of the blood-brain barrier. These general reasons can explain some of the vulnerability of the developing CNS to thyroid insults, but more important is the fact that optimal amounts of thyroid hormone are specifically required for normal CNS development.

Response of the Developing Brain to Thyroid Disruption

Several thorough reviews of thyroid hormone (TH) and CNS development are available (Anand and Nemeroff 1996; Bernal and Nunez 1995; DeGroot et al. 1996; DeLong 1996; Dratman 1993; Dussault and Ruel 1987; Morreale de Escobar et al. 1983; Porterfield and Hendrich 1993; Walker 1983). The neurodevelopmental functions of thyroid hormone are briefly examined here.

The Thyroid and Normal Brain Development

Human and experimental animal studies have established that adequate amounts of TH are required for normal brain development, but the studies have not yet identified TH-dependent rate-limiting steps for brain maturation (DeGroot et al. 1996). The developmental effects of TH are thought to be essentially mediated through regulation of DNA transcription and, ultimately, protein synthesis (Farwell and Braverman 1995). The developmental effects of TH are most dramatically seen in amphibians. As a result of TH action, a tadpole is changed into a frog (Farwell and Braverman 1995). In the absence of TH, tadpole-to-frog metamorphosis does not occur and the tadpoles just continue to grow bigger and bigger.

In humans, developmental effects are less dramatic but are still profound. Cell biology and molecular biology data suggest that TH is a major physiological regulator of CNS development: an epigenetic signal required to orchestrate the elaborate step-by-step construction of a normal neuronal network during development (Bernal and Nunez 1995). Animal data suggest that TH has both organizational and developmental effects on multiple and varied CNS developmental events (Hendrich and Porterfield 1992; Mellström et al. 1991; Munoz et al. 1991; Pipaon et al. 1992). Tightly controlled amounts of TH during developmental periods fine-tune specific neurodevelopmental events leading to the creation of neuronal networks (Bernal and Nunez 1995).

The effects of thyroid hormone vary depending on the region of the brain, specific cell type, neural system, and developmental phase of the organism. Although the effects of TH on the developing CNS are still not completely understood, animal and human research data support three principles (DeLong 1996). First, thyroid-dependent brain development is determined primarily by the availability of thyroxine (T_4) and not that triiodothyronine (T_3). This is because T_4 is the primary form of TH taken up by the fetal or neonatal CNS. In rodents, replacement with T_4 (but not T_3) was found to elevate fetal thyroid hormone concentrations (Calvo et al. 1990). In the brain, T_4 is deiodinated intracellularly to T_3. T_3 so generated initiates TH action by binding to the thyroid hormone receptor (TR), controlling thyroid-sensitive gene expression (Mellström et al. 1991). Both neurons and oligodendrocytes contain developmentally regulated TRs and are direct cellular targets of T_3 (Bernal and Nunez 1995).

Second, although TH plays a role in a variety of developmental processes—including gene expression, growth factors, and cell proliferation—its more important and pervasive CNS effect appears to be on postproliferation events, such as differentiation, neurite growth, gliogenesis, synaptogenesis, process formation, and myelination (Hendrich and Porterfield 1992; Walker 1983).

Third, TH influences the developmental timing and alters the pace of some CNS developmental events. TH is required to synchronize a number of development events. The onset time or rate of such developmental events is accelerated by TH excess and is retarded by TH deficiency. In either case, the result is generally disordered CNS development (Dratman 1993).

Role of Thyroid Hormone During Critical Developmental Periods

Although thyroid hormones are essential throughout life for normal functioning of the CNS, they are especially needed during fetal and neonatal life for normal neurodevelopment to occur. The developing CNS during this critical period is highly vulnerable to any insults to the thyroid system, and both thyroid deficiency and thyroid excess in this period may produce irreversible, profound, and lasting brain and CNS effects (Porterfield 1994). Animal and human data indicate that this critical period extends from birth to postnatal day 21 (P-21) in mice and up to 2 years in humans (Anand and Nemeroff 1996). Neurodevelopmental effects of thyroid hormone during this period may be subdivided into three phases (Porterfield and Hendrich 1993).

In phase 1, maternal thyroid hormones play the predominant role. For years, it was assumed that the developmental fetal CNS was independent of thyroid hormone, because earlier studies (Grumbach and Werner 1956; Myant 1958) suggested poor placental transfer of TH. However, the results of these studies were suspect because they were conducted in late pregnancy, and placental transfer of TH may vary during pregnancy (Burrow 1997). More recent studies suggest that significant maternal-fetal transport of thyroid hormone does occur (Bernal and Pekonen 1984); rat and human fetal tissues during the early stages of development contain significant amounts of T_4 and T_3 and many T_3 receptors (deVijlder et al. 1996). This makes it very likely that thyroid hormone receptors are functional during the fetal period and maternal thyroid hormones have a role in the fetal brain. Thyroid hormones found in fetal tissues are thought to be of maternal origin because fetal thyroid is incapable of producing thyroid hormone (Ferreiro et al. 1988).

Another study found that in infants with congenital absence of thyroid peroxidase (and thus inability to synthesize T_4), T_4 concentrations in the cord serum were 25%–50% of normal (Vulsma et al. 1989). Currently, maternal thyroid status is regarded as an important determinant in fetal development, but the importance of maternal contribution of TH in early pregnancy has yet to be defined (Burrow 1997). Experimental data from rodents and sheep also support the hypothesis that maternal thyroid function may play an important role in the development of the fetal brain (DeGroot et al. 1996; Piosik et al. 1997). Although its neurodevelopmental effects remain unclear, maternal TH could be important for brain stem and cerebral neurogenesis in this phase.

In phase 2 (12–40 weeks of fetal life in humans and 17–21 postnatal days in rats), neurodevelopment is affected by both maternal and fetal thyroid hormones. Several neurodevelopmental events occurring during this period—including neurogenesis, neuronal migration, neurite formation, and synaptogenesis—are extremely sensitive to TH.

In phase 3 (the period after birth: up to 2 years in humans and day 21 in rats), TH is supplied by the neonatal thyroid gland. In this phase, TH affects myelination and glial cell proliferation and maturation throughout the brain. TH also affects neuronal maturation and cerebellar development. A major role of TH in the early postnatal period is to function as a time clock, terminating neuronal proliferation and stimulating neuronal differentiation. TH has an important role in the synchronization and coordination of various developmental events by specific effects on cell differentiation and gene expression. Several T_3-dependent genes have been identified in the rat brain, such as myelin protein–encoding genes and specific neuronal genes. However, thyroid hormone response elements (TREs) have been found only in the regulatory region of the myelin-based protein gene (Farsetti et al. 1991).

Neurodevelopmental Effects of Thyroid Disruption

TH deficiency or excess during the first 2 years of life is associated with alterations of cell differentiation, migration, or gene expression in the CNS (Porterfield 1994). Generally, perturbations of TH economy that occur during the critical period of neural differentiation and CNS development (in utero to 2 years of age) can produce permanent and severe alterations in CNS anatomy and function (Dussault and Ruel 1987; Porterfield and Hendrich 1993), although some effects may be transient. For instance, even in the absence of TH treatment there is spontaneous recovery in the growth of Purkinje cell dendrites in the cerebellum (Bernal and Nunez 1995). The neurodevelopmental effects of thyroid excess are discussed in Chapter 7; neurodevelopmental changes associated with hypothyroidism are briefly discussed below.

Hypothyroidism in Animals

If the developing CNS is exposed to too little TH, the rate of neuronal proliferation decreases but the period of proliferation is increased, resulting in delayed CNS development (Porterfield and Hendry 1998). Experimental animal data demonstrate irreversible changes in neuronal connectivity associated with TH deficiency during the early developmental period (Morreale de Escobar et al. 1983). When rat embryos are made thyroid deficient experimentally or are inbred as genetically hypothyroid mice ("hyt-hyt" mice), the final CNS cell number may be normal, but the rate of cell acquisition and neuronal differentiation is slowed (Anthony et al. 1993; Porterfield 1994). An inspection of brain tissues in such animals usually reveals normal gross anatomy, but cytoarchitecture of the neocortex and the cerebellum appears disorganized (Lauder 1977). In the cerebral cortex, alterations of neuronal differentiation and derangement of lamination and axonal projections are found. TH deficiency is associated with retardation of cell migration, neurite outgrowth, synaptogenesis, and neurotransmitter synthesis. Neuronal cell death and astrocyte proliferation (gliosis) is accelerated (Bernal and Nunez 1995). The neurons do not develop enough processes to make appropriate connections (Eayrs 1955). Experimentally induced hypothyroidism in rats is associated with delayed cell accumulation in mesencephalic and motor nuclei. Brain electrical activity, oligodendrocyte differentiation, myelin synthesis, and Purkinje cell differentiation are also impaired (Anand and Nemeroff 1996; Bernal and Nunez 1995). Some of these effects result from direct T_3 action (decreased neurite growth, myelin synthesis, and Purkinje cell differentiation), but in other cases the mechanism is not known (Bernal and Nunez 1995). Thus, not only does the CNS maturation appear to be delayed, it also appears to show deficits and derangements (DeGroot et al. 1996).

Hypothyroid animals show decreased messenger ribonucleic acid (mRNA) and protein synthesis in the CNS (Farsetti et al. 1991). Because myelin basic protein is the product of a specific gene that is regulated by TH during development, brains of hypothyroid animals show defective myelinization (Porterfield and Hendrich 1993). However, the genetic expression is not permanently blocked but merely delayed. The normal level of myelinization is eventually achieved in hypothyroid animals (Farwell and Braverman 1995). In addition, impairments of microtubule polymerization have been shown in congenitally hypothyroid rats (Bernal and Nunez 1995). Correlating with these CNS changes in animals is developmental slowing of innate behavior patterns and impairments in performance tests of adaptive behavior (Anthony et al. 1993).

Human Data (Congenital Hypothyroidism)

See Rovet, Chapter 4 in this volume, for a complete discussion of this topic.

*Effects of Maternal Hypothyroidism
During Pregnancy on the Offspring*

Limited amounts of TH cross the placenta throughout pregnancy in humans. This maternal contribution appears to be important for early fetal development (Porterfield and Hendry 1998). Subtle problems of cognition, attention, and behavior are overrepresented in the offspring of mothers who were hypothyroid during pregnancy (Jones and Man 1969; Man et al. 1971). However, before any firm conclusions are drawn, it should be noted that these studies by Jones and Man were undertaken before the availability of sensitive thyroid function tests and should be replicated using current psychiatric diagnostic terminology.

Thyroid System Disrupters: An Overview

Numerous factors can adversely affect thyroid functions, particularly in developing organisms (Dratman 1993). However, the full range of substances that disrupt the natural endocrine modulation of neurobehavioral development cannot be entirely defined at present (Alleva et al. 1998). Table 8–1 lists selected thyroid disrupters by their presumed mechanism of action (Green 1996; Kaplan 1981; Meier and Burger 1996; Smallridge 1995).

TDs may be classified into two groups. The first group, natural TDs, consists of natural substances, such as iodine, that have been present in the environment since ancient times. The second group, synthetic TDs, includes such recently introduced synthetic compounds as dioxins and polychlorinated biphenyls (PCBs). In this chapter, we shall briefly discuss the effects of common natural TDs, but our main focus will be on a group of synthetic TDs referred to as dioxin-like compounds (DLCs).

Common Natural Thyroid Disrupters

Iodine Excess

Although iodine deficiency is a major cause of thyroid dysfunction in large geographical areas of the world, including parts of Western Europe (reviewed by Delange and Ermans 1996), in other regions (North America, Scandinavia, Britain, and Japan) daily adult iodine intake may exceed the recommended daily intake of 150 µg daily. For instance, in the United States the average daily iodine intake is 150–250 µg, and excessive iodide intake is a known disrupter of thyroid homeostasis (Roti and Vagenakis 1996).

Adult Response to Iodine Excess

If the iodine intake is persistently increased in normal euthyroid adult volunteers, glandular iodine uptake is initially increased and

Table 8–1. Some thyroid disrupters listed by their presumed mechanism

Mechanism	Examples
Alteration of immunity	Interferon alfa, *Yersinia enterocolitica*
Inhibition of thyroid hormone synthesis	Inhibition of iodine uptake by dietary iodine deficiency (endemic cretinism) and competitive inhibitors of iodine uptake (perchlorate, thiocyanate, and pertechnetate)
	Inhibition of thyroid peroxidase by thionamides (thioureas, thiouracil, propylthiouracil, methimazole, carbimazole, and goitrin), aniline derivatives and related compounds (paraaminobenzoic acid and sulfonamides), and others (iodoantipyrine and antipyrine)
Decreased thyroid secretion	Excessive iodine (failure to "escape" from Wolff-Chaikoff effect), aminoglutethimide, lithium
Iodine-induced thyrotoxicosis	Jodbasedow phenomenon
Alteration of T_4/T_3 transport in serum	Increased serum TBG concentration by estrogens, tamoxifen, heroin, methadone, mitotane, and fluorouracil
	Decreased serum TBG concentration by androgens, anabolic steroids (e.g., danazol), slow-release nicotinic acid, and glucocorticoids
	Displacement from protein-binding sites by furosemide, fenclofenac, mefenamic acid, polyhalogenated biphenyls (PCBs, PBBs), chlorinated dibenzo-*p*-dioxins (TCDD), and salicylates
Altered T_4 and T_3 metabolism	Increased hepatic metabolism by anticonvulsants (phenobarbital, phenytoin, and carbamazepine), rifampin, steroids (spironolactone), chlorinated hydrocarbons (chlordane, DDT), and PCBs.
	Decreased T_4 5′-deiodinase activity by β-adrenergic-antagonistic drugs, propylthiouracil, amiodarone, and glucocorticoids

Inhibition of T_4 to T_3 conversion	Glucocorticoids, propylthiouracil, propranolol, ipodate, iopanoic acid, and amiodarone
Altered TSH	Increased TSH concentration by lithium, dopamine antagonists, cimetidine, PCBs, and iodine
	Decreased TSH concentration by glucocorticoids, lead, dopamine agonists, and somatostatin
Potentiation/inhibition of T_3/T_4 at T_3 receptor	In lower doses, PCBs and TCDD, meat contaminated by animal thyroid tissue
Thyromimetic effect	In higher doses, PCBs, TCDD, and meat contaminated by animal thyroid tissue
Decreased T_4 absorption	Colestipol, cholestyramine, aluminum hydroxide, ferrous sulfate, sucralfate

Note. DDT = dichlorodiphenyl trichloroethane; PBBs = polybromated biphenyls; PCBs = polychlorinated biphenyls; T_3 = triiodothyronine; T_4 = thyroxine; TBG = thyroxine-binding globulin; TCDD = 2,3,7,8-tetrachlorodibenzo-*p*-dioxin; TSH = thyroid-stimulating hormone.

more organic iodine compounds are formed. At first, TH secretion may increase, but subsequently a number of autoregulatory events occur that act to inhibit TH synthesis and release (Farwell and Braverman 1995). Thus, normal persons without underlying thyroid dysfunction remain euthyroid even when they are administered large quantities of iodine (Roti and Braverman 1996). This temporary (2-day) blockade of TH synthesis by iodine load is called the Wolff-Chaikoff effect (Surks and Sievert 1995; Wolff and Chaikoff 1948). However, this effect is short-lived, and with time there is "escape" from the Wolff-Chaikoff effect (Woeber 1991; Wolff and Chaikoff 1948).

By contrast, in euthyroid persons with autoimmune disease and in those with a history of treated Graves' disease, postpartum lymphocytic thyroiditis, and subacute thyroiditis, escape from the Wolff-Chaikoff effect may not occur. Thus, such persons may develop hypothyroidism from iodine (Roti and Braverman 1996; Woeber 1991). Excessive iodide may also produce hyperthyroidism in euthyroid patients who live in areas of severe iodine deficiency (jodbasedow phenomenon) or in other instances of thyroid autonomy: multinodular goiter, hyperfunctioning thyroid adenoma, and Graves' disease (Surks and Sievert 1995). Iodine-induced thyrotoxicosis is also described in Chapter 7.

Iodine Excess in the Perinatal and Neonatal Periods

In the fetal and neonatal years, thyroid autoregulation is defective, and escape from the Wolff-Chaikoff effect may not occur (Woeber 1991). Moreover, the fetal thyroid gland may be exquisitely sensitive to the inhibitory effects of iodides, and iodides readily cross the placenta and are secreted in milk (Roti and Braverman 1996). Therefore, excessive maternal iodine intake can induce goiter in the fetus or newborn (transplacentally or through breast milk) with or without hypothyroidism (Delange et al. 1988; DiGeorge and LaFranchi 1996; Theodoropoulos et al. 1979). Similarly, applications of povidone iodine in pregnant women or in neonates can cause transient neonatal hypothyroidism (Smerdely et al. 1989). It is possible that iodine contamination is a major cause of transient neonatal hypothyroidism (Chanoine et al. 1988; L'Allemand et al. 1987). Parenteral administration of small amounts of iodinated contrast dye through nonradiopaque Silastic catheters in premature infants may produce hypothyroidism in some cases (Ares et al. 1995). Children may also be directly exposed to excessive iodine through iodine-rich products available from health food stores such as vitamin preparations containing iodine, kelp, and dulse (Roti and Vagenakis 1996).

Drugs containing iodine may also induce fetal or neonatal thyroid dysfunctions. Amiodarone, an iodine-containing antiarrhythmic, can cause either hypothyroidism or hyperthyroidism in patients receiving it (reviewed by Harjai and Licata 1997; Lombardi et al. 1990). It is an inhibitor of type 1 5'-deiodinase and pituitary TSH secretion (Roti and Vagenakis 1996). In the absence of hyperthyroidism or hypothyroidism, amiodarone can cause increases in serum T_4, reverse T_3, and thyroid-stimulating hormone (TSH) concentrations and decreases in serum T_3 concentrations (Harjai and Licata 1997).

In areas of low iodine intake, amiodarone-induced thyrotoxicosis is prevalent and can occur in up to 23% of patients receiving the drug (Lombardi et al. 1990). Although the factors that trigger the development of thyrotoxicosis in patients receiving amiodarone are not completely understood, the condition is frequently caused by iodine-induced increased synthesis of thyroid hormone, particularly in individuals with underlying thyroid disease (Harjai and Licata 1997). Several other mechanisms have also been proposed, such as the disturbance of thyroid iodine regulation and preexisting susceptibility due to thyroid autoimmunity (Lombardi et al. 1990). Another hypothesis (the destruction inflammation theory) proposes that amiodarone has a direct, dose-dependent cytotoxic effect on thyroid follicles (Harjai and Licata 1997). It is likely that the thyrotoxicosis is related to several pathogenic mechanisms.

Amiodarone-induced hypothyroidism is more likely to occur in areas of high iodine intake such as the United States. Its incidence has been reported to be between 1% and 32% (Martino et al. 1987). Unlike thyrotoxicosis, amiodarone-induced hypothyroidism is related to a lack of release from Wolff-Chaikoff effect (attributed to a subtle defect in thyroid hormone synthesis) (Harjai and Licata 1997). Whereas thyrotoxicosis is quite dramatic in its presentation, the symptoms of amiodarone-induced hypothyroidism may be vague. A case of congenital goiter was reported in a neonate whose mother was treated with amiodarone during pregnancy (De Wolf et al. 1988).

Lithium

Lithium interacts with the thyroid system in a complex manner that may result in the development of euthyroid goiter, hypothyroidism with or without goiter, or altered thyroid function tests within a euthyroid range (for a more detailed review see Joffe and Levitt 1993). Rarely, lithium may produce hyperthyroidism (Reus et al. 1979). Long-term lithium treatment is associated with several thyroid abnormalities. Common effects of lithium on thyroid function include goiter (in up to 50% of patients), subclinical hypothyroidism (in up to 20% of patients), overt hypothyroidism (in up to 20% of patients), and a higher incidence of antithyroid antibodies than in the normal population (Bocchetta et al. 1991; Perrild et al. 1990; Spaulding et al. 1972). Among lithium-treated patients having antithyroid antibodies, nearly 50% show subclinical hypothyroidism (compared with only 15% of patients with no antithyroid antibodies). The high incidence of antithyroid antibodies suggests a predisposition to an autoimmune thyroid disease, increasing vulnerability to the antithyroid actions of lithium. Alternatively, increased autoimmunity could be induced by lithium (Surks and Sievert 1995).

Lithium impairs the synthesis and secretion of TH (Surks and Sievert 1995). It affects thyroid function at a number of sites, but the most consistent and significant effect of a therapeutic dosage is that it inhibits the release of iodine, T_3, and T_4 (Bagchi et al. 1982; Burrow et al. 1971; Jefferson and Griest 1977). In vitro studies have demonstrated that lithium inhibits colloid droplet formation stimulated by cyclic adenosine monophosphate, which is a critical step in TH secretion (Mannisto 1973). Consequently, the circulating TH level drops, in turn stimulating TSH release and restoring euthyroidism. Goiter may occur as part of a compensatory process, or hypothyroidism may result if decreased TH release is not adequately compensated. This agent inhibits monodeiodination of T_4 to T_3.

In addition to its direct effects on the thyroid gland (synthesis and secretion of TH), lithium may also decrease circulating levels of TSH and thyrotropin-releasing hormone (TRH), suggesting that lithium can disrupt thyroid homeostasis at multiple levels (Joffe and Levitt 1993).

Goitrogens

The term *goitrogen* refers to a number of compounds that can inhibit TH synthesis, causing decreased T_3 and T_4 serum levels. These compounds are called goitrogens because, as a result of decreased serum T_3 and T_4, TSH secretion is increased, causing the formation of a goiter (Green 1996). Some goitrogens occur naturally in food; others are drugs with goitrogenic side effects. The latter group includes drugs used in the treatment of thyrotoxicosis.

Dietary Goitrogens

Throughout the world, iodine deficiency is the major cause of endemic goiter and cretinism. However, dietary goitrogens may be an important contributing factor in some areas (Green 1996). Some of the widely eaten plant groups contain goitrogens. For instance, cyanogenic glycosides (thiocyanate precursors) are present in almonds, cassava, sorghum, maize, and millet. On hydrolysis by glycosidases, these foods release free cyanide (an inhibitor of iodine uptake). Similarly, hydrolysis of thioglycosides in plants of the Cruciferae family (cabbage, cauliflower, kohlrabi, and broccoli) produce thiocyanates and isothiocyanates. Such thiocyanates inhibit peroxidase activity and organification of iodine and can produce goiters in animals (Dratman 1993). Outbreaks of goiters have been reported in people who drank milk from cows feeding on plants from the cabbage family containing thiocyanate (Welch 1995).

Goitrogenic Drugs

A number of drugs, such as thionamides (see Table 8–1), decrease thyroid hormone synthesis primarily through inhibition of thyroid peroxidase, decreasing the organification of iodine (Farwell and Braverman 1995). Some of these drugs have multiple effects and affect thyroid physiology at several levels (Meier and Burger 1996). For example, thionamides also block coupling of iodotyrosines and may inhibit extrathyroidal conversion of T_4 to T_3 (Kaplan 1981). The presence of goitrogenic substances in the environment can increase the risk of hypothyroidism.

Exogenous Thyroid Hormones

During the past two decades at least two epidemics of thyrotoxicosis due to ingestion of meat contaminated by animal thyroid have been well documented (Hedberg et al. 1987; Kinney et al. 1988). *Thyrotoxicosis factitia* is the term used to describe such exogenous thyrotoxicosis caused by ingestion of excessive quantities of thyroid hormones (see Bhatara and McMillin, Chapter 7 in this volume).

Natural Thyroid System Disrupters and Developmental Neurotoxicity

In infants and children, iatrogenic maternal exposure to some TDs (radioiodine, antithyroid drugs) is a known cause of transient or permanent congenital hypothyroidism (Foley 1996). In such cases, the signs and symptoms vary according to cause, severity, and duration of thyroid deficiency or excess before birth (see Rovet, Chapter 4 in this volume). Long-term consequences of such thyroid disruptions are not known, and the effects of alterations in the organization of brain deserve further study.

Synthetic Thyroid Disrupters

A growing list of synthetic compounds appear to have a potential for disrupting hypothalamic-pituitary-thyroid function (Table

8–2), but dioxin-like compounds (DLCs) have received the most attention as a possible major public health hazard (DeGroot et al. 1996; Gaitan 1994; Welch 1995). This section presents DLCs as prototypical synthetic environmental contaminants.

DLCs are a disparate group of compounds of halogen-substituted multiring structures including polychlorinated dibenzodioxins (PCDDs), polychlorinated dibenzofurans, hexachlorobenzene (HCB), and polychlorinated biphenyls (PCBs). The toxicity of DLCs depends on the dose and the structure of the congener; the most toxic and most well-studied DLC is 2,3,7,8-tetrachlorodibenzo-p-dioxin (TCDD, or dioxin) (Lindstrom et al. 1995). Despite their structural differences, it is useful to review the general action of DLCs as a group for two reasons. First, DLCs have similar biochemical properties, perhaps because of their ability to bind to the aryl hydrocarbon (Ah) receptor (Vanden Heuvel and Lucier 1993; Whitlock 1990). Second, because of their structural similarity and lipid solubility, DLCs are usually found as complex mixtures of multiple congeners in almost all compartments of the biosphere, including animal and human tissues as well as body fluids.

Threat Posed by Universal Exposure to Dioxin-Like Compounds

In their book *Our Stolen Future,* Colborn et al. (1996) warned about the threat posed by universal exposure to DLCs. On the basis of data from wildlife studies, animal experiments, and human studies, they present evidence suggesting that synthetic compounds may be covertly undermining the future of humans by disrupting their endocrine systems.

To date, DLCs have not been shown to cause an increase in the incidence of any disease state in the general population. However, data from several sources support the view that the general public is at risk for toxicity from DLCs. Furthermore, the data for developmental toxicity from current levels of exposure appear especially persuasive; a literature review found evidence for several subtle adverse effects of DLCs on neurobehavioral development and thy-

Table 8–2. Some synthetic thyroid disrupters

Flavonoids (polyphenols)
  Aglycones
  C-ring fission metabolites (phloroglucinols and phenolic acids)
  Glycosides
Phthalate esters and metabolites
  3,4-Dihydroxybenzoic acid (DHBA)
  3,5-Dihydroxybenzoic acid
  Diisobutyl phthalate
  Dioctyl phthalate
  0-Phthalic acid
  m-Phthalic acid
Polychlorinated and polybrominated biphenyls (PCBs and PBBs)
  PBBs and PBB oxides
  PCBs (Aroclor)
Polycyclic aromatic hydrocarbons (Pahs)
  3,4-Benzpyrene (BaP)
  7,12-Dimethylbenzanthracene (DMBA)
  3-Methylcolanthrene (MCA)
Polyhydroxyphenols and phenol derivatives
  Catechol (1,2-dihydroxybenzene)
  3-Chloro-4-hydroxbenzoic acid
  4-Chlororesorcinol
  m-Dihydroxyacetophenones
  2,4-Dinitrophenol
  Hydroquinone (1,4-dihydroxybenzene)
  4-Methylcatechol
  2-Methylresorcinol
  5-Methylresorcinol (orcinol)
  Phenol
  Phloroglucinol (1,3,5-trihydroxybenzene)
  Pyrogallic acid (1,2,3-trihydroxybenzene)
  Resorcinol (1,3-dihydroxybenzene)
Pyridines
  Dihydroxypyridines
  3-Hydroxypyridine
Other organochlorines
  Dichlorodiphenyldichloroethane (*p,p'*-DDE) and dieldrin
  Dichlorodiphenyltrichloroethane (*p,p'*-DDT)
  2,3,7,8-Tetrachlorodibenzo-*p*-dioxin (TCDD)

roid homeostasis in infants and children exposed to background levels of DLCs. Several studies suggest that prenatal exposure to these compounds affects reproductive, endocrine, neurodevelopmental, and immune systems of the progeny (Brouwer et al. 1995; Lindstrom et al. 1995). The case for recent concern about DLC-induced neural toxicity is summarized in Table 8–3 (Colborn et al. 1996).

More than 90% of human exposure is estimated to occur through these three food groups: meat (50%), milk and dairy products (35%), and fish (7%). The source of over 96% of dioxin-like compounds in the atmosphere is hospital and municipal incinerators, with nonferrous metal smelting and refining and diesel vehicle fuels accounting for the rest. From these sources, TCDD and related compounds enter the food chain by deposition on plants or soil.

However, despite the potential for adverse effects to date, there is little definitive information linking DLCs with disease states (e.g., thyroid disease) in the general population. Because this failure to demonstrate a DLC exposure–disease state link may be due to insensitivity of current detection methodology, further studies are needed, especially in high-risk groups (children and individuals occupationally or accidentally exposed to DLCs).

Disproportionate Pediatric Impact

Data from human studies and experimental animal studies suggest that the embryo/fetus is more sensitive than the adult to adverse effects caused by DLCs. Although transplacental transfer of DLCs is incomplete and maternal DLC levels are higher than those found in the fetus, the fetus is still at significant risk. A study found that nursing infants retain almost all of the DLCs present in breast milk. Although a few neurodevelopmental effects can be attributed to lactational exposure to DLCs, the benefits of breast-feeding are still judged to outweigh by far the risks from low-level exposure to DLCs (Jacobson and Jacobson 1996; Koopman-Esseboom et al. 1996). In general, exposed children are at a much higher risk for neurodevelopmental and other toxic effects of DLCs because of several factors (summarized in Table 8–4) (Carlson and Harvey 1995; Damstra and McMohan 1994).

Table 8-3. The case for neurodevelopmental toxicity from dioxin-like compounds: supporting evidence

Feature	Description
Extent of exposure	Exposure is universal, particularly in the industrialized countries. DLCs are present in almost all compartments of the biosphere, including animal and human tissues.
Level of exposure	Current background body burdens of DLCs in the general population are within the range of lowest observable adverse effect levels (LOAELs) for developmental, neurobehavioral, and reproductive toxicity. Estimates of LOAELs were based on body burden of TCDD-toxic equivalents in animals.
Time of exposure	At conception and during development, when the organism is highly vulnerable to toxic effects. DLCs are stable in biological systems because animals as well as plants do not appear to have mechanisms to detoxify or excrete these compounds. This results in accumulation and intergenerational transfer of DLCs, resulting in a continued future threat. DLCs can cross the placenta and are concentrated in milk; the fetus and newborn may be exposed through both the placenta and mother's milk.
Chronicity of exposure	Many DLCs appear to be persisting in the environment. For example, after an initial reduction in human tissue concentrations, PCB levels have held steady in recent years.
Lipid solubility and sequential bioconcentration	Because of their lipid solubility, DLCs accumulate in adipose tissue. They can be sequentially bioconcentrated in the environment. As DLCs move up the food chain, their concentrations can be magnified a million-fold.
Experimental animal and wildlife data	A cross-species comparison of DLC effects reveals commonalities across species in the endocrine mechanisms controlling CNS development and function. This means that toxic effects observed in wildlife and in laboratory animals may also occur in humans, although specific effects may differ from species to species.
Between 1972 and 1976, when Great Lakes PCB and TCDD contamination was increasing, there was a parallel increase in the incidence of goiter in coho salmon (from 44% to 79.5%).

Human studies	Described in the text.
Effects of endocrine disruption	Animal and human data suggest that DLCs are endocrine disrupters that are associated with neurodevelopmental alterations. For example, any disruptions in thyroid economy before 2 years of age in humans is known to cause neurodevelopmental toxicity.

Note. CNS = central nervous system; DLCs = dioxin-like compounds; PCBs = polychlorinated biphenyls; TCDD = 2,3,7,8-tetrachlorodibenzo-*p*-dioxin.

Table 8–4. Factors leading to disproportionate impact of exposure to dioxin-like compounds in children

Factor type	Description
Physiological	Higher CNS sensitivity (critical period from in utero to 2 years), immature HPT axis, lower absorption barriers (through the skin, gastrointestinal tract, and lungs), higher retention of DLCs by nursing infants, lower level of detoxifying enzymes at birth
Nutritional	In the very young, nursing is the primary mode of food intake; high calorie intake per kilogram of body weight
Behavioral	Closer contact with outside environment, hand-to-mouth exploratory behavior
Food chain status	A child, being at the top of food chain, may be exposed to highly magnified DLC levels. For example, as PCBs work their way up the food chain (from contaminated lake water to zooplankton to fish), their levels are magnified several millionfold by bioconcentration in the food web. The PCB concentration will be further elevated in the child consuming the lake fish.

Note. CNS = central nervous system; DLCs = dioxin-like compounds; HPT = hypothalamic-pituitary-thyroid; PCBs = polychlorinated biphenyls.

DLC Exposure and the Thyroid System

DLCs are capable of producing alterations in both the thyroid system and the developing CNS. Theoretically, these toxins could be either direct-acting thyroid disrupters (affecting the thyroid before the CNS) or, conversely, indirectly acting thyroid disrupters, causing neurotoxicity first, which in turn may cause thyroid changes (Kavlock et al. 1996). Experimental animal and human data suggest that DLCs may have both direct and indirect toxic effects on the thyroid gland (Schantz, quoted in Feeley 1995).

The effects of DLCs are complex and vary with the structure and the dose of congener used, the species, and the age of the animal at the time of exposure (Ness et al. 1993). For example, large doses of TCDD in experimental animals produce a fatal toxic syndrome suggestive of thyroid dysfunction. This syndrome is characterized by anorexia, transient hyperlipidemia, hyperkeratosis, and thyroid hyperplasia (Akoso et al. 1982; Bastomsky 1977). Rozman et al. (1984) demonstrated that thyroidectomy can partially protect experimental animals from TCDD toxicity. They found that nearly 75% of euthyroid animals expired within 45 days of treatment with 100 μg/kg of TCDD, but none of the thyroidectomized animals died at this dose.

The embryo/fetus is more sensitive to thyroid-disrupting effects of DLCs than adults (Brouwer et al. 1995). Most data are derived from studies in animals, particularly rodents. These animal studies are reviewed with special reference to effects in the developmental period; the data on DLC exposure in adult animals are reviewed as a background against which the effects of prenatal and perinatal exposure can be highlighted.

Studies in Adult Animals

Exposure to DLCs frequently results in reduced peripheral concentrations of total T_4 (TT_4), but total T_3 (TT_3) levels are not usually affected (Feeley 1995; Porterfield 1994). Some studies have also reported circulating levels of free T_4 (FT_4) to be reduced (Bastomsky 1977; Bastomsky et al. 1976; Spear et al. 1990). From 1972 to 1976, when the Great Lakes DLC contamination was increasing, there was a parallel increase in the incidence of goiter in coho salmon, from 44% to 79.5% (Moccia et al. 1977; Sonestegard and Leatherland 1979). When rats were fed Great Lakes fish for a period of 2 months, this resulted in a significant decrease in serum TT_4 levels without any change in TT_3 levels (Sonestegard and Leatherland 1979). Circulating levels of thyrotropin (TSH) have been found to be elevated (Bastomsky et al. 1976; Spear et al. 1990).

Schantz (quoted in Feeley 1995) summarized the thyroid response to a commercial PCB mixture (Aroclor 1254) in rats as follows: metabolism of T_4 is accelerated, serum T_4 is reduced, the response of TH level to external TSH is decreased, the binding of congeners and/or metabolites to transthyretin (TTH; the main TH transporting protein in rats) is diminished, and there are indirect and direct toxic effects on the thyroid gland.

Several other effects of DLCs on thyroid function have also been shown. TCDD can cause increased expression of the gene encoding the T_3 receptor (Bombick et al. 1988). Exposure to DLCs may be associated with increases in the turnover and biliary excretion of TH (Bastomsky 1977; Bastomsky et al. 1976; Spear et al. 1990) and increased weight of the thyroid gland. Microscopically, changes suggestive of sustained TSH stimulation are seen, including increased development of endoplasmic reticulum, vacuolization of mitochondria, and a decrease in the colloid droplet–lysozyme interaction needed for TH release. DLCs probably impair the release of thyroid hormones (Welch 1995).

Studies in Developing Animals

Morse and Brouwer (1994) studied perinatal alterations in thyroid function following maternal exposure to Aroclor 1254 in rats. They did not find any changes in plasma TSH levels at any time during the study. However, fetal TT_4 and FT_4 concentrations decreased by 50% and 80% in the low-dose and the high-dose groups, respectively; maternal plasma TT_4 and FT_4 were reduced (50%) in only the high-dose group. In the neonates receiving high doses, TT_4 and TT_3 were reduced (50%) 4 days after birth. In female neonates (but not in male neonates), decreased plasma FT_4 concentrations were found in both the high-dose and low-dose groups. On day 21 postpartum, maternal thyroid function tests were normal in both high-dose and low-dose groups, but in the neonates exposed to the high Aroclor dose, TT_4, FT_4, and TT_3 were decreased. T_4 levels in fetal cerebella were reduced and not detectable by the assay in the high-dose group. T_3 concentrations in the fetal cerebella were only minimally affected; fetal forebrain T_3 concentrations were decreased.

These findings are consistent with those of earlier studies in rats that examined the effects of perinatal exposure to PCB congeners commonly found in human tissue and breast milk (Brouwer et al. 1995; Morse et al. 1992, 1993; Ness et al. 1993). As a group, these studies are in agreement that DLCs produce decreases in fetal and neonatal TT_4 and FT_4 levels, T_4 depletion, and increased activity of type II thyroxine 5′-deiodinase (5′D-II) in the brain. Nonetheless, in contrast to Morse and Brouwer (1994), who found TT_3 levels to decrease in rat pups, Ness et al. (1993) did not find any changes in TT_3 values in their sample. They found that rats with in utero and lactational exposure to two PCB congeners (118 and 153) had lower T_4 values and growth retardation. They also observed histological changes suggestive of sustained TSH stimulation in fetal/neonatal thyroid glands. These included increased follicular cell vacuolization, increased follicular cell height, nuclear vesication, and decreased colloid in PCB-118–exposed thyroid. Despite these histological changes, Morse and Brouwer (1994) did not find serum TSH levels to increase. Therefore, they suggested that pituitary feedback regulation of TH homeostasis may be impaired by Aroclor 1254.

Human Studies: Perinatal DLC Exposure and the Thyroid

Several studies have demonstrated that exposure to DLCs in utero or via lactation may be associated with alterations of thyroid homeostasis in the absence of overt signs of maternal toxicity (Feeley 1995). Generally, reduced T_4 and increased TSH levels have been reported (Dewailly et al. 1993; Koopman-Esseboom et al. 1994; Murai et al. 1987; Pluim et al. 1993a, 1993b).

Pluim and colleagues (1993a, 1993b) examined the effects of prenatal and postnatal exposure to chlorinated dioxins and furans on neonatal TH concentrations. They divided their sample of 38 healthy breast-fed infants into two groups according to the dioxin concentrations in the milk fat of the mothers. The authors measured TT_4 and TSH levels sequentially in infants at birth, at 1 week of age, and at 11 weeks of age. They found TT_4 concentration to be elevated in the high-exposure group with breast milk TCDD toxic equivalent (TEQ) values of 37.5 ng per kilogram of milk fat. TSH concentrations were increased in the high-exposure group at the age of 11 weeks, but not at birth or at 1 week of age.

Koopman-Esseboom et al., in a workshop on perinatal exposure to DLCs (quoted in Feeley 1995), described an ongoing study of the effects of perinatal exposures to low levels of DLCs in Dutch children (100 breast fed, 100 formula fed). They obtained infant (10 days and 3 months postpartum), maternal, and umbilical cord blood samples, which were analyzed for TT_3, TT_4, TSH, and FT_4. They found that neonatal TSH levels were elevated at 10 days and at 3 months, but FT_4 and TT_4 values were not affected. The increased TSH levels (but not T_4 levels) correlated with increased breast milk dioxin and coplanar PCB values.

In an earlier report, the same group (Koopman-Esseboom et al. 1994) studied the effects of DLCs on TH levels in 105 Dutch mother-infant pairs. Higher DLC concentrations in human milk, expressed as TEQs, correlated with elevated infant plasma TSH (at 2–3 weeks postpartum) and reduced maternal T_3 and T_4 values. At 2–3 weeks after birth, infants with high TEQs had reduced TT_4 and FT_4, but within the euthyroid range. Although changes in TH values were small, it was concluded that such small changes may have developmental effects.

Dewailly et al. (1993) studied the effects of perinatal DLC exposure on TSH concentrations of Inuit children. They reported that in male infants, the birth length was inversely related to the PCB level in breast milk of the mother. However, there was no correlation between the TSH and DLC levels.

Synthesis of Findings From Animal and Human Data

Developmental exposure to DLCs results in alterations in TH homeostasis (Brouwer et al. 1998). Several recent reviews on DLCs and TH-directed brain development are available (Leatherland 1998; Porterfield and Hendry 1998; Sher et al. 1998). Some of the effects that have been reported for DLCs on the thyroid function are summarized in Table 8–5. Exposure to DLCs frequently results in reduced peripheral concentrations of TT_4, but total TT_3 levels are not usually affected (Feeley 1995; Porterfield 1994). These findings suggest that DLCs act preferentially on T_4. Some studies have also reported circulating levels of FT_4 to be reduced (Bastomsky 1977; Bastomsky et al. 1976; Spear et al. 1990). Doses of DLC that did have adverse effects in adult rats produced reduction in fetal TT_4 and FT_4 levels.

The mechanism by which DLCs may disrupt the thyroid system has not been established, but it is likely that thyroid dysregulation is produced by multiple mechanisms. Molecular and theoretical modeling data suggest that certain DLCs, T_3, and T_4 have similar structures: they all have phenol rings and are halogenated (McKinney 1989; McKinney et al. 1985). Perhaps because of this structural similarity, DLCs can act as agonists, partial agonists, and antagonists of TH, depending on the species, dosage, and congener used (Porterfield and Hendry 1998). The binding affinities to thyroid hormone transport protein, or transthyretin (TTR), of many DLC congeners are several times higher than that of T_4 itself (Rickenbacher et al. 1986). Competition of DLCs with T_4 for binding sites on serum TTR and CSF TTR can interfere with TH transport in the circulation and into brain cells, respectively (Rickenbacher et al. 1986). DLCs could also compete with TH for membrane transport and thus decrease intraneuronal TH level (Porterfield 1994). Although it is conceivable that DLCs might also compete with TH for binding to the T_3 receptor, these binding experiments have not yet been conducted. The question remains whether the thyroid toxicity of DLCs is partly or predominantly mediated by changes in hormone binding to TR (Hauser et al. 1998).

DLCs may reduce circulating T_4 by multiple mechanisms (Ness et al. 1993). First, they may displace T_4 from TTR by competing for its binding sites and by accelerating T_4 metabolism and excretion (Brouwer 1989; Brouwer and van den Berg 1986; Brouwer et al. 1990). Second, they may also increase TH metabolism by inducing hepatic T_4-UDPGT (uridine 5′-diphosphate-glucuronyltransferase) (Feeley 1995), thereby facilitating biliary excretion of T_4. Morse et al. (1993) studied the effects of DLCs on TH metabolism in rats. For PCB congener 169, they described increased hepatic T_4-UDPGT activity to be a probable cause of reduced neonatal and maternal, but not fetal, plasma TT_4 levels.

DLCs can decrease the availability of TH at T_3 receptor sites in the CNS by several mechanisms. The preferential effect of DLCs on

Table 8–5. Effects on the thyroid system of exposure to dioxin-like compounds

Effect on the thyroid system	Animal studies	Human studies
A fatal toxic syndrome in rodents, induced by large doses of TCDD, was characterized by anorexia, transient hyperlipidemia, hyperkeratosis, and thyroid hyperplasia. Thyroidectomy was shown to partially protect experimental animals from TCDD toxicity.	Akoso et al. 1982 Bastomsky 1977 Rozman et al. 1984	
Reduced serum TT_4	Bastomsky et al. 1976 Brouwer 1989	Koopman-Esseboom et al. 1994
Elevated serum TT_4	Henry and Gasiewicz 1987	Pluim et al. 1993a, 1993b
Reduced serum FT_4	Bastomsky 1977 Bastomsky et al. 1976 Spear et al. 1990	Emmet et al. 1988
Increased serum TT_3 and TT_4 without changes in FT_4	Murai et al. 1987	
Increased serum TSH	Bastomsky et al. 1976 Spear et al. 1990	Koopman-Esseboom et al. 1994 Pluim et al. 1993a, 1993b
No change in TSH		Dewailly et al. 1993
Decreased T_4 and T_3 in brain	Morse and Brouwer 1994	
Increased thyroid weight, thyroid hyperplasia, hypertrophy of follicular cells, and probably decreased TH release	Ness et al. 1993	

Mechanism	References
Competition for binding to TH transport proteins in blood (particularly transthyretin)	Brouwer et al. 1995
Induction of microsomal phase II enzyme UDP-glucuronosyltransferase	Morse et al. 1992, 1993
Increased biliary excretion of T_4	Bastomsky 1977; Bastomsky et al. 1976; Spear et al. 1990
Increased TH turnover	Bastomsky 1977; Bastomsky et al. 1976; Spear et al. 1990
Increased expression of the gene encoding the T_3 receptor: v-erb-A	Bombick et al. 1988
Effects of perinatal exposure in the fetus or the neonate: reduced or increased serum TT_4, increased TT_4:TBG ratio (an indicator of FT_4), decreased FT_4, increased serum TSH, increased activity of type II thyroxine 5′-deiodinase (5′D-II) in brain, and histological changes suggestive of sustained TSH stimulation in the thyroid gland	Brouwer et al. 1995; Collins and Capen 1980; Morse and Brouwer 1994; Morse et al. 1992, 1993; Ness et al. 1993; Koopman-Esseboom et al. 1994; Murai et al. 1987; Pluim et al. 1993

Note. FT_4 = free T_4; T_3 = triiodothyronine; T_4 = thyroxine; TBG = thyroxine-binding globulin; TCDD = 2,3,7,8-tetrachlorodibenzo-*p*-dioxin; TSH = thyroid-stimulating hormone; UDP = uridine 5′-diphosphate.

T_4 levels may reduce the availability of thyroid hormone in the CNS. This is because CNS development is dependent on the availability of T_4 and not T_3 (80% of TH in the brain comes from serum T_4) (Calvo et al. 1990). Possible disruptions in TH availability in the CNS may be further aggravated by two other actions of DLCs: competition for binding to TH carrier proteins (particularly transthyretin) and competition for binding to T_3 receptor (Heussen Kikspoors et al. 1992). TTH may have an important role in transporting TH to neurons, and competitive inhibition of this or other CNS transport mechanisms may alter CNS thyroid homeostasis. The activity of brain 5'D-II (the enzyme responsible for local deiodination of T_4 to T_3) was significantly induced in the fetal forebrain in a dose-dependent manner by maternal Aroclor 1254 exposure (Morse and Brouwer 1994). However, unexpectedly, in neonatal forebrain homogenates, 5'D-II activity was significantly decreased in the low-exposure group but was unchanged in the high-exposure group. These reductions in enzyme activity suggest that 5'D-II activity was not able to compensate for low T_4 uptake in the CNS.

In susceptible individuals, exposure to DLCs can induce lymphocytic autoimmune thyroiditis that can lead to primary hypothyroidism (Bahn et al. 1980; Rao and Banerji 1990). Thus, it is possible that DLC toxicity may increase the incidence of autoimmune thyroid diseases. Porterfield (1994) speculated that a preexisting thyroid disorder could exacerbate the effects of DLCs.

Neurodevelopmental and Behavioral Effects of DLC Exposure

Neurological data in adults exposed to DLCs appears inconclusive, but neurodevelopmental toxicity of DLCs is well known (Birnbaum 1995; de Duffard and Duffard 1996; Golub and Jacobson 1995; Rogan and Gladen 1992).

Neurotoxicity in Adults Versus Developmental Neurotoxicity

Human and animal studies suggest that DLCs are neuroteratogens—that is, agents that can produce anatomic or physiological changes in the developing CNS but have little or no effect in adult animals (Seegal and Schantz 1994). In utero or fetal exposure to DLCs has usually been associated with impairments of cognition and psychomotor activity (Tilson et al. 1990), but exposed adult animals did not demonstrate neurotoxicity (Tilson et al. 1979).

In humans, there have been two recorded incidents of mass poisoning caused by ingestion of cooking oil contaminated with PCBs, polychlorinated dibenzofurans (PCDFs), and polychlorinated naphthalenes. The congener usually hypothesized to be most responsible for neurotoxicity is PCDF (James et al. 1993), but this hypothesis must be tested (Hartman 1995). The first incident, called "yusho," occurred in Japan during 1968. In 1978, a similar incident occurred in Taiwan and was named "yu-cheng" (Chen et al. 1994; Hsu et al. 1985; Rogan et al. 1988). Neurological studies in the adult yu-cheng patients did not reveal any clear signs of CNS toxicity, although many patients had peripheral sensory neuropathy, headaches, and dizziness (Chia and Chu 1984, 1985). The neurological symptoms did not correlate with blood PCB levels. By contrast, perinatal exposures in children with yu-cheng were demonstrated to cause developmental delays and impaired cognition (Chen et al. 1992, 1994). It is possible that subtle neurotoxicity in adults with yu-cheng was missed because neuropsychological measures were not used (Hartman 1995).

Perinatal Exposure to DLCs: Animal Studies

Several cognitive and behavioral paradigms have been used to demonstrate the developmental neurotoxicity of DLCs in many species, including mice, rats, monkeys, and humans. The actual effects depend on the dose, the structure of the congener, and the species and age of the animal at the time of exposure. There is a variability of response even within the same species, suggesting differences in susceptibility to DLC toxicity. Despite this variability, a cross-species comparison by Tilson and associates (1990) revealed that data on developmental neurotoxicity across various animal species were generally consistent with each other and with the findings from human studies. Animal models are available for most, if not for all, human responses to DLCs (Porterfield 1994; Tilson et al. 1990). For example, growth retardation and spatial learning/memory deficits demonstrated in humans have also been observed in monkeys and rats in the laboratory setting. Inspired by the article by Tilson et al. (1990), we tabulated the neurodevelopmental effects of DLCs across several animal species (Table 8–6).

Perinatal Exposure to DLCs: Human Studies

Data from epidemiological studies in cohorts that have had in utero or lactational exposure to DLCs, either accidentally or through contaminated food, are summarized in Table 8–7. Even prenatal exposures to levels of DLCs considered to be background or several times higher in the United States can produce neurotoxic effects in some children (Jacobson et al. 1985). Whereas fatalities and overt signs and symptoms of acute poisoning were observed in Asian (yusho and yu-cheng) cohorts, subtler effects of low-level and long-term DLC exposure were seen in the European and North American studies.

One of the original prospective United States studies is from Michigan. The findings of this Michigan study (Jacobson and Jacobson 1996; Jacobson et al. 1985, 1990a, 1990b) indicate that perinatal exposures to DLCs are associated with poorer intellectual function in school-age children and poorer short-term memory and developmental delays during infancy and early childhood. On retesting 212 of these children at age 11 years, Jacobson and Jacobson (1996) demonstrated that the neurocognitive effects of DLC exposure persisted through the school years. The data from IQ and achievement tests revealed that the transplacental (but not lactational) exposure was associated with lower full-scale and verbal IQs after controlling for confounding variables (such as socioeconomic status and in utero exposure to nicotine and alcohol). The strongest cognitive effects of low-level exposure were related to short-term memory, long-term memory, focused attention, and sustained attention. Children with high exposure tended to be at least 2 years behind in their reading comprehension. Jacobson and

Table 8–6. A cross-species comparison of neurodevelopmental effects of dioxin-like compounds

Species	Motor activity	Cognition	Neurological development	References
Mice	Hyperactivity, stereotypical spinning	Impaired active avoidance acquisition	Decreased coordination	Chou et al. 1979 Storm et al. 1981 Tilson et al. 1979
Rats	Hyperactivity or hypoactivity, decrease in hyperactivity after dextroamphetamine challenge, reduced grip strength of forelimbs and hindlimbs, impaired inclined screen, impaired swimming	Impaired active avoidance acquisition and t-maze learning, impaired discrimination learning (manifested by perseveration and incorrect and unnecessary responses of animal that did not lead to reinforcement), no deficits in object recognition (comparable to the short-term memory measures for humans)	Stereotypical spinning, altered swimming, no changes in startle response, impaired neurological development	Holene et al. (cited in Brouwer et al. 1995) Koja et al. 1978, 1979 Lilienthal et al. 1990 Overmann et al. 1987 Panteleoni et al. 1988 Sauer et al. 1994 Shiota 1976

(continued)

Table 8–6. A cross-species comparison of neurodevelopmental effects of dioxin-like compounds (continued)

Species	Motor activity	Cognition	Neurological development	References
Monkeys	Hyperactivity or hypoactivity	On Wisconsin General Test Apparatus, impairments on two cognitive paradigms—delayed spatial alternation and discrimination-reversal learning (RL)—reflecting dysfunctions of learning and memory, were shown. These dysfunctions may reflect changes in prefrontal cortex, frontal cortex, and temporal lobes.	On a series of fixed-interval reinforcement schedules of food reinforcement, PCB-treated monkeys showed decreased index of curvature, suggesting an altered pattern of operant response.	Bowman et al. 1981a, 1981b Levin et al. 1988, 1992 Mele et al. 1986 Schantz and Bowman 1989 Schantz et al. 1989

Note. PCB = polychlorinated biphenyl.

Table 8–7. Neurodevelopmental effects of perinatal exposure to dioxin-like compounds: selected human studies

Study and design	Neuromotor effects	Cognitive effects	Effects on neurological development	Conclusions
Yusho (Japan) cohort: Developmental effects of in utero exposure to heat-degraded PCBs (PCDFs and polychlorinated naphthalenes) through contaminated rice oil were studied.	Hypoactivity and delayed neuromotor development	Severe, clinically apparent cognitive impairments	Hypotonia, apathy, delayed speech and language development	It remains unclear which compounds were responsible for severe neurodevelopmental toxicity.
Yu-cheng cohort (Taiwan, N = 118): Developmental effects of in utero exposure to heat-degraded PCBs (PCDFs and polychlorinated naphthalenes) through contaminated rice oil were studied.	On Rutter scale, exposed children showed hyperactivity.	The exposed children showed short- and long-term cognitive impairments, including about 5-point drop on standardized IQ tests lasting until 7 years of age.	Delayed neurological development	Although it remains unclear which compounds caused toxicity, PCB exposure was associated with decreased growth, impaired cognitive abilities, and skin abnormalities.

(continued)

Table 8–7. Neurodevelopmental effects of perinatal exposure to dioxin-like compounds: selected human studies *(continued)*

Study and design	Neuromotor effects	Cognitive effects	Effects on neurological development	Conclusions
Lake Michigan Maternal-Infant Cohorts ($N = 242$): Cognitive and neurobehavioral effects of in utero exposure to PCBs (and related lake contaminants) in children of mothers eating Lake Michigan fish were assessed. The children were retested at the age of 11 years with a battery of IQ and achievement tests.	Hypoactivity in 4-year-olds and delayed neuromotor development in infants	The exposed children showed impaired attention, short-term memory, and cognitive efficiency. At 4 and 11 years of age, a higher PCB level predicted poorer verbal and memory scores on tests.	Hypotonia and hyporeflexia at birth, and a deficit in visual recognition memory in 7-month-olds	Developmental exposure to low levels of PCBs (and other lake contaminants) may cause short- and long-term deficits in cognition, attention, and activity levels. Lower full-scale and verbal IQs in 11-year-olds were found, suggesting that the deficits in intellect, memory, and attention persist through school years.

North Carolina Cohort ($N \geq 800$): Children born to mothers who had no unusual PCB exposure were followed through 5 years of age. Levels of PCB exposure and development (using Brazelton Neurobehavioral Development Scale [NBAS], the Bayley Scales, and the McCarthy Scales) were assessed.	Hypoactivity and delayed neuromotor development with prenatal (but not postnatal) exposure lasting until 12 months of age.	No association was found between prenatal exposure and cognitive functions evaluated by McCarthy scores.	At birth, the more highly exposed were hypotonic and hyporeflexic. In 3- to 5-year-olds, no effects were observed.	Transplacental (but not lactational) PCB exposures were associated with hypoactivity and developmental delays lasting until 2 years of age.

(continued)

Table 8–7. Neurodevelopmental effects of perinatal exposure to dioxin-like compounds: selected human studies *(continued)*

Study and design	Neuromotor effects	Cognitive effects	Effects on neurological development	Conclusions
Dutch Cohort Studies (N = 207): Neurobehavioral effects of PCB or dioxin exposure (transplacental or lactational) in Dutch children born to mothers who had no unusual DLC exposure were evaluated. Psychomotor and mental scores on Bayley Infant Development Scales were measured at 3, 7, and 18 months of age.	In 3-month-old children higher in utero exposure was associated with lower psychomotor scores.	In utero exposure did not influence mental scores on the Bayley Scale at any age.	Prenatal exposure was not related to outcome on Fagan Visual Memory Recognition Test.	Background developmental exposure of Dutch infants to DLCs, which may affect thyroid function of mother and infant, is not related to a serious delay in development. At 7 months of age, DLC exposure through lactation had an adverse effect on psychomotor outcome and outweighed the positive effect on mental outcome of breast feeding. At 18 months of age, DLC exposure (transplacental or lactational) did not have any developmental consequences.

Oswego Newborn and Infant Development Project, New York ($N = 395$; 152 in high-exposure group and 243 in low-exposure group): Neurobehavioral effects of exposure to PCBs and other DLCs (and other lake contaminants) in children born to mothers eating Lake Ontario fish were evaluated. NBAS assessments were given at 12–24 hours after birth, and again at 25–48 hours after birth.	No abnormalities of motor function were detected.	No data available.	The more highly exposed neonates had poorer scores on the habituation, autonomic, and reflex cluster of NBAS (suggesting hyperreactivity, autonomic immaturity, and a greater number of abnormal reflexes).	This study replicated and extended the neonatal results of Lake Michigan, Maternal Infants cohorts study (Jacobson and Jacobson 1996; Jacobson et al. 1985).

Note. DLCs = dioxin-like compounds; NBAS = Brazelton Neurobehavioral Development Scale; PCBs = polychlorinated biphenyls; PCDFs = polychlorinated dibenzofurans.

Jacobson concluded that the fetal CNS was exquisitely sensitive to PCBs and that in utero PCB exposure can have a long-term impact on general intellectual function, memory, and attention.

A large-scale prospective study in the United States has also been undertaken in North Carolina (Gladen and Rogan 1991; Gladen et al. 1988; Rogan et al. 1986, 1987). Unlike the Michigan children, the North Carolina children did not show any neurodevelopmental or cognitive abnormalities at 3–5 years of age. The reasons for this disagreement between the Michigan and North Carolina studies are not known, but a possible explanation is that the Michigan cohort, but not the North Carolina cohort, was exposed to all the contaminants in the lake. Another reason may be that in these two studies children were tested at different ages.

The findings of Jacobson et al. (1990a) have been generally extended and replicated by ongoing Dutch studies (Koopman-Esseboom et al. 1996) and by the Oswego Newborn and Infant Development Project in New York (Lonky et al. 1996). Not presented in Table 8–7 is a study by Schantz et al. (1990), who observed decreased activity level in a cohort of children born to mothers exposed to PCBs through contaminated beef and dairy products. Also not tabulated are the preliminary results of a small Times Beach, Missouri, study that examined the quantitative electroencephalographs of 15 children born to TCDD-exposed mothers. Frontal and prefrontal lobe abnormalities suggestive of impaired attention were found (G. Smoger; findings reported in Golub and Jacobson 1995).

Synthesis of Findings From Human and Animal Data

The experimental animal and human data reviewed in this section lead to the conclusion that DLCs are developmental neurotoxicants. Transplacental exposure to DLCs may produce an array of short- or long-term impairments in a variety of neuropsychological domains, including effects on behavior, learning, memory, attention, sensory function, and psychomotor development (Bowman et al. 1989, 1990). The magnitude and nature of response may depend on the dose and the structure of the congener, the species, and the age of the animal at the time of exposure, but there is considerable biological variability even within the same species. These individual differences in response to similar doses of the congener within the same species suggest biological differences in vulnerability to DLC effects. Of these, the timing of exposure is a critical variable; adults appear to be tolerant to the neurotoxic effects of DLCs.

Acute perinatal exposures to relatively high levels of DLCs (e.g., yusho and yu-cheng) cause a severe and potentially fatal syndrome. The neurotoxic effects of such developmental exposures are manifested by a spectrum of cognitive manifestations, ranging from subtle dysfunctions of intellect and achievement to learning disorders and mental retardation. The neuromotor effects of such perinatal DLC exposures range from hypoactivity or hyperactivity to delayed neuromotor development and cerebral palsy.

Low-level in utero exposures (slightly higher than the current background level in the United States) are not associated with any gross brain malformations or mental retardation, but several prospective studies have linked such exposures to adverse effects on neural development (Jacobson and Jacobson 1996). Such exposures also produce an array of neuropsychological abnormalities, including lower performance on IQ and achievement tests, psychomotor changes, and developmental delays. A deficit of 6.2 in full-scale IQ scores was found to persist at the age of 11 years in patients who were transplacentally exposed to DLCs. The most frequent manifestations of DLC-induced neurodevelopmental toxicity are disturbances in neuromotor activity and attention, impairments of higher cognitive functions and learning, and neurodevelopmental delays. Disturbances in all these domains may potentially persist through the school years (Jacobson and Jacobson 1996) and possibly into adulthood.

Disturbances in neuromotor activity and attention. Most human studies have reported alterations in neuromotor activity. In a majority of samples, the level of activity appeared to be reduced in the DLC-exposed children (Jacobson et al. 1990a, 1990b), but children with yu-cheng were hyperactive. Whereas earlier studies in mice reported hyperactivity (Agrawal et al. 1981; Chou et al. 1979; Tilson et al. 1979), more recently hypoactivity has been reported in rats exposed to PCBs (Schantz et al. 1992). Perhaps this variability in neuromotor toxic responses is related to differences in the dose and the structure of the congeners used across studies. The earlier studies (such as yusho and yu-cheng) focused on high-dose perinatal DLCs exposures, which were fetotoxic (Chou et al. 1979; Seegal and Schantz 1994; Tilson et al. 1979). Conceivably, high-level perinatal exposures are more likely to be associated with hyperactivity, whereas low-level in utero exposures are associated with hypoactivity (Erickson 1988; Erickson et al. 1991; Jacobson et al. 1990a, 1990b; Schantz et al. 1992).

Longitudinal follow-up by Jacobson and Jacobson (1996) suggests that DLC-exposed children may have deficits in focused and sustained attention and that these deficits may persist during the school years. On the basis of the neurobehavioral data from epidemiological studies reviewed in Table 8–7, it may be hypothesized that like lead, DLC neurotoxicity in some children may mimic symptoms of attention-deficit/hyperactivity disorder (ADHD). However, these children need to be assessed systematically for ADHD-like symptoms before any conclusions are drawn.

Impairments of higher cognitive functions and learning. Higher cognitive functions and learning were evaluated in DLC-exposed monkeys by a commonly used monkey test apparatus called the Wisconsin General Testing Apparatus (WGTA). Profound decrements in performance on two cognitive tasks—delayed spatial alternation (DSA) and discrimination-reversal learning (RL)—reflecting dysfunctions in learning and memory, were demonstrated (Bowman and Heironimus 1981; Bowman et al. 1978, 1981; Levin et al. 1988, 1992; Schantz and Bowman 1989; Schantz et al. 1989). Similarly, studies in humans have linked in utero DLC exposure with poorer short-term and long-term memory during infancy and early childhood and in 11-year-olds. Such children tend to score poorly on achievement tests (Jacobson and Jacobson 1996). They may be found to have learning disabilities, particularly language disorders.

Neurodevelopmental delays. Although mental retardation is rare, neurodevelopmental delays are frequently seen in DLC-exposed animals and children (Fein et al. 1984). Delays may be observed in the ontogeny of reflexes and acquisition of complex movements. Delays in language and speech development, as well as development of visual recognition memory, have also been described.

Mechanism of DLC-Induced Developmental Neurotoxicity

Many biological effects of DLCs are believed to be mediated by Ah receptors. However, PCB congeners with low affinity for Ah receptors can cause neurotoxic effects, and it is likely that mechanisms independent of Ah receptors are involved in the developmental neurotoxicity. It is possible that complex interactions between neuroendocrine (particularly thyroid system) and neurophysiological (particularly dopamine) systems in a developing CNS lead to neural toxicity. Based on the resemblance between neurodevelopmental changes induced by DLCs and those secondary to hypothyroidism and resistance to thyroid hormone, disruption of CNS and peripheral thyroid homeostasis has been proposed to be the major mechanism underlying adverse neurodevelopmental effects from DLCs (Brouwer et al. 1998; Hauser et al. 1998; Porterfield and Hendry 1998). Thyroid disruption of the developing CNS can permanently change behavior, whereas a fully differentiated brain may be unaffected by the thyroid-disrupting effects of DLCs.

According to a model of DLC-induced neurodevelopmental toxicity (Sher et al. 1998), DLC-induced changes in fetal or neonatal brain T_3/T_4 levels may alter TH receptor regulation (and subsequent expression or stability of mRNAs) of genes critical for neuroanatomic and behavioral development. It is possible that even transient decreases in the availability of T_4 in the CNS during the critical developmental periods produce alterations in neuronal branching and brain cytoarchitecture (Porterfield 1994). Competition by DLCs and T_4 for binding to transthyretin in cerebrospinal fluid can interfere with TH transport into the CNS. Competition with thyroid hormones for membrane transport would also decrease brain intracellular TH levels.

Because of the plasticity of the developing brain, even temporary alterations in the thyroid system can cause permanent changes in CNS organization and thyroid homeostasis. Therefore, even transient perinatal DLC toxicity may lead to long-term disturbances. It might be speculated that these changes in the anatomy and physiology of the brain, in turn, could produce cognitive and behavioral deficits.

Low-level DLC neurotoxicity is not known to be associated with any changes in the gross anatomy of the brain. Such exposures can still have a long-term effect on both cognitive function and circulating thyroid hormone concentrations. Alterations in neuronal connectivity could explain subtle neurobehavioral deficits in such cases. By contrast, more severe cases of perinatal DLC exposure in Asian cohorts resulted in mental retardation and gross malformations of the brain. It is possible that high-dose perinatal exposure to DLCs produces neurobehavioral and neuromotor changes through both direct toxicity to CNS regulators of motor activity (such as the corticospinal tract and cerebellum) and thyroid toxicity. The eventual results of moderate to severe disturbances of fetal TH economy include cerebral palsy, mental retardation, learning disability, ADHD, hydrocephalus, seizures, and other permanent neurological abnormalities (Alleva et al. 1998).

Similarity of the CNS effects of DLCs and thyroid disorders. Some key similarities and differences exist between physiological and neurodevelopmental effects of DLCs and those of thyroid disorders; the similarities have been highlighted by Porterfield (1994). She pointed out that both hypothyroidism and exposure to DLCs are physiologically associated with low T_4, no change in T_3, and elevated TSH in rodents. Some of the similar neurodevelopmental changes in both hypothyroidism and DLC toxicity are delayed acquisition of auditory startle, cliff avoidance, negative geotaxis, and air-righting. Neuromotor disturbances (hypoactivity and hyperactivity), pervasive developmental disorders, and cognitive impairments (impaired learning and memory) have been also demonstrated in both conditions. Like children perinatally exposed to DLCs, children with congenital hypothyroidism who are inadequately treated have lower scores on intellectual, achievement, and memory tests. On the basis of this similarity, Porterfield (1994) hypothesized that very low body concentrations (lower than those usually thought to be toxic) of DLCs can cause neurodevelopmental toxicity by disrupting both maternal and fetal thyroid function at particular times during critical periods of CNS development. Small disturbances in thyroid function during development can lead to profound and lasting effects.

However, the studies that have focused on thyroid function tests in DLC exposure have produced inconsistent results. Although most of these studies are in agreement that exposure to DLCs may lead to reduced T_4, TSH levels have been variously described as elevated or unchanged.

An alternative proposal linking thyroid dysfunction with DLC-induced neurotoxicity was offered by Hauser et al. (1998). They observed that both the syndrome of resistance to thyroid hormone (RTH) and DLC-induced neurodevelopmental changes were similarly associated with mild cognitive and behavioral disturbances (e.g., decreases in full-scale IQ). They speculated that by comparing and contrasting the neurodevelopmental effects of mild to moderate thyroid dysfunction (such as is observed in resistance to thyroid hormone) with those of DLCs, it may be possible to generate new hypotheses to develop new insights into developmental neurotoxicity associated with DLCs.

Role of dopamine. It has been hypothesized that alterations of dopamine levels in the prefrontal cortex are also related to neurobehavioral toxicity, particularly neuromotor abnormalities associated with perinatal DLC exposure (Seegal et al. 1991). Dopamine is involved in the initiation and control of motor behavior. Chou et al. (1979) exposed mice on gestational days 10–16 to high doses of tetrachlorobiphenyl (TCB). Some pups were stillborn. Of those who survived, nearly 50% exhibited rapid spinning, hyperactivity, and head bobbing. When dextroamphetamine (an indirect dopamine agonist) was given to these mice, their hyperactivity decreased considerably. These findings suggest that dopamine plays a role in locomotor changes associated with PCB toxicity.

Similarly, in experimental animals, exposure to PCBs produces alterations in CNS dopamine. The direction of dopamine change is age and time dependent (Seegal 1994). Whereas perinatal exposures produce elevated dopamine concentrations in the brain, PCB exposures in adults result in decreased CNS dopamine (Seegal and Schantz 1994). These results indicate that PCB exposure of both the developing and the adult CNS causes long-term alterations in brain dopamine levels. Similarly, time- and dose-dependent decreases in cellular dopamine content were also observed with in vitro exposure to Aroclor 1254 by Seegal et al. (1989). These findings demonstrate that PCBs reduced dopamine levels by a direct effect, perhaps through decreased dopamine synthesis. Another possibility is that PCB-induced neuromotor effects occur through a combination of changes in both thyroid and dopamine systems.

Dopamine may also be involved in deficits of performance in two learning paradigms (DSA and RL). DSA impairments have been related to lesions of the hippocampus and frontal cortex or to depletion of dopamine in the frontal cortex (Goldman et al. 1971). Reversal of frontal cortical DA depletion by administration of L-dopa enhanced DSA performance. Decrements in RL tasks are observed with specific lesions of frontal and temporal lobes and the mammillary bodies (Holmes et al. 1983; Mahut 1971). These learning deficits in monkeys persist long after the perinatal exposure. These long-term alterations in dopamine function may be the mechanism by which DSA and RL task impairments occur (Seegal and Schantz 1994).

Conclusions and Future Directions

Thyroid system disrupters (TDs) have been present in the environment throughout history, and biological systems have evolved in their presence. Over a period of several millennia, humans and other animals have successfully adapted to naturally occurring TDs. However, the introduction of a multitude of synthetic TDs during the 20th century has created a different situation. Not only humans but also many other biological systems lack the capacity to degrade and excrete DLCs. As a result of bioaccumulation, the general population is exposed to levels of DLCs that are estimated to be potentially neuroteratogenic and endocrine disruptive (Alleva et al. 1998). It is likely that DLCs and some other TDs produce both organizational and activational neurodevelopmental effects (Guillette et al. 1995).

Recent reviews from the U.S. Environmental Protection Agency (EPA) and the European Environmental Research Organization are in agreement that the current level of exposure to DLCs is potentially hazardous, particularly to children. This consensus is based on the estimation that the average human daily intake of dioxins is between 3 and 6 picograms of TCDD equivalent per kilogram of body weight, leading to an average body burden of 30–60 picograms per gram of lipid. At this or the corresponding level of exposure in animals, several effects have been demonstrated in humans and animals. These include enzyme induction, altered cell function (reduced glucose tolerance), and altered circulating hormone (reproductive and thyroid) levels. On the basis of these observations, it has been suggested that persons with body burdens three to seven times higher than the average might be at risk for developmental toxicity and a decreased ability to withstand immunological challenge.

A consensus appears to be emerging that children below 2 years of age may be at risk for neurodevelopmental toxicity from DLCs, with the greatest risk occurring during gestation. A panel of international experts meeting in Erice, Sicily (Alleva et al. 1998) estimated that "every pregnant woman in the world has endocrine disrupters in her body that are transferred to the fetus." She also has "measurable concentrations of endocrine disrupters in her milk that are transferred to the infant." Similarly, a consensus report of the EPA-sponsored workshop on endocrine disrupters concluded that the endocrine disrupter hypothesis was of sufficient concern and that concerted efforts should be undertaken to evaluate the validity of the hypothesis (Kavlock et al. 1996). It was noted that the embryo, fetus, and neonate may be especially susceptible to brief periods of thyroid and other types of endocrine disruptions.

Although the subtle effects of DLCs may not be observed in an individual child, the epidemiological and experimental animal data have implications at a population level. There is evidence suggesting that low-level perinatal exposure to DLCs can impair motor function, spatial perception, learning memory, auditory development, fine motor coordination, balance, and attentional processes. In cases of high-level DLC exposures during the perinatal period, mental retardation may result.

Even minimal and transient decreases in thyroid hormone secretion during the first few months of life can cause neurological deficits (Calaciura et al. 1995; Vulsma and Kok 1996). For example, premature infants will sometimes have a transient decrease in levels of thyroid hormone following birth. Physicians have not been concerned about this because the levels always increase to normal over time. However, a study by Reuss et al. (1996) found that premature infants who have this transient hypothyroxinemia have a fivefold increase in cerebral palsy at 2 years of age. They also have, on average, a decrease of 10 IQ points compared with premature infants with normal thyroid hormone levels.

Recommendations and Research Implications

So far, DLCs have not been shown to be a specific etiological factor in diseases of the thyroid or CNS (including neuropsychiatric disorders). However, given the widespread occurrence and persistence of DLCs in the environment and the potential seriousness of the problem, it is important to fill the most critical gaps in our knowledge base. The critical issue is whether sufficiently high levels of TDs exist in the ambient environment to exert adverse neurodevelopmental or thyroid toxic effects in the general population. Although the definitive evidence linking environmental TDs with any specific disease in the general population is still lacking, the evidence for a possible threat from environmental TDs is sufficiently compelling to necessitate specific interventions. Guidelines should be developed to identify groups of children who are at high risk for toxicity from DLCs. Both the level of exposure (e.g., maternal consumption of contaminated fish or milk) and vulnerability factors (e.g., a family history of thyroid disease) should be considered. Although it is premature to offer any specific guidelines, clinicians might consider screening for hypothyroidism at 3 and 6 weeks of age in children suspected of having moderate to high DLC exposure and intervene if low values are found. Studies should examine whether intervention is helpful in infants with low thyroid hormone levels. We hypothesize that DLCs and other TDs contribute to an array of long- and short-term neuropsychiatric problems in children. These include learning disorders (particularly language disorders), ADHD, cerebral palsy, hearing loss, and other cognitive-behavioral problems associated with disturbances of thyroid economy.

We suggest that research studies be conducted that elucidate the mechanisms of action of DLC-induced developmental neurotoxicity in humans with a particular emphasis on the role of thyroid hormone. Data that definitively link exposure to low levels of DLCs during the perinatal period with specific long-term thyroid or neurobehavioral disturbance are also of importance. Studies of the delayed effects on neurobehavioral and thyroid systems— especially in postpubertal cohorts exposed perinatally to DLCs— are needed. A recently held environmental health summit identified endocrine modifiers and neurodevelopmental outcomes in children exposed perinatally to DLCs as a priority research area (Baldwin 1996). Those attending expressed special interest in the possible relationship of DLC exposure with such diverse psychiatric disorders as ADHD, depression, delinquency, and pervasive developmental disorders. The effects of DLCs on autoimmunity and reproduction must also be elucidated.

Above all, strategies for reducing population exposure to DLCs and other potential synthetic TDs are needed. DLCs will continue to be present in the food chain and endanger yet another generation. Not only must we find ways to decrease the levels of DLCs in the environment, but we should also develop systems that can help humans and other biological systems reduce their burdens of DLCs.

References

Agrawal AK, Tilson HA, Bondy SC: 3,4,3',4'-tetrachlorobiphenyl given to mice prenatally produces long-term decreases in striatal dopamine and receptor binding sites in the caudate nucleus. Toxicol Lett 7:417–424, 1981

Akoso BT, Sleight RF, Nachreiner RF, et al: Effects of purified polybrominated biphenyl congeners on the thyroid and pituitary glands in rats. Journal of the American College of Toxicologists 1:23–36, 1982

Alleva E, Brock J, Brouwer A, et al: Statement from the work session on environmental endocrine disrupting chemicals: neural, endocrine, and behavioral effects. Toxicol Ind Health 14:1–8, 1998

Anand KJS, Nemeroff CB: Developmental psychoneuroendocrinology, in Child and Adolescent Psychiatry: A Comprehensive Textbook, 2nd Edition. Edited by Lewis M. Baltimore, MD, Williams & Wilkins, 1996, pp 64–86

Anthony A, Adams PM, Stein SA: The effects of congenital hypothyroidism using the hyt/hyt mouse on locomotor activity and learned behavior. Horm Behav 27:418–433, 1993

Ares S, Pastor I, Quero J, et al: Thyroid complications including overt hypothyroidism, related to the use of non-radiopaque Silastic catheters for parenteral feeding in prematures requiring injection of small amounts of an iodinated contrast medium. Acta Pediatr 84:579–582, 1995

Bagchi N, Brown TR, Mack RE: Effects of chronic lithium treatment on hypothalamic-pituitary regulation of thyroid function. Horm Metab Res 14:92–93, 1982

Bahn A, Mills J, Snyder P, et al: Hypothyroidism in workers exposed to polybrominated biphenyls. N Engl J Med 302:31–33, 1980

Baldwin CM: Environmental health summit report: research blueprint for the 21st century. Environ Health Perspect 104:210–213, 1996

Bastomsky CH: Enhanced thyroxine metabolism and high uptake goiters in rats after a single dose of 2,3,7,8-tetrachlorodibenzo-p-dioxin. Endocrinology 101:292–296, 1977

Bastomsky CH, Murthy PVN, Banovac K: Alterations in thyroxine metabolism produced by cutaneous application of microscope immersion oil: effects due to polychlorinated biphenyls. Endocrinology 98:1309–1314, 1976

Bernal J, Nunez J: Thyroid hormones and brain development. Eur J Endocrinol 133:390–398, 1995

Bernal J, Pekonen F: Ontogenesis of the nuclear 3,5,3'-triiodothyronine receptor in the human fetal brain. Endocrinology 114:677–679, 1984

Birnbaum LS: Workshop on perinatal exposure to dioxin-like compounds, V: immunologic effects. Environ Health Perspect 103 (suppl 2):157–160, 1995

Bocchetta A, Bernardi F, Pedditzi M, et al: Thyroid abnormalities during lithium treatment. Acta Psychiatr Scand 83:193–198, 1991

Bombick DW, Jankum J, Tullis K, et al: 2,3,7,8-Tetrachlorodibenzo-*p*-dioxin causes increases in expression of c-erb-A and levels of protein-tyrosine kinases in selected tissues of responsive mouse strains. Proc Natl Acad Sci U S A 85:4128–4132, 1988

Bowman RE, Heironimus MP: Hypoactivity in adolescent monkeys perinatally exposed to PCBs and hyperactivity as juveniles. Neurobehavioral Toxicology and Teratology 3:15–18, 1981

Bowman RE, Heironimus MP, Allen JR: Correlation of PCB body burden with behavioral toxicology in monkeys. Pharmacol Biochem Behav 9:49–56, 1978

Bowman RE, Heironimus MP, Barsotti DD: Locomotor hyperactivity in PCB exposed rhesus monkey. Neurotoxicology 2:251–268, 1981

Bowman RE, Schantz SL, Gross ML, et al: Behavioral effects of monkeys exposed to 2,3,7,8-TCDD transmitted maternally during gestation and for four months of nursing. Chemosphere 18:235–242; 1989

Bowman RE, Schantz SL, Ferguson SA, et al: Gross, controlled exposure of female rhesus monkeys to 2,3,7,8-TCDD; cognitive behavioral effects in their offspring. Chemosphere 20:1103–1108, 1990

Brouwer A: Inhibition of thyroid hormone transport in plasma of rats by polychlorinated biphenyls. Arch Toxicol Suppl 13:440–445, 1989

Brouwer A, van den Berg KJ: Transthyretin (prealbumin) binding of PCBs, a model for the mechanism of interference with vitamin A and thyroid metabolism. Chemosphere 15:1699–1706, 1986

Brouwer A, Klasson-Wehler E, Bodkam M, et al: Competitive inhibition of thyroxin binding to transthyretin by monohydroxy metabolites of 3,4,3',4'-tetrachlorobiphenyl. Chemosphere 20:1257–1262, 1990

Brouwer A, Ahlborg UG, Van den Berg M, et al: Functional aspects of developmental toxicity of polyhalogenated aromatic hydrocarbons in experimental animals and human infants. Eur J Pharmacol 293:1–40, 1995

Brouwer A, Morse D, Lans M, et al: Interaction of persistent environmental organohalogens with the thyroid system: mechanisms and possible consequences for animal and human health. Toxicol Ind Health 14:59–84, 1998

Burrow GN: Mothers are important (editorial). Endocrinology 138:3–4, 1997

Burrow GN, Burke WR, Himmelhoch JM, et al: Effect of lithium on thyroid function. J Clin Endocrinol Metab 32:647–652, 1971

Calaciura F, Mendorla G, Distefano M, et al: Childhood IQ measurements in infants with transient congenital hypothyroidism. Clin Endocrinol 43:473–477, 1995

Calvo R, Obregon MJ, Ruiz de Ona C, et al: Congenital hypothyroidism studied in rats. J Clin Invest 86:889–899, 1990

Carlson JE, Harvey B: Environmental health during childhood: pediatrician advocacy. Pediatr Ann 24:624–628, 1995

Carson R: Silent Spring. Boston, MA, Houghton Mifflin, 1962

Chanoine JP, Boulvain M, Bourdoux P, et al: Increased recall rate at screening for congenital hypothyroidism in breast fed infants born to iodine overloaded mothers. Arch Dis Child 63:1207–1210, 1988

Chen YC, Guo YL, Hsu CC, et al: Cognitive development of yu-cheng ("oil disease"): children prenatally exposed to heat-degraded PCB's. JAMA 268:3213–3218, 1992

Chen YC, Yu ML, Rogan WJ, et al: A 6-year follow-up of behavior and activity disorders in the Taiwan yu-cheng children. Am J Public Health 84:415–421, 1994

Chia LG, Chu F: Neurological studies on polychlorinated biphenyl (PCB)-poisoned patients. Am J Ind Med 5:117–126, 1984

Chia LG, Chu F: A clinical and electrophysiological study of patients with polychlorinated biphenyl poisoning. J Neurol Neurosurg Psychiatry 48:894–901, 1985

Chiovato L, Tonacchera M, Lapi P, et al: Thyroid autoimmunity and neuropsychological development. Acta Med Austriaca 19 (suppl 1):91–95, 1992

Chou SM, Miike T, Payne WM, et al: Neuropathology of "spinning syndrome" induced by prenatal intoxication with a PCB in mice. Ann N Y Acad Sci 320:373–396, 1979

Colborn T, Dumanoski D, Myers JP: Our Stolen Future. New York, Dutton/Penguin Books, 1996

Collins W, Capen C: Fine structural lesions and hormone alterations in thyroid glands of perinatal rats exposed in utero and by milk to polychlorinated biphenyls. Am J Pathol 99:125–142, 1980

Damstra T, McMohan A: Introduction to symposium: tots and toxins-altered brains. Environ Health Perspect 102 (suppl 2):115, 1994

de Duffard AM, Duffard R: Behavioral toxicology, risk assessment, and chlorinated hydrocarbons. Environ Health Perspect 104 (suppl 2): 353–360, 1996

DeGroot LJ, Larsen PR, Henneman G: The Thyroid and Its Diseases, 6th Edition. New York, Churchill Livingstone, 1996

Delange F, Ermans A: Iodine deficiency, in Werner and Ingbar's The Thyroid: A Fundamental and Clinical Text, 7th Edition. Edited by Braverman L, Utiger R. Philadelphia, PA, JB Lippincott, 1996, pp 296–315

Delange F, Chanoine JP, Abrassart C, et al: Topical iodine, breastfeeding, and neonatal hypothyroidism. Arch Dis Child 63:106–110, 1988

DeLong GR: The neuromuscular system and brain in hypothyroidism, in Werner and Ingbar's The Thyroid: A Fundamental and Clinical Text, 7th Edition. Edited by Braverman L, Utiger R. Philadelphia, PA, JB Lippincott, 1996, pp 826–835

deVijlder JM, Vulsma T, Kooistra L, et al: The importance of partial deprivation of iodine and thyroid hormone during pregnancy for the offspring. Abstracts from the Merck European Thyroid Symposium, Warsaw, Poland, May 16–18, 1996. Thyroid 6:667, 1996

Dewailly E, Bruneau S, Ayotte P: Health status at birth of Inuit newborn prenatally exposed to organochlorines. Chemosphere 27:359–366, 1993

De Wolf D, De Schepper J, Verhaaren H, et al: Congenital hypothyroid goiter and amiodarone. Acta Paediatr Scand 77:616–618, 1988

DiGeorge AM, LaFranchi S: Hyperthyroidism, in Nelson's Textbook of Pediatrics, 15th Edition. Edited by Nelson WE, Behrman RE, Kleigman RM, Arvin AM. Philadelphia, PA, WB Saunders, 1996, pp 1600–1602

Dratman MB: Cerebral versus peripheral regulation and utilization of thyroid hormones, in The Thyroid Axis and Psychiatric Illness. Edited by Joffe R, Levitt A. Washington, DC, American Psychiatric Press, 1993, pp 1–94

Dussault JH, Ruel J: Thyroid hormones and brain development. Annu Rev Physiol 49:321–334, 1987

Eayrs JT: The cerebral cortex of normal and hypothyroid rats. Acta Anat 25:160–183, 1955

Emmet E, Maroni M, Jefferys J, et al: Studies of transformer repair workers exposed to PCBs. Am J Ind Med 14:47–62, 1988

Ericksson P: Effects of 3,3', 4,4'-tetrachlorobiphenyl in the brain of the neonatal mouse. Toxicology 49:43–48, 1988

Ericksson P, Lundkvist U, Fredrickson A: Neonatal exposure to 3,3',4,4'-tetrachlorobiphenyl: changes in spontaneous behavior and cholinergic muscarinic receptors in the adult mouse. Toxicology 69:27–34, 1991

Farsetti A, Mitsuhashi T, Desvergne B, et al: Molecular basis of thyroid hormone regulation of myelin basic protein gene expression in rodent brain. J Biol Chem 266:23226–23232, 1991

Farwell A, Braverman L: Thyroid and antithyroid drugs, in Goodman and Gilman's The Pharmacological Basis of Therapeutics, 9th Edition. Edited by Hardman G, Limbird LE. New York, McGraw-Hill, 1995, pp 1383–1409

Feeley MM: Workshop on perinatal exposure to dioxin-like compounds, III: endocrine effects. Environ Health Perspect 103 (suppl 2):147–150, 1995

Fein G, Jacoboson JL, Jacoboson S, et al: Prenatal exposure to polychlorinated biphenyls: effects on birth size and gestational age. J Pediatr 105:315–320, 1984

Ferreiro B, Bernal J, Goodyer G, et al: Estimation of nuclear thyroid hormone saturation in human fetal brain and lung during early gestation. J Clin Endocrinol Metab 67:853–856, 1988

Foley TP: Congenital hypothyroidism, in Werner and Ingbar's The Thyroid: A Fundamental and Clinical Text, 7th Edition. Edited by Braverman L, Utiger R. Philadelphia, PA, JB Lippincott, 1996, pp 988–994

Fry DM: Reproductive effects in birds exposed to pesticides and industrial chemicals. Environ Health Perspect 103 (suppl 7):165–171, 1995

Gaitan E: Environmental aspects, in Diseases of The Thyroid. Edited by Wheeler MH, Lazarus JH. London, Chapman & Hall, 1994, pp 73–84

Ginsburg J: Tackling Environmental Endocrine Disrupters. Lancet 347:1501–1502, 1996

Gladen BC, Rogan WJ: Effects of perinatal polychlorinated biphenyls and dichlorodiphenyl dichloroethene on later development. J Pediatr 119:58–63, 1991

Gladen BC, Rogan WJ, Hardy P, et al: Development after exposure to polychlorinated biphenyls and dichlorodiphenyl dichloroethene transplacentally and through breast milk. J Pediatr 113:991–995, 1988

Goldman PS, Rosvold HE, Vest B, et al: Analysis of delayed-alternation deficit produced by dorsolateral prefrontal lesions in the rhesus monkey. Journal of Comparative and Physiological Psychology 77:212–220, 1971

Golub MS, Jacobson SW: Workshop on perinatal exposure to dioxin-like compounds, IV: neurobehavioral effects. Environ Health Perspect 103 (suppl 2):151–155, 1995

Green WL: Antithyroid compounds, in Werner and Ingbar's The Thyroid, 7th Edition. Edited by Braverman L, Utiger R. Philadelphia, PA, JB Lippincott, 1996, pp 266–276

Grumbach MM, Werner SC: Transfer of thyroid hormone across the human placenta at term. J Clin Endocrinol Metab 16:1392–1395, 1956

Guillette LJ, Crain A, Rooney AA: Organization versus activation: the role of endocrine-disrupting contaminants (EDCs) during embryonic development in wildlife. Environ Health Perspect 103 (suppl 7): 157–164, 1995

Harjai KJ, Licata AA: Effects of amiodarone on thyroid function. Ann Intern Med 126:63–73, 1997

Hartman DE: Neuropsychological Toxicology: Identification and Assessment of Human Neurotoxic Syndromes, 2nd Edition. New York, Plenum, 1995, pp 401–404

Hauser P, McMillin JM, Bhatara VS: Resistance to thyroid hormone: implications for neurodevelopmental research on the effects of thyroid hormone disruptors. Toxicol Ind Health 14:85–101, 1998

Hedberg CW, Janssen RS, Meyers B, et al: An outbreak of thyrotoxicosis caused by the consumption of bovine thyroid gland in ground beef. N Engl J Med 316:993–998, 1987

Hendrich CE, Porterfield SP: Serum growth hormone levels in hypothyroid and GH-treated thyroidectomized rats and their progenies. Proc Soc Exp Biol Med 201:296, 1992

Henry E, Gasiewicz T: Changes in thyroid hormones and thyroid glucuronidation in hamsters compared with rats following treatment with 2,3,7,8-tetrachlorodibenzo-dioxin. Toxicol Appl Pharmacol 89: 165–174, 1987

Heussen Kikspoors ML, Spenkelink A, Brouwer A, et al: Inhibition of binding of thyroxin to transthyretin by outdoor and indoor airborne particulate matter and effects on thyroid hormone and vitamin A metabolism in rats. Arch Environ Contam Toxicol 23:6–12, 1992

Holmes EJ, Butters N, Jacobson S, et al: An effect of mammary-body lesions on reversal learning sets in monkeys. Physiological Psychology 11:159–165, 1983

Hsu ST, Ma CI, Hsu SK, et al: Discovery and epidemiology of PCB poisoning in Taiwan: a four year follow-up. Environ Health Perspect 59:5–10, 1985

Jacobson JL, Jacobson SW: Intellectual impairment in children exposed to polychlorinated biphenyls in utero. N Engl J Med 335:783–789, 1996

Jacobson JL, Jacobson SW: Evidence for PCBs as neurodevelopmental toxicants in humans. Neurotoxicology 18:415–424, 1997

Jacobson JL, Jacobson SW, Fein CG, et al: Prenatal exposure to an environmental toxin: a test of the multiple effects model. Dev Psychol 20:523–532, 1984

Jacobson SW, Fein G, Jacoboson JL, et al: The effects of intrauterine PCB exposure on visual recognition memory. Child Dev 56:853–860, 1985

Jacobson JL, Jacobson SW, Humphrey H: Effects of in utero exposure to polychlorinated biphenyls and related contaminants on cognitive functioning in young children. J Pediatr 116:38–45, 1990a

Jacobson JL, Jacobson SW, Humphrey H: Effects of exposure to PCBs and related compounds on growth and activity in children. Neurotoxicol Teratol 12:319–326, 1990b

James RC, Busch H, Tamburro CH, et al: Polychlorinated biphenyl exposure and human diseases. Journal of Occupational Medicine 35:136–148, 1993

Jefferson JW, Griest JH: Primer of Lithium Therapy. Baltimore, MD, Williams & Wilkins, 1977

Joffe R, Levitt A: The thyroid and depression, in The Thyroid Axis and Psychiatric Illness. Edited by Joffe R, Levitt A. Washington DC, American Psychological Press, 1993, pp 195–253

Jones WS, Man EB: Thyroid function in human pregnancy, VI: premature deliveries and reproductive failures of pregnant women with low serum butanol-extractable iodines. Maternal serum TBG and TBPA capacities. Am J Obstet Gynecol 104:909–914, 1969

Kaplan MM: Interactions between drugs and thyroid hormones. Thyroid Today 4(5):1–6, 1981

Kavlock RJ, Daston GP, De Rosa C, et al: Research needs for risk assessment of health and environmental effects of endocrine disruptors: a report of the US EPA–sponsored workshop. Environ Health Perspect 104 (suppl 4):715–740, 1996

Kinney JS, Hurwitz ES, Fishbein DB, et al: Community outbreak of thyrotoxicosis: epidemiology, immunogenetic characteristics, and long-term outcome. Am J Med 84:10–18, 1988

Koja T, Fujisaka T, Shimizu T, et al: Changes of gross behavior with polychlorinated biphenyls (PCBs) in immature rats [in Japanese]. Kagoshima Daigaka Igaka Zasshi 30:377–381, 1978

Koja T, Kishita C, Shimizu T, et al: Effects of polychlorinated biphenyls (PCBs) on the gross behavior of immature rats and the influence of drugs upon them [in Japanese]. Kagoshima Daigaka Igaka Zasshi 31:315–319, 1979

Koopman-Esseboom C, Morse DC, Weisglas-Kuperus N, et al: Effects of dioxins and polychlorinated biphenyls on thyroid hormone status of pregnant women and their infants. Pediatr Res 36:468–473, 1994

Koopman-Esseboom C, Weisglas-Kuperus N, de Ridder MAJ, et al: Effects of polychlorinated biphenyl/dioxin exposure and feeding type on infants' mental and psychomotor development. Pediatrics 97:700–706, 1996

L'Allemand D, Gruters AJ, Beyer P, et al: Iodine in contrast agents and skin disinfectants is the major cause for hypothyroidism in premature infants during intensive care. Horm Res 28:42–49, 1987

Lauder JM: The effects of early hypo- and hyperthyroidism on the development of rat cerebellar cortex: kinetics of cell proliferation in the external granular layer. Brain Res 126:31–51, 1977

Leatherland JF: Changes in thyroid hormone economy following consumption of environmentally contaminated Great Lakes fish. Toxicol Ind Health 14:41–58, 1998

Levin ED, Schantz SL, Bowman RE: Delayed spatial alternation deficits resulting from perinatal PCB exposure of monkeys. Arch Toxicol 62:267–273, 1988

Levin ED, Schantz SL, Bowman RE: The lesion model of neurotoxic effects on cognitive function in monkeys. Neurotoxicol Teratol 14:131–141, 1992

Lilienthal H, Neuf M, Munoz C, et al: Behavioral effects of pre- and postnatal exposure to a mixture of low chlorinated PCBs in rats. Fundamental and Applied Toxicology 33:282–293, 1990

Lindstrom G, Hooper K, Petreas M, et al: Workshop on perinatal exposure of dioxin-like compounds: summary. Environ Health Perspect 103 (suppl 2):135–142, 1995

Lombardi A, Martino E, Braverman LE: Amiodarone and the thyroid. Thyroid Today 13(2):1–7, 1990

Lonky E, Reihman J, Darvill T, et al: Neonatal behavioral assessment scale performance influenced by maternal consumption of environmentally contaminated Lake Ontario fish. Journal of Great Lakes Research 22:198–212, 1996

Mahut H: Spatial and object reversal learning in monkeys with partial temporal lobe ablations. Neuropsychologica 9:409–424, 1971

Man EB, Holden RH, Jones WS: Thyroid function in human pregnancy, VII: development and retardation of 4-year-old progeny of euthyroid and of hypothyroxinemic women. Am J Obstet Gynecol 109:12–19, 1971

Mannisto PT: Thyroid iodine metabolism in vitro, II: effect of lithium ion. Annales Medicinae Experimentalis et Biologiae Fenniae 51:42–45, 1973

Martino E, Aghini-Lombardi F, Mariotti S, et al: Amiodarone-induced hypothyroidism: risk factors and follow-up in 28 cases. Clin Endocrinol 26:227–237, 1987

McKinney JD: Multifunctional receptor model for dioxin and related compound toxic action: possible thyroid hormone-responsive effector-linked site. Environ Health Perspect 82:323–336, 1989

McKinney JD, Chae K, Oatley SJ, et al: Molecular interactions of toxic chlorinated dibenzo-p-dioxins and dibenzofurans with thyroxine binding prealbumin. J Med Chem 28:375–381, 1985

Meier CA, Burger AG: Effects of pharmacologic agents on thyroid hormone homeostasis, in Werner and Ingbar's The Thyroid, 7th Edition. Edited by Braverman L, Utiger R. Philadelphia, PA, JB Lippincott, 1996, pp 276–286

Mele P, Bowman R, Levin E: Behavioral evaluation of perinatal PCB exposure in rhesus monkeys: fixed-interval performance and reinforcement omission. Neurobehav Toxicol Teratol 8:131–138, 1986

Mellström B, Naranjo JR, Santos A, et al: Independent expression of the α and β c-erb A genes in developing rat brain. Mol Endocrinol 5:1339–1350, 1991

Moccia RD, Leatherland JF, Sonstegard RA: Increasing frequency of thyroid goiters in coho salmon (*Oncorhynchus kisutch*) in the Great Lakes. Science 198:425–426, 1977

Morreale de Escobar G, Escobar del Rey F, Ruiz-Marcos A: Thyroid hormone and the developing brain, in Congenital Hypothyroidism. Edited by Dussault JH, Walker P. New York, Marcel Dekker, 1983, pp 85–127

Morse DC, Brouwer A: Perinatal alterations of thyroid homeostasis and long-term neurochemical alterations in rats following Aroclor 1254 exposure. Organohalogen Compounds 21:439–443, 1994

Morse DC, Koeter HB, van Prooijen AE, et al: Interference of polychlorinated biphenyls in thyroid hormone metabolism: possible neurotoxic consequences in fetal and neonatal rats. Chemosphere 25 (1,2):165–168, 1992

Morse DC, Groen D, Veerman M, et al: Interference of polychlorinated biphenyls in hepatic and brain thyroid metabolism in fetal and neonatal rats. Toxicol Appl Pharmacol 122:27–33, 1993

Munoz A, Rodriguez-Peña A, Perez-Castillo A, et al: Effects of neonatal hypothyroidism on rat brain gene expression. Mol Endocrinol 5: 273–280, 1991

Murai K, Okamura K, Tsuji E, et al: Thyroid function in "yusho" patients exposed to polychlorinated biphenyls (PCBs). Environ Res 44: 179–187, 1987

Myant NB: Passage of thyroxine and triiodothyronine from mother to fetus in pregnant women. Clin Sci 17:75–79, 1958

Ness DK, Schantz SL, Moshtaghian J, et al: Effects of perinatal exposure to specific PCB congeners on thyroid hormone concentrations and thyroid histology in the rat. Toxicol Lett 68:311–323, 1993

Overmann S, Kostas J, Wilson L, et al: Neurobehavioral and somatic effects of perinatal PCB exposure in rats. Environ Res 44:56–70, 1987

Panteleoni G, Fannini D, Sponta A, et al: Effects of maternal exposure to PCBs on F1 generation behavior of rats. Fundamental and Applied Toxicology 11:440–449, 1988

Perrild H, Hegedus L, Baastrup PC, et al: Thyroid function and ultrasonically determined thyroid size in patients receiving long-term lithium treatment. Am J Psychiatry 147:1518–1521, 1990

Piosik PA, van Groenigen M, van Doorn J, et al: Effect of maternal thyroid status on thyroid hormones and growth in congenitally hypothyroid goat fetuses during the second half of gestation. Endocrinology 138:5–11, 1997

Pipaon C, Santos A, Perez-Castillo A: Thyroid hormone up-regulates NGFI-A gene expression in rat brain during development. J Biol Chem 267:21–23, 1992

Pluim HJ, Koope JG, Olie K: Effects of dioxins and furans on thyroid hormone regulation in the human newborn. Chemosphere 27:391–394, 1993a

Pluim HJ, de Vijlder JJ, Olie K, et al: Effects of pre- and postnatal exposure to chlorinated dioxins and furans on human neonatal thyroid hormone concentrations. Environ Health Perspect 101:504–508, 1993b

Porterfield SP: Vulnerability of the developing brain to thyroid abnormalities: environmental insults to the thyroid system. Environ Health Perspect 102 (suppl 2):125–130, 1994

Porterfield SP, Hendrich CE: The role of thyroid hormones in prenatal and neonatal neurological development—current perspectives. Endocr Rev 14:94–106, 1993

Porterfield SP, Hendry L: Impact of PCBs on thyroid hormone–directed brain development. Toxicol Ind Health 14:103–120, 1998

Rao CV, Banerji SA: Effect of polychlorinated biphenyl (Aroclor 1260) on histology of kidney and thyroid of rats. Indian J Exp Biol 28:152–154, 1990

Rattner BA: Endocrine responses to avian environmental pollutants. J Exp Zool 232:683–685, 1984

Reus VI, Gold P, Post R: Lithium-induced thyrotoxicosis. Am J Psychiatry 136:724–725, 1979

Reuss ML, Paneth N, Pinto-Martin JA, et al: The relation of transient hypothyroxinemia in preterm infants to neurologic development at two years of age. N Engl J Med 334:821–827, 1996

Rickenbacher U, McKinney JD, Oatley SJ, et al: Structurally specific binding of halogenated biphenyls to thyroxine transport protein. J Med Chem 29:641–648, 1986

Rodier PM: Vulnerable periods and processes during central nervous system development. Environ Health Perspect 102 (suppl 2):121–124, 1994

Rogan WJ, Gladen BC: Neurotoxicity of PCBs. Neurotoxicology 13:27–39, 1992

Rogan WJ, Gladen BC, McKinney JD, et al: Neonatal effects of transplacental exposure to PCBs and DDE. J Pediatr 109:335–341, 1986

Rogan WJ, Gladen BC, McKinney JD, et al: Polychlorinated biphenyls (PCBs) and dichlorodiphenyl dichloroethene (DDE) in human milk: effects on growth, morbidity, and duration of lactation. Am J Public Health 77:1294–1297, 1987

Rogan WJ, Gladen BC, Hung K, et al: Congenital poisoning by polychlorinated biphenyls and their contaminants in Taiwan. Science 241:334–336, 1988

Roti E, Braverman LE: Iodine excess and thyroid function. Abstracts from the Merck European Thyroid Symposium, Warsaw, Poland, May 16–18, 1996. Thyroid 6:663, 1996

Roti E, Vagenakis AG: Effects of excess iodide: clinical aspects, in Werner and Ingbar's The Thyroid, 7th Edition. Edited by Braverman L, Utiger R. Philadelphia, PA, JB Lippincott, 1996, pp 316–327

Rozman K, Rozman T, Graham H: Effects of thyroidectomy and thyroxine on 2,3,7,8-tetrachlorodibenzo-p-dioxin induced toxicity. Toxicol Appl Pharmacol 72:372–379, 1984

Sauer P, Huisman M, Koopman-Esseboom C, et al: Effects of polychlorinated biphenyls (PCBs) and dioxins on growth and development. Hum Exp Toxicol 13:901–906, 1994

Schantz SL, Bowman RE: Learning in monkeys exposed perinatally to 2,3,7,8-tetrachlorodibenzo-p-dioxin (TCDD). Neurotoxicol Teratol 11:13–19, 1989

Schantz SL, Levin ED, Bowman RE, et al: Effects of perinatal PCB exposure on discrimination-reversal learning in monkeys in peer group. Neurotoxicol Teratol 11:243–250, 1989

Schantz SL, Levin ED, Bowman RE: Long-term neurobehavioral effects of perinatal PCB exposure in monkeys. Environmental Toxicology and Chemistry 10:747–756, 1992

Schultz M, Muller R, Von Zur Muhlen A, et al: Induction of hyperthyroidism by interferon-alpha-2b. Lancet 1:1452, 1989

Seegal RF: The neurochemical effects of PCB exposure are age-dependent. Arch Toxicol Suppl 16:128–137, 1994

Seegal RF, Schantz SL: Neurochemical and behavioral sequelae of exposure to dioxins and PCBs, in Dioxins and Health. Edited by Schecter A. New York, Plenum, 1994, pp 136–144

Seegal RF, Brosch K, Bush B, et al: Effects of Aroclor 1254 on dopamine and norepinephrine concentrations in pheochromocytoma (PC-12) cells. Neurotoxicology 10:757–764, 1989

Seegal RF, Bush B, Brosch K: Comparison of effects of Aroclor 1016 and 1260 on catecholamine function in nonhuman primates. Toxicology 66:145–163, 1991

Sher ES, Xu XM, Adams P, et al: The effects of thyroid hormone level and action in developing brain: are these targets for actions of polychlorinated biphenyls and dioxins? Toxicol Ind Health 14:121–158, 1998

Shiota K: Postnatal behavioral effects of prenatal treatment with PCBs (polychlorinated biphenyls) in rats. Okajimas Folia Anat Jpn 53: 105–144, 1976

Smallridge RC: Thyroid function tests, in Principles and Practice of Endocrinology and Metabolism, 2nd Edition. Edited by Becker KL. Philadelphia, PA, JB Lippincott, 1995, pp 299–307

Smerdely P, Lim A, Boyages SC, et al: Topical iodine-containing antiseptics and neonatal hypothyroidism in very-low-birth-weight infants. Lancet 2:661–662, 1989

Sonestegard RA, Leatherland JF: Hypothyroidism in rats fed Great Lakes coho salmon. Bull Environ Contam Toxicol 22:779–784, 1979

Spaulding SW, Burrow GN, Bermudez F, et al: The inhibitory effect of lithium on thyroid hormone release in both euthyroid and thyrotoxic patients. J Clin Endocrinol Metab 35:905–911, 1972

Spear PA, Higueret P, Garcis H: Increased thyroxine turnover after 3,3',4,4',5,5'-hexabromobiphenyl injection and lack of effect on peripheral triiodothyronine production. Can J Physiol Pharmacol 68: 1079–1084, 1990

Storm J, Hart J, Smith R: Behavior of mice after pre- and postnatal exposure to Aroclor 1254. Neurobehav Toxicol Teratol 3:5–9, 1981

Surks MS, Sievert R: Drugs and thyroid function. N Engl J Med 333: 1688–1694, 1995

Theodoropoulos T, Braverman LE, Vagenakis AG: Iodine-induced hypothyroidism: a potential hazard during fetal life. Science 205: 502–504, 1979

Tilson HA, Davis GJ, Mclachlan JA, et al: The effects of polychlorinated biphenyls given prenatally on the neurobehavioral development of mice. Environ Res 19:466–474, 1979

Tilson HA, Jacobson JL, Rogan WJ: Polychlorinated biphenyls and developing nervous system: cross-species comparisons. Neurotoxicol Teratol 12:239–248, 1990

Vanden Heuvel JP, Lucier G: Environmental toxicity of polychlorinated dibenzo-*p*-dioxins and polychlorinated dibenzofurans. Environ Health Perspect 100:189–200, 1993

Vulsma T, Kok JH: Prematurity-associated neurologic and developmental abnormalities and neonatal thyroid function. N Engl J Med 334: 857–858, 1996

Vulsma T, Gons MH, de Vijlder JJ: Maternal-fetal transfer of thyroxine in congenital hypothyroidism due to a total organification defect or thyroid dysgenesis. N Engl J Med 321:13–16, 1989

Walker P: Developmental actions of thyroid hormones, in Congenital Hypothyroidism. Edited by Dussault JH, Walker P. New York, Marcel Dekker, 1983, pp 63–85

Welch LS: Environmental toxins and endocrine functions, in Principles and Practice of Endocrinology and Metabolism, 2nd Edition. Edited by Becker KL. Philadelphia, PA, JB Lippincott, 1995, pp 1900–1907

Whitlock JP: Genetic and molecular toxicity of 2,3,7,8-tetrachlorobenzo-*p*-dioxin action. Annu Rev Pharmacol Toxicol 30:251–261, 1990

Woeber KA: Iodine and thyroid disease. Med Clin North Am 75:169–178, 1991

Wolff J, Chaikoff IL: Plasma inorganic iodide as homeostatic regulator of thyroid function. J Biol Chem 174:555–564, 1948

Conclusions

Peter Hauser, M.D., and Joanne Rovet, Ph.D.

Thyroid hormone is an extremely important hormone for children's intellectual functioning and behavior. This volume has demonstrated that thyroid hormone has a multiplicity of effects on different organ systems, primary of which is the brain. The role of thyroid hormone in major neurodevelopmental processes is well described by the authors contributing chapters to this book. They have shown that when thyroid hormone levels are too high or too low, especially during gestation and early life, important structural processes, such as neuronal migration, myelination, or synaptogenesis, will be disrupted. There also may be effects on different neurotransmitter systems, and the timing of the thyroid hormone abnormality is key to the type of abnormality that occurs.

Part I of this volume, which presented a comprehensive description of the mechanisms of thyroid hormone action at the molecular and physiological levels, described the complexity of the actions of thyroid hormone and their biological significance. Part II described the major pediatric disorders associated with abnormalities of thyroid hormone synthesis and regulation. Part II, which has been organized to describe the behavioral consequences of thyroid hormone disruption at different stages of development, provided information about both congenital and acquired disorders of both deficiency and excess of thyroid hormone. Collectively, the chapters in Part II convey the message that abnormalities in behavior or cognitive functioning, sometimes severe, occur if thyroid hormone production is altered. The final chapter—on how environmental contaminants disrupt thyroid hormone production—has provided a timely and shocking discussion showing the necessity of this hormone for human development and the dire consequences of tampering with it in utero or in early life.

Part I—Thyroid Hormone Physiology and Function

In the first chapter of Part I, Dr. Lash, who examines the thyroid system globally in terms of hormone synthesis and regulation, has outlined how the hypothalamic-pituitary-thyroid axis functions to maintain thyroid hormone homeostasis in the body. His description of the role of deiodinase enzymes and their developmental regulation in allowing appropriate thyroid hormone levels within the cell shows how appropriate thyroid concentrations might be maintained at critical times in the brain when the thyroid supply is abnormal. Dr. Lash thereby set the stage for the chapters that follow on primary pediatric disorders of fetal, infant, and later childhood thyroid dysfunction as well as on disorders that are secondary to abnormal maternal supply in utero. His message calling for timely and alternative therapies and stating the critical importance for early treatment of congenital hypothyroidism is a prelude to the first chapter in Part II on newborn screening.

In Chapter 2, Dr. Meier has provided a comprehensive review of the molecular actions of thyroid hormone and thyroid hormone receptors. He has described how thyroid hormone is synthesized, its mode of action at the nuclear level in brain cells, and its time course of action on the developing brain. He has also provided evidence concerning the need for timely expression of thyroid-responsive genes in the production of essential proteins for normal brain development. His descriptions of thyroid hormone–regulated target genes and their mutations and of thyroid hormone receptors have set the stage for the discussions later in this volume on resistance to thyroid hormone (RTH) and its associated sequelae. Dr. Meier's review of alternative mechanisms for modulating thyroid hormone action subsequent to thyroid receptor mutations, such as the "dominant negative effect," conveys a potential mechanism of action for physiological adaptation and neuroplasticity.

Part II—Clinical Studies of Thyroid Diseases in Infancy and Childhood

The first chapter in Part II is on newborn screening for metabolic disorders. In this chapter, Dr. Pass has provided a historical overview of newborn screening and its suitability for diagnosing congenital hypothyroidism in the neonate before the appearance of any clinical symptoms. Because early diagnosis following newborn screening has allowed for prompt treatment, it was recognized that mass screening of neonates might prevent the tragic and devastating effects of cretinism. Dr. Pass, who is one of the North American leaders in the newborn screening arena, has enlightened the reader concerning current practices regarding specimen collection, laboratory techniques, notification, and diagnosis. Problems with early discharge, missed cases, and false-positive reporting are highlighted, and guidelines for treatment and management are presented. Capitalizing on the author's experience, this chapter has provided important clinical information for the treatment and management of children with congenital hypothyroidism (CH) and has additionally described several new and exciting screening techniques for diseases beyond CH. These include screening for HIV, for single-gene disorders (e.g., sickle cell disease, cystic fibrosis, Duchenne muscular dystrophy, and thalassemia), and for diseases that present in later life (e.g., Huntington's chorea, diabetes, Alzheimer's dementia). In addition, the expansion of newborn thyroid screening programs to assess for high levels of thyroid hormone has opened up the possibility of screening for RTH and, quite possibly, congenital Graves' disease. The efforts of Drs. Pass, Hauser, and Mizejewski in their recent collaboration have shown the potential of newborn screening for identifying attention-deficit/hyperactivity disorder (ADHD) at birth in a segment of the affected population. By having an early impact on ADHD symptomatology, newborn screening may benefit the emotional and social development of affected children and their families.

In the chapter on congenital hypothyroidism by Dr. Rovet, the findings on early-treated CH—now possible with newborn screening—are summarized. Despite significantly reduced morbidity of this once devastating pediatric disorder, these children remain at risk for lower IQs and selective cognitive, hearing, and neuromotor impairments. The timing and severity of neonatal thyroid hormone deficiency are shown to be critical for the types of neurocognitive impairment that persist. This chapter serves to sensitize the reader to the fact that the different findings among the various research programs may reflect the specific screening techniques, because different diagnostic criteria can result in the inclusion of children with different CH etiologies. It also represents the first attempt to describe the clinical picture of early-treated CH, which was until now based mainly on group or subgroup averages of children studied prospectively. The consequences of thyroid hormone replacement dosage and the need for continuous later monitoring are stressed, particularly to ensure normal thyroid hormone levels and prevent attentional dysfunction associated with high levels of thyroid hormone.

The chapter by Dr. Hauser on resistance to thyroid hormone has synthesized existing knowledge on this recently described disorder. RTH represents the first known association between an autosomal dominant single-gene disorder and ADHD. The sequelae of RTH have relevance for specific neuropsychological and psychoeducational deficits, as well as for attentional disorders, and RTH represents a human model for studying the effects of thyroid disruption on brain development. Indeed, this has been supported in the recent studies by Hauser and colleagues using magnetic resonance imaging (MRI) and positron-emission tomography (PET) technologies. These studies showed that patients with RTH have structural anomalies of the corpus callosum and Sylvian fissure as well as abnormalities of anterior cingulate and right parietal lobe metabolism, which are relevant structures for attentional and language processing. As Hauser has aptly pointed out, a comparison of the findings between CH and RTH conditions may ultimately reveal a more refined picture of the neurodevelopmental effects of moderate impairments in thyroid function on the brain.

Next, a clinical portrait of acquired hypothyroidism in childhood was provided by Drs. Rovet and Daneman. This disorder was poorly studied from a behavioral perspective until these authors observed three adolescents who developed severe and persisting behavioral pathology following the initiation of thyroxine replacement therapy. Unlike CH and RTH, juvenile hypothyroidism has few behavioral sequelae; however, significant iatrogenic effects may occur after the initiation of therapy in a small proportion of affected children. When Rovet and Daneman subsequently studied 23 newly diagnosed and treated cases prospectively, they observed less severe iatrogenicity, with only about 25% of children affected and to a much milder degree. Their discussions of the etiology of these behavioral disturbances have implications for the role of thyroid hormone in neurotransmitter regulation.

Drs. Bhatara and McMillin, in their chapter on the disorders associated with elevations of thyroid hormone, have provided an elegant and thorough review of the clinical picture, including cognitive and behavioral manifestations, of such conditions as congenital Graves' disease, thyrotoxicosis factitia, and neonatal thyrotoxicosis. A pediatric neuropsychiatrist with a deep-seated interest in thyroid hormone, Dr. Bhatara has provided descriptions and findings of psychiatric conditions mimicking thyrotoxicosis as well as speculation (and findings) that an underlying abnormality in thyroid hormone regulation may be contributing to certain disorders. In particular, he and Dr. McMillin have presented exciting findings on different thyroid hormone abnormalities among different subgroups of patients with ADHD. This chapter has served to increase our awareness of the need to rule out thyrotoxicosis in diagnosing pediatric psychiatric disorders and of the high-risk situations in which conducting thyroid function tests may be indicated.

A central feature among all the pediatric disorders sampled in this book is that thyroid hormone appears to play an important role in attentional cognitive processing. Just as the sex hormones are often linked to cognitive behavior associated with verbal and spatial processing while the adrenal hormones are associated with stress and its management, it may be that thyroid hormone is the hormone regulating human attention. In light of recent studies demonstrating thyroid hormone's involvement in neurotransmitter regulation, the current, ongoing, and proposed work in our laboratories, as well as the laboratories of other investigators, may help to clarify more precisely the role of thyroid hormone in attention. The sensitive and astute acumen of clinicians like Drs. Daneman and Bhatara has opened our eyes to the possibility of thyroid disorders masking as psychopathology as well as psychopathology arising from thyroid disorders.

The study of environmental contaminants and toxins such as polychlorinated biphenyls (PCBs) signifies that not all thyroid disorders are caused endogenously. Indeed, findings of effects from ingestion of contaminated beef in the midwestern United States and the potential for acute thyrotoxic-linked psychopathology in young children suggest the need for adequate controls within the food industry. Similarly, the effects of intrauterine and postnatal PCB exposure on neurobehavioral functioning are alarming, although control of these substances may come too late to prevent the risk of attention, cognitive, and somatic disorders. There is a growing consensus that certain PCBs bear a striking resemblance to thyroid hormone and may compete with it at the receptor site, thereby disabling critical genes. Thus, although PCBs are no longer produced, the facts that they remain in the environment and appear to be potentiated in the food chain are frightening. Similar implications for other toxicants magnify the enormity of the problem. The final chapter by Drs. Bhatara, Hauser, and McMillin on thyroid disrupters therefore offers a timely treatise on this alarming issue. These authors enlighten the reader concerning the potential hazards to intellectual and behavioral development from exposure to these omnipresent synthetic substances, particularly during and shortly after gestation. Because most of the current research is based on animals, these authors have sensitized us to the fact that the time has now come to devote greater study to children with such exposures. With statistics showing annual increments in the rates of learning disabilities, ADHD, and pediatric anxiety disorders in the general population increasing annually, one wonders about the role of environmental contaminants in adversely shaping the neurodevelopment of today's youth and of our future progeny. We have just begun to realize that we may only be seeing the tip of the iceberg. The new research directions, to which the authors allude, must be addressed.

When we originally conceived of this volume, we did not consider problems associated with iodine deficiency because we did not see it as a North American issue. Nevertheless, we do recognize that lack of iodine—which still exists in developed countries such as Belgium, as well as in much of the underdeveloped world—may cause the most severe form of thyroid hormone deficiency, neurological cretinism. However, as Dr. Bhatara has pointed out, the potential for iodine excess does exist in North America because of the use of food products (e.g., kelp), medications (e.g., amiodarone), and topical preparations (e.g., povidone iodine) that can predispose a child to thyrotoxicosis and possibly hypothyroidism.

Future Directions

Where do we go from here? Although there is little disagreement about the findings from studies of children exposed to too much or too little thyroid hormone, we do not know the precise mechanism of action of thyroid hormone on human brain development. Animal studies have shown marked pathology secondary to thyroid hormone lack or excess at critical stages of development. In vitro studies have shown, for example, that myelin synthesis may be normalized in thyroid-deficient animals following treatment with thyroid hormone.

Although studies of children with CH identified by screening indicate that subtle selective deficits may persist despite early treatment, there are no neuroimaging studies on this population to suggest that abnormalities in brain development occur. The only neuroimaging research is on late-treated and severely affected patients, who were normalized following the initiation of therapy. However, as the methods in these studies were relatively gross and did not allow for observation of more subtle effects, the jury is still not in. On the other hand, Hauser has described permanent structural and functional abnormalities in the RTH population, and his most recent studies of the corpus callosum have shown that the formation of white matter (myelin) is indeed impaired. Comparable studies are needed in early-treated CH, including newer and more sensitive qualitative studies of myelin abnormalities as well as volumetric MRI and PET.

An early study by Moschini and colleagues found abnormalities in electroencephalograms and event-related potentials in children with CH (see Rovet, Chapter 4 in this volume). However, this line of research was never continued. Just as recent studies indicate electrophysiological abnormalities in children with ADHD, might the same be true for children with congenital hypothyroidism or with severe juvenile hypothyroidism who acquire learning problems iatrogenically? This line of research is also clearly warranted in children with these thyroid abnormalities.

Drs. Bhatara, Rovet, and Daneman have shown that there may be significant behavioral sequelae associated with thyroxine therapy. This is based mostly on anecdotal evidence and a preliminary small-scale study by the latter two authors. It is important to cull the information on these cases, which have frequently been described by other clinicians. The need clearly exists for a multicenter study of treatment for acquired thyroid disorders, as well as for studying the adequacy of thyroxine replacement and possibly other pharmacotherapies. In our experience, methylphenidate was found to reverse the iatrogenic effects of thyroxine replacement in a child with severe acquired hypothyroidism. The possibility that subclinical hypothyroidism may co-occur in some children with ADHD also attests to the usefulness of further studies of thyroid function in this population.

The role of thyroid hormone in pregnancy is certainly an issue of intense interest, yet the existing literature is limited or inconsistent. Further studies of the offspring of mothers with hypothyroidism or treated hyperthyroidism are clearly indicated. The initiatives by Dr. Pop in The Netherlands and by Dr. Haddow in Maine, who are following the offspring of mothers with subclinically low levels of thyroid hormone or thyroid antibodies early in pregnancy, are important first steps in evaluating the effects of this hormone on the fetal brain. Similarly, the studies of thyroid function in premature infants, who lack the maternal contribution of thyroid hormone in the last trimester of pregnancy, also indicate the need for further studying the relations between thyroid hormone levels before expected term and later abilities. The pioneering work of Dr. van Wassenaer and her colleagues in The Netherlands showing the efficacy of thyroid hormone replacement in some premature infants before term is extremely exciting and begs further investigation on this side of the Atlantic. The potential for this therapy to improve intelligence and cognitive abilities, including attention, in this highly prevalent population has enormous societal implications.

This volume has attempted to help readers understand how thyroid hormone affects children. It represents the collaboration of two behavioral scientists with an unusual curiosity and passion for understanding how thyroid hormone affects the human brain and behavior. We have both dedicated significant portions of our research careers to this cause and now, in collaboration, may have partially succeeded. Future efforts and collaborations with the other authors in this volume as well as others elsewhere will add to this understanding. Our volume, we hope, will provide the impetus to advance this science. Certainly, initiatives such as those currently being pursued by the American Thyroid Association in funding research in this area will make this a reality.

We sincerely hope the information contained in this volume will serve as a practical and essential guide for treating and managing children with thyroid disorders and for providing better health care. Also, as our knowledge expands of newer and effective therapies for children with thyroid disease and of the role of environmental factors in affecting the juvenile thyroid system, we hope this book will be a start in improving the quality of life of future children. If so, we will have achieved our goals.

Index

*Page numbers printed in **boldface** type refer to tables or figures.*

Achenbach's Child Behavior
  Checklist, 172
Acquired immunodeficiency
  syndrome (AIDS), 73
Acquired thyroid disease, 20–22.
  See also Juvenile acquired
  hypothyroidism
Adolescence. *See also* Age
  age-related manifestations of
    hypothyroidism and, 21
  compliance with medication
    and, 72, 114
  eating disorders and thyroid
    hormone abuse, 189
  juvenile acquired
    hypothyroidism and, 165
  thyrotoxicosis and, 188
Adults
  thyroid-disrupting
    contaminants and,
    250–251, 266
  thyrotoxicosis in, 193–195
Age. *See also* Adolescence; Bone
  age; Infants
  clinical manifestations of
    hypothyroidism and, 20–21
  onset of attention-deficit/
    hyperactivity disorder and,
    210, 211
  onset of juvenile acquired
    hypothyroidism and, 165
  thyrotoxicosis and, 188, 210
Aggression, and thyrotoxicosis, 206
AGGTCA site, 37, 40
Agranulocytosis, and
  thionamides, 22
Ah receptors, 263
Albumin, 8
Aluminum hydroxide, **231**
American Academy of Pediatrics
  (AAP), 72, 96
Aminoglutethimide, **230**
Amiodarone, as thyroid-
  disrupting contaminant, 190,
  230, 231, 233–234
Amphibians, and developmental
  effects of thyroid hormone,
  223–224
Anabolic steroids, **230**
ANALYZE (software program), 146
Androgens, **230**
Aniline derivatives, **230**
Animal studies
  thyroid-disrupting contaminants
    and, 227–228, 242–245,
    251–252, 260–261, **253–254**
  thyroid hormone and brain
    development, 90–92

Animal studies *(continued)*
  thyroid hormone and neurotransmitter systems, 146
Anorexia nervosa, 200
Antibodies, congenital hypothyroidism and maternal, 18, 71–72
Anticonvulsants, **230**
Antidepressants, 199
Antipyrine, **230**
Antiseptics, and iodine, 69
Antisocial personality disorder, and resistance to thyroid hormone (RTH), **135,** 139
Anxiety, and thyrotoxicosis, 194–195, 205–207, 210. *See also* Anxiety disorders
Anxiety disorders. *See also* Anxiety
  resistance to thyroid hormone (RTH) and, **135**
  thyrotoxicosis and, 194, 195, 207
Apathetic thyrotoxicosis, **197,** 198
Aplasia cutis, 17
Aroclor 1254, 244–245
Athyrosis
  congenital hypothyroidism and, 88
  maternal supply of thyroid hormones and, 89
  motor skills and, 99, **100, 101**
Attention. *See also* Attention-deficit/ hyperactivity disorder; Behavior; Cognitive deficits
  congenital hypothyroidism and resistance to thyroid hormone (RTH) as genetic models for study of, 154–155
  juvenile acquired hypothyroidism and, **178**
  thyroid-stimulating hormone and thyroxine levels and, 110–112
  thyrotoxicosis and, 195
Attention-Deficit Disorder with Hyperactivity (ADD-H) Comprehensive Teachers Rating Scale (ACTeRS), **111**
Attention-deficit/hyperactivity disorder (ADHD). *See also* Attention; Behavior; Cognitive deficits
  congenital hypothyroidism and, 110
  dioxin-like compounds (DLCs) and neurotoxicity, 262
  juvenile acquired hypothyroidism and, 167, 180, 181–182
  neurotransmitter systems and, 129
  resistance to thyroid hormone (RTH) and, 22, 74, 134–141, 151–155
  stimulant medications and cerebral metabolism in, 142
  structural imaging studies and, 144–150
  thyrotoxicosis and, 193, 196, 200, 202–205, 210, 211
Autoimmune thyroid disease, 20, 189, 250
Avoidant personality disorder, and resistance to thyroid hormone (RTH), **135**

Bacteria, in groundwater, 164
Bacterial inhibition assay (BIA), 61

Behavior and behavioral
  abnormalities. *See also*
  Attention; Attention-deficit/
  hyperactivity disorder;
  Cognitive deficits
  congenital hypothyroidism and,
    97–115
  juvenile acquired
    hypothyroidism and, 110,
    114, 166–180
  resistance to thyroid hormone
    (RTH) and, 134–141
  thyroid-disrupting
    contaminants and, **242**,
    250–266
  thyrotoxicosis and, 193–211
Beta-adrenergic-antagonistic
  drugs, **230**
Beta-blockers, 19
Bioaccumulation, of
  thyroid-disrupting
  contaminants, 267
Bipolar disorder, 198, 206
Blood transfusions, 70
Bone age
  congenital hypothyroidism and,
    70
  juvenile acquired
    hypothyroidism and, 165
Bovine thyroid hormone, 199,
  206
Brain and brain development. *See
  also* Development;
  Neurodevelopment
  attention-deficit/hyperactivity
    disorder and, 145
  resistance to thyroid hormone
    (RTH) and, 45–46, 142–151
  thyroid-disrupting
    contaminants and, 223–229

thyroid hormone
  deficiency of, 90–94
  effects of on cells in vivo
    and in vitro, 33–35
  modulation of action, 43–45
  molecular basis of action,
    35–45
  receptors for, 10, 38–39
  regulation of target genes,
    39–43
  synthesis, uptake, and local
    deiodination of, 29–32
  time course of effects on,
    32–33
Breast feeding and breast milk
  congenital hypothyroidism and,
    71, 96
  thyroid-disrupting
    contaminants and, 239
Bruininks-Oseretsky Test of
  Neuromotor Proficiency, 99,
  100, 101
Buck, Pearl, 60, 62

CAMP-response element binding
  protein (CREB), 42
Canada, and government budgets
  for health care, 115
Carbamazepine, **230**
Carbimazole, **230**
Cardiac malformations, and
  congenital hypothyroidism,
  65, **66**
Carson, Rachel, 221
Carter, Thomas, 63
Case studies, of behavioral
  problems in juvenile acquired
  hypothyroidism, 168–171
Catecholamine. *See*
  Neurotransmitter systems

Centers for Disease Control and
    Prevention, 68
Central nervous system (CNS). *See
    also* Neurodevelopment
  attention-deficit/hyperactivity
    disorder and thyroid
    hormone metabolism,
    204–205
  thyroid-disrupting
    contaminants and, 223,
    263–265
  thyroid hormone and fetal
    development of, 10, 129,
    224
  thyrotoxicosis and normal
    development of, 208–209
Cerebral palsy, 268
Chernobyl nuclear accident (1986),
    22
Child Behavior Checklist (CBCL),
    111
Childbirth. *See also* Pregnancy;
    Prematurity
  length of hospital stay and
    screening for
    hypothyroidism, 14,
    75–76
  thyroid physiology in neonate
    and, 10–12
Children. *See* Adolescence; Age;
    Infants; Thyroid diseases;
    Thyroid hormones
Children's Personality
    Questionnaire, 206
Chlorinated hydrocarbons, **230**
Cholestyramine, **231**
Chorionic gonadotropin (CG), 4
Choroid plexus, 30
Chronic lymphocytic autoimmune
    thyroiditis, 164

Cimetidine, **231**
Clioquinol, 190
Cognitive deficits. *See also*
    Attention; Attention-deficit/
    hyperactivity disorder;
    Behavior; Memory
  congenital hypothyroidism and,
    97–106, 113–115
  dioxin-like compounds (DLCs)
    and, 262
  thyrotoxicosis and,
    193–211
Compliance, with treatment of
    congenital hypothyroidism,
    72, 98, 114
Conduct disorder, and resistance
    to thyroid hormone (RTH),
    135
Congenital hypothyroidism (CH)
  behavioral and cognitive
    abnormalities associated
    with
    characteristic types of,
      108–113
    demographic factors in,
      94–95
    diagnosis and treatment of,
      95–97
    growth and development,
      97
    hearing problems and,
      107–108
    history of, 85–87
    psychometric studies of,
      97–106
    treatment and management
      issues in, 113–115
  dioxin-like compound (DLC)
    exposure compared with,
    264–265

as genetic model for study of attention, 154–155
maternal thyroid hormone and, 10, 17–18
residual deficits from, 128
screening programs for, 12–16, 59, 63–77, 128
thyroid dysgenesis and, 16
thyroid physiology and, 18–20
Congenital malformations, and congenital hypothyroidism, 65, **66**
Corpus callosum, and resistance to thyroid hormone (RTH), 145, 146–150
Corticosteroids, 19. *See also* Steroids
Council of Regional Networks for Genetics Services (CORN), 76
CREB-binding protein (CBP), 42
Cretinism, 64, 235. *See also* Mental retardation
Criminal behavior, and thyrotoxicosis, 195
Cruciferae family (plants), 235
Cyanide, and iodine uptake, 235
Cyanogenic glycosides, 235

Dairy products and thyroid-disrupting contaminants, 239
Danazol, **230**
DDT. *See* Dichlorodiphenyl trichloroethane
Deiodinase enzymes, 88, 90. *See also* 5′-deiodinases
Delirium, and thyrotoxicosis, 198
Depression. *See also* Major depression
resistance to thyroid hormone (RTH) and, 139
thyrotoxicosis and, 194
De Quervain's thyroiditis, 189
Development, and thyroid hormones. *See also* Brain and brain development; Growth; Neurodevelopment
congenital hypothyroidism and, 14, 97, 128
fetal thyroid function in utero, 9–10
role of thyroid hormone during critical periods of, 225–226
Diabetes mellitus, 164
Diagnosis, of thyroid diseases. *See also* Differential diagnosis
congenital hypothyroidism and, 18–19, 67–73, 95–97
thyrotoxicosis and, 21
Dichlorodiphenyl trichloroethane (DDT), 221, **230**
Diesel fuels, as source of DLCs in atmosphere, 239
Diet. *See* Foods; Meat
Dietary goitrogens, 235
Differential diagnosis. *See also* Diagnosis
behavioral or cognitive syndromes and thyrotoxicosis, 200–211
of hypothyroidism in infants and children, 20
of juvenile acquired hypothyroidism, 165
Diiodotyrosine (DIT), 6, **7**

Dioxin-like compounds (DLCs), as thyroid-disrupting contaminants, 221, 237–266. *See also* Dioxins
Dioxins. *See also* Dioxin-like compounds (DLCs)
  congenital hypothyroidism and, 95
  as thyroid-disrupting contaminants, 221, 222
Disruptive behavior disorders, and resistance to thyroid hormone (RTH), **135**
DLCs. *See* Dioxin-like compounds
DNA-based tests, and newborn screening programs, 76–77
DNA-binding domain (DBD), 36, 130
Dopamine agonists, **231**
Dopaminergic system
  perinatal dioxin-like compound (DLC) exposure, 265–266
  thyroid hormones and, 92
Dosage, of thyroxine for replacement therapy. *See also* Thyroxine replacement therapy
  congenital hypothyroidism and, 19, 71, 72, 96–97
  juvenile acquired hypothyroidism and, 110, 114, 166, **177**, 181–182
  TSH assays and, 13
DSM-III, DSM-III-R, and DSM-IV diagnostic criteria
  for attention-deficit/hyperactivity disorder, 136, 138
  differential diagnosis of thyrotoxicosis and, 211
  for psychosis and delirium, 198
Dulse (seaweed), as source of excess iodine, 190, 233
Dyshormonogenesis, 88, 94
Dysphoria, and thyrotoxicosis, 194, 205–207, 210
Dysplastic glands, 94
Dysthymic disorder, and resistance to thyroid hormone (RTH), **135**

Eating disorders, 189, 200
Ectopic thyroid, 88, 94
Einstein Assessment of School-Related Skills, 105
Electroencephalography, and congenital hypothyroidism, 93
Emotional lability, and thyrotoxicosis, 205–207
Encephalopathy, and thyrotoxicosis, 198
Enuresis, and resistance to thyroid hormone (RTH), **135**
Environmental Protection Agency (EPA), 267
Environmental toxins. *See also* Thyroid-disrupting contaminants
  congenital hypothyroidism and, 95
  juvenile acquired hypothyroidism and, 164
Equilibrium dialysis, and free thyroid hormone measurement, 13
Estrogen, **230**

Ethnicity, and congenital
  hypothyroidism, 94
European Environmental Research
  Organization, 267
Exogenous thyroid hormones, 236

Fenclofenac, **230**
Ferrous sulfate, **231**
Fetus. *See also* Infants; Pregnancy;
    Prematurity
  dioxin-like compounds (DLCs)
    and, 245–246, 251–252,
    255–259, 260–261
  excess iodine and, 232–234
  maternal-fetal thyroid hormone
    relationships, 89–90
  maternal hypothyroidism and,
    228–229
  neurodevelopment of, 225–226
  physiology of thyroid function
    in utero, 9–10
  perinatal exposure to excess
    iodine, 69
Fish, and thyroid-disrupting
  contaminants, 239, **242,** 243,
  256, 259
5'-deiodinases, 6, 9, 10–12, 30. *See
  also* Deiodinase enzymes
Flavonoids, **238**
Fluorouracil, **230**
Follicle-stimulating hormone
  (FSH), 4
Fölling, Asbjörn, 60–61
Foods. *See also* Meat
  excess iodine in, 190
  thyroid-disrupting
    contaminants and, 233,
    239, **242**
Free thyroid hormone
  measurement, 12–13, 67–68

Free thyroid index, 13
Functional imaging studies, of
  resistance to thyroid hormone
  (RTH), 142–144
Furans, and congenital
  hypothyroidism, 95
Furosemide, **230**

Gender
  congenital hypothyroidism and,
    65, 94
  juvenile acquired
    hypothyroidism and, 164
  resistance to thyroid hormone
    (RTH) and, 151
  thyrotoxicosis and, 188, 211
Generalized anxiety disorder
  resistance to thyroid hormone
    (RTH) and, **135**
  thyrotoxicosis and, 194, 195,
    207
Genetic disorders. *See also*
    Genetics
  congenital hypothyroidism as,
    20
  newborn screening for, 59,
    76–77
  resistance to thyroid hormone
    (RTH) as, 22, 128
Genetics. *See also* Genetic
    disorders
  brain development and thyroid
    hormones, 33–45
  of resistance to thyroid
    hormone (RTH), 45–46,
    128, 131–134, 151–155
  subunits of thyroid-stimulating
    hormone, 5
  thyrotoxicosis and, 189
Glucocorticoids, **230, 231**

Goiter. *See also* Iodine
  congenital hypothyroidism and, 88
  excess maternal iodine and fetal or neonatal, 232–234
  history of, 64
  iodine deficiency and endemic, 16, 20, 235
  juvenile acquired hypothyroidism and, 165
  lithium and, 235
  thyrotoxicosis and, **192**
Goitrin, **230**
Goitrogenic drugs, 236
Goitrogens, 235–236
Goitrous hypothyroidism, 64
"Good baby" syndrome, 109
Graves' disease
  congenital hypothyroidism and maternal, 18, 19
  iodine and hypothyroidism, 232
  pregnancy and thionamides, 17
  thyroid function tests and, 12
  thyrotoxicosis and, 21–22, 188–189, 190, 191, 194
Great Britain, prevalence of thyrotoxicosis in, 188
Great Lakes, thyroid-disrupting contaminants in fish from, 242, **256, 259**
Groundwater bacteria, and juvenile acquired hypothyroidism, 164
Growth, and congenital hypothyroidism, 97. *See also* Development
Guidelines, for exposure to thyroid-disrupting compounds, 267, 268–269

Guthrie, Robert, 61, 62
Guthrie spot test, 62, 67–68, 73
Hashimoto's thyroiditis, 20, 164
Health care. *See* Health maintenance organizations; Insurance; Physicians
Health maintenance organizations (HMOs), and monitoring of thyroxine replacement therapy, 115
Hearing problems, and congenital hypothyroidism, 107–108
Heroin, **230**
Hexachlorobenzene (HCB), 237
Histopathological studies, of congenital hypothyroidism, 93
Homeostasis, of thyroid hormone and hypothalamic-pituitary-thyroid axis, 3, **4**
Hospital and municipal incinerators, as source of DLCs in atmosphere, 239
Hospital for Sick Children (Toronto), 87, 171
Human Genome Project, 77
Hyperactivity. *See* Attention-deficit/hyperactivity disorder
Hyperactivity Index of Conners Rating Scales, **111, 112**
Hyperfunctioning thyroid adenoma, 232
Hyperthyroidism, and thyrotoxicosis, 188–189, **197**, 202
Hypoplasia, 88
Hypothalamic hypothyroidism, 14, 15

Hypothalamic-pituitary-thyroid axis, and physiology and function of thyroid hormone, 3–10
Hypothyroxinemia, 90

Iatrogenic central hypothyroidism, 20
Illinois, and educational programs on hypothyroidism, 115
Immunology, and juvenile acquired hypothyroidism, 164–165
Incinerators, hospital and municipal, as source of DLCs in atmosphere, 239
Infants. *See also* Fetus; Pregnancy; Prematurity
  birth and thyroid function in neonate, 10–12
  excess iodine and, 232–234
  neurological development and thyroid hormones, 32–33
  screening programs for thyroid diseases, 12–16, 59–77
  thyrotoxicosis in, 190, 191
Insurance, and length of hospitalization for childbirth, 75–76. *See also* Health maintenance organizations
Intelligence quotient (IQ)
  congenital hypothyroidism and, 14, **15**, 97–98
  juvenile acquired hypothyroidism and, 166, 172, **173, 174,** 175
  perinatal exposure to dioxin-like compounds and, 252, 260, 261
  resistance to thyroid hormone (RTH) and, 140–141
  thyrotoxicosis and, 207
  transient hypothyroxinemia and, 268
Interferon alpha, **230**
Iodide molecules, and synthesis of thyroid hormone, 6
Iodine. *See also* Goiter
  congenital hypothyroidism and, 16
  endemic goiter and, 16, 20
  thyroid-disrupting contaminants and, 229, 232–234
  thyrotoxicosis and, 190, **197,** 200, **230**
Iodine-induced thyrotoxicosis, 190, **197,** 200, **230**
Iodoantipyrine, **230**
Iodotyrosines, 236
Iopanoic acid, **231**
Iothalamate, 190
Ipodate, **231**
Irritability, and thyrotoxicosis, 205–207
Isothiocyanates, 235

Japan, and thyroid-disrupting contaminants, 251, 252, **255**
Jodbasedow phenomenon, **230,** 232
Juvenile acquired hypothyroidism. *See also* Acquired thyroid disease
  behavioral manifestations of, 166–180
  characteristics of, 164–166
  definition of, 163

Juvenile acquired hypothyroidism *(continued)*
 thyroxine therapy and behavior problems, 110, 114, 166
 treatment and management of, 181–182

Kelp (seaweed), as source of excess iodine, 190, 200, 233
Kentucky, and prevalence of hypothyroidism, 164
Kidney, and thyroid hormones, 30

Language disorders
 congenital hypothyroidism and, 101, 102
 and, 262, 263
 resistance to thyroid hormone (RTH) and, 141, 150
 thyroid hormone receptor and, 22
Lead, as thyroid-disrupting contaminant, **231**
Leakage thyrotoxicosis, 189
Learning disabilities
 congenital hypothyroidism and, 105–106, **107**
 dioxin-like compounds (DLCs) and, 262
 dopamine and, 266
Levothyroxine. *See* Thyroxine replacement therapy
Ligand-binding domain (LBD), 36
Lithium, as thyroid-disrupting contaminant, **230, 231,** 234–235
Liver, and thyroid hormones, 30
Luteinizing hormone (LH), 4

Magnetic resonance imaging (MRI) and magnetic resonance spectroscopy (MRS)
 congenital hypothyroidism and, 93
 resistance to thyroid hormone (RTH) and, 144–151
 thyrotoxicosis and, 208
Major depression, and resistance to thyroid hormone (RTH), **135,** 139. *See also* Depression
Mania, and thyrotoxicosis, 198
Masked thyrotoxicosis, 198
Matching Familiar Figures Test, 172
McCune-Albright syndrome, 21
Meat, contamination of with thyroid hormones, 189–190, 199, 206, **231,** 236, 239. *See also* Foods
Mefenamic acid, **230**
Memory. *See also* Cognitive deficits
 dioxin-like compounds (DLCs) and, 262
 thyrotoxicosis and, 195
Mental retardation. *See also* Cretinism
 juvenile acquired hypothyroidism and, 166
 thyroid deficiency and, 64
Messenger RNAs (mRNAs), 130–131
Metal smelting and refining, as source of DLCs in atmosphere, 239
Methadone, **230**
Methimazole, 17, **230**

Methylphenidate, and attention-deficit/hyperactivity disorder, 110, 180, 181–182
Michigan
 dioxin-like compounds (DLCs) and neurotoxicity in children, 252, **256**
 educational programs on congenital hypothyroidism, 115
Microtubule-associated proteins (MAPs), 33–34
Mitotane, **230**
Monoiodotyrosine (MIT), 6, **7**
Mood disorders, and resistance to thyroid hormone (RTH), **135**
Motor skills, and congenital hypothyroidism, 99, **100, 101,** 102
Multinodular goiter, 232
Multiple Heschl's gyri, and reading disability, 150, 151
Myelin basic protein (MBP), 34

National Institutes of Health, 75
Neonatal thyrotoxicosis, 190, 191, **197,** 198
Nerve growth factor, 35
Netherlands, and thyroid-disrupting contaminants, **258**
Neurocognitive deficits, and congenital hypothyroidism, 99
Neurodevelopment. *See also* Brain and brain development; Central nervous system; Development
 thyroid-disrupting contaminants and, 236, 250–266
 thyroid hormone and normal, 129–131
 thyrotoxicosis and, 208–209
Neurological cretinism, 89
Neuronal proteins, regulation of by thyroid hormones, 34–35
Neurotransmitter systems
 attention-deficit/hyperactivity disorder and, 129, 146
 brain development and thyroid hormone, 92
 juvenile acquired hypothyroidism and, 179–180
Neurotropin-3, 35
New England Congenital Hypothyroidism Collaborative, 98, 103–104
New York
 newborn screening programs in, 62–63, 73
 thyroid-disrupting contaminants and, **259**
NGFI-A gene, 129, 146
Nongoitrous myxedema, 18
Norway, and newborn screening programs, 60
North Carolina, and thyroid-disrupting contaminants, **257**
Nuclear hormone receptor superfamily, 35–37
Nuclear receptor corepressor (N-CoR), 43

Oligodendrocytes, 34
Ontario, and newborn screening programs, 87
Oppositional defiant disorder, and resistance to thyroid hormone (RTH), **135**

Organochlorines, **238**
Our Stolen Future (Colborn et al. 1996), 222, 237

Panhypopituitarism, 15
Panic disorder, and resistance to thyroid hormone (RTH), **135**
Paraaminobenzoic acid, **230**
Paranoia, and thyroxine replacement therapy, 110
Parry, Caleb, 187, 188–189
PCBs. *See* Polychlorinated and polybrominated biphenyls
PCP-2 gene, 34, 35
Pendred's syndrome, 107
Perchlorate, **230**
Peroxisome proliferator-activated receptors (PPARs), 34, 35, 37, 44–45
Pertechnetate, **230**
Phenobarbital, **230**
Phenylketonuria (PKU), 59, 60–62
Phenytoin, **230**
Phthalate esters and metabolites, **238**
Physicians, primary. *See also* Health maintenance organizations; Insurance
  late-appearing forms of congenital hypothyroidism and, 70
  quality of care and monitoring of thyroxine replacement therapy, 115
Physiology, of thyroid hormones
  birth and thyroid function in neonate, 10–12
  brain development and, 29–46
  congenital hypothyroidism and, 88
  fetal thyroid function in utero, 9–10
  hypothalamic-pituitary-thyroid axis and, 3–9
  overview of, 286
  pregnancy and thyroid abnormalities, 16–18
  screening programs for infants and, 12–16
Pituitary hypothyroidism, and neonatal screening, 14, 15
Placenta, crossing of by maternal thyroid hormones, 9, 90
Plants, as dietary goitrogens, 235
Polychlorinated and polybrominated biphenyls (PCBs, PBBs)
  congenital hypothyroidism and, 95
  as thyroid-disrupting contaminants, **230**, **231**, 237, **238**, 242, 244–245, 246, 251, **255**, **256**, **257**, **258**, **259**, 262, 265–266
Polychlorinated dibenzodioxins (PCDDs), 237
Polychlorinated dibenzofurans (PCDFs), 237, 251
Polychlorinated naphthalenes, 251, **255**
Polycyclic aromatic hydrocarbons (Pahs), **238**
Polyhydroxyphenols, **238**
Polyphenols, **238**
Positron emission tomography, and studies of resistance to thyroid hormone (RTH), 142–144
Postpartum lymphocytic thyroiditis, 232

Povidone, 190, 232
Prefrontal lobe dysfunction, and thyrotoxicosis, 208
Pregnancy. *See also* Childbirth; Fetus; Infants; Prematurity
  dioxin-like compounds (DLCs) and, 245–246, 251–252, **255–259,** 260–261
  excess iodine and fetus, 69, 232–234
  maternal-fetal thyroid hormone relationships, 89–90
  maternal hypothyroidism and fetal development, 228–229
  neurodevelopment of fetus and, 32, 225–226
  physiology of fetal thyroid function, 9–10
  thyroid abnormalities in, 16–18
  thyroid-stimulating hormone assays and, 14
  thyroid-stimulating hormone in second and third trimesters of, **11**
Prematurity, of neonates. *See also* Fetus; Infants; Pregnancy
  cognitive problems and thyroid hormone deficiency, 90
  postpartum rise in TSH, 10
  transient hypothyroidism and, 68–69
  transient hypothyroxinemia and, 268
Primary fetal hypothyroidism, 16–17
Primary sporadic congenital hypothyroidism, 88
Propranolol, 182, 202, 207, **231**
Propylthiouracil (PTU), 17, **230, 231**

Proton magnetic resonance spectroscopy, 93
Psychometric studies, of congenital hypothyroidism, 97–106
Psychosis
  juvenile acquired hypothyroidism and, 169
  thyrotoxicosis and, 194, 198, 199
Puberty, hypothyroidism and precocious or delayed, 21, 165
Public health
  newborn screening programs and, 60
  thyroid-disrupting contaminants and, 221–222
Pyridines, **238**

Race, and congenital hypothyroidism, 94
Radiation
  acquired thyroid disease and, 20
  thyroid cancer and, 22
Radioactive iodine therapy, during pregnancy, 18
Radiocontrast materials, 190
Radiological studies, of congenital hypothyroidism, 93
RC3 gene, 34–35
Receptors, thyroid hormone
  brain development and, 10, 38–39, 91–92
  dioxin-like compounds (DLCs) and, 263
  language development and, 22
  neurodevelopment and, 130–131
  resistance to thyroid hormone (RTH) and, 146

Resistance to thyroid hormone (RTH)
   attention-deficit/hyperactivity disorder and, 22, 74, 134–141, 151–155
   behavioral studies and, 134–141
   description of, 131
   dioxin-like compound–induced neurotoxicity and, 265
   function imaging studies of, 142–144
   genetics of, 22, 45–46, 131–134, 151–155
   Guthrie spot test and, 74–75
   structural imaging studies of, 144–151
Retinoic acid receptors (RARs and RXRs), 37, 130
Reverse triiodothyronine (rT_3), 6
Rifampin, **230**

Salicylates, **230**
Schizophrenia, 92
School performance
   congenital hypothyroidism and, 103–106
   juvenile acquired hypothyroidism and, 166, 175, 178, 179
   thyrotoxicosis and, 196, 207–208, 212–213
Screening programs, for infants
   congenital hypothyroidism and, 59–77, 95
   differential diagnosis of thyrotoxicosis and, 209–211
   physiology and function of thyroid hormones and, 12–16
   resistance to thyroid hormone (RTH) and, 140

Secondary hypothyroidism, and neonatal screening, 14, 15
Selenium, 30
Selenocysteine, 30
Severe thyrotoxicosis, 198
Sickle cell disease, 77
Silencing mediator for RARs and TRs (SMRT), 43
Silent Spring (Carson 1962), 221
Slow-release nicotinic acid, **230**
Somatostatin, **231**
Spatial ability, and cognitive hypothyroidism, 102, **104**
Speech development
   congenital hypothyroidism and, 101
   dioxin-like compounds (DLCs) and, 263
Spironolactone, **230**
Steroids, as thyroid-disrupting contaminants, **230**. *See also* Corticosteroids
Structural imaging studies, of resistance to thyroid hormone (RTH), 144–151
Subacute thyroiditis, 189, 232
Substance abuse, and resistance to thyroid hormone (RTH), **135**
Sucralfate, **231**
Sulfonamides, **230**
Sylvian fissure, and resistance to thyroid hormone (RTH), 150, 151, **152**
Synthetic thyroid disrupters, 236–266

T_3. *See* Triiodothyronine
T_4. *See* Thyroxine
Tachycardia, and thyrotoxicosis, 191, **192**

Taiwan, and thyroid-disrupting contaminants, 251, 252, **255**
Tamoxifen, **230**
TCDD. *See* Dioxin-like compounds
Technetium scans, 70
Tertiary hypothyroidism, and neonatal screening, 15
Testing. *See* Screening
Thiocyanates, **230,** 235
Thionamides
  Graves' disease in children and, 22
  pregnancy and fetal hypothyroidism, 17–18, 19
  as thyroid-disrupting contaminants, **230,** 236
Thiouracil, **230**
Thioureas, **230**
Thyroglobulin, 6
Thyroid adenomas, 20
Thyroid cancer
  radiation and, 22
  thyroxine replacement therapy and, 13
Thyroid diseases. *See also* Thyroid gland; Thyroid hormones
  acquired forms of, 20–22, 163–182
  clinical studies of, 287–291
  congenital hypothyroidism
    behavioral and cognitive abnormalities associated with, 85–116
    newborn screening programs for, 59–77
    thyroid physiology and function, 18–20
  future directions for research on, 291–293
  juvenile acquired hypothyroidism and behavioral or cognitive abnormalities, 163–182
  resistance to thyroid hormone (RTH)
    Attention-deficit/hyperactivity disorder and, 22, 74
    child psychiatric research and, 127–155
    genetics of, 22, 45–46
    Guthrie spot test and, 74–75
  thyroid-disrupting contaminants and neurodevelopmental changes, 221–269
  thyrotoxicosis
    behavioral and cognitive abnormalities associated with, 187–213
    maternal Graves' disease and neonatal, 18, 19
    overview of, 21–22
    TSH assays and, 13
Thyroid-disrupting contaminants, and neurodevelopment. *See also* Environmental toxins
  brain development and, 223–229
  common natural forms of, 229–236
  definition of, 222–223
  future directions for research on, 266–269
  public health and, 221–222
  synthetic forms of, 236–266

Thyroid gland. *See also* Thyroid
diseases; Thyroid hormones
leakage thyrotoxicosis and,
189
thyroid-stimulating hormone
and regulation of, 5
Thyroid hormone response
elements (TREs), 130, 131, 133
Thyroid hormone– and retinoic
acid–associated corepressors
(TRACs), 43
Thyroid hormones. *See also*
Receptors; Thyroid diseases;
Thyroid gland
future directions for research
on, 291–293
importance of in developmental
processes, 285
maternal-fetal relationships
and, 89–90
neurodevelopment and,
129–131, 223–226
physiology and function of
birth and thyroid function in
neonate, 10–12
brain development and,
29–46
congenital hypothyroidism
and, 88
fetal thyroid function in
utero, 9–10
hypothalamic-pituitary-
thyroid axis, 3–9
overview of, 286
pregnancy and thyroid
abnormalities, 16–18
screening programs for
infants and, 12–16
thyrotoxicosis of extrathyroidal
origin and, 189–190, 199

Thyroid peroxidase (TPO), **7**
Thyroid-stimulating hormone
(TSH)
attention in children and levels
of, 110–112, 138, **139**
birth and, 10, **11**
fetus in utero and, 9, **11**
measurement of, 13–14
newborn screening programs
and, 67–68, 95
synthesis, structure, and
function of, 3, 4–6
Thyrotoxicosis
amiodarone-induced, 233–234
behavioral and cognitive
abnormalities associated
with, 193–200
behavioral and cognitive
syndromes resembling,
200–211
etiology and pathophysiology
of, 188–190
general clinical features of,
191–193
history of, 187
maternal Graves' disease and
neonatal, 18, 19
overview of, 21–22
prevalence of, 188
TSH assays and, 13
Thyrotoxicosis factitia, 190, 191,
197, 199–200, 206, 236
Thyrotoxic storm, 191, 193, **197,**
198
Thyrotropin-releasing hormone
(TRH), 3, **4, 5**
Thyroxine (T_4). *See also* Dosage;
Thyroxine replacement
therapy
assay for, 67–68

attention and levels of, 110–112, 138, **139**
birth and, 10–12
brain development and, 224
liver and kidney and conversion of, 30
synthesis and function of, 6–9, **88**
Thyroxine replacement therapy. *See also* Dosage; Treatment
adverse behavioral reactions to, 110, 114, 167–168
congenital hypothyroidism and, 14, 19, 70–71, 96–97
juvenile acquired hypothyroidism and, 110, 114, 166, **177,** 181–182
TSH assays and adjustment of dose, 13
Thyroxine-binding globulin (TBG), 7
Thyroxine-binding prealbumin (TBPA), 8
Toronto protocol, for treatment of congenital hypothyroidism, 71
Transient hypothyroxinemia, 268
Transient neonatal hypothyroidism, 68–69, 232–233
Transthyretin, 30
Treatment, of thyroid diseases. *See also* Dosage; Thyroxine replacement therapy
congenital hypothyroidism and, 19, 67–73, 95–97
Graves' disease and, 21–22
juvenile acquired hypothyroidism and, 166, 181–182

Triiodothyronine (T_3)
attention-deficit/hyperactivity disorder and levels of, 138, **139**
birth and, 10–12
liver and kidney and conversion of, 30
NGFI-A gene and, 129
synthesis and function of, 6–9, 88
TSH. *See* Thyroid-stimulating hormone
TSH-secreting pituitary tumors, 21
Turner's syndrome, 106

Ultrasonography, 70
U.S. Department of Agriculture, 190

Visual evoked potential testing, and congenital hypothyroidism, 93–94
Visuomotor and visuospatial skills
congenital hypothyroidism and, **100,** 102–103, **104**
juvenile hypothyroidism and, 175, 178
Vitamin D receptors (VDRs), 37
Vitamin supplements, and iodine, 190
"Vulnerable child" syndrome, 109

Wechsler Intelligence Scale for Children (WISC), 140, **174**
Wechsler Preschool and Primary Scale of Intelligence (WPPSI), **174**
Wet diaper test, 61
Wide Range Achievement Test—Revised (WRAT-R), 140, 172, **174**

Wisconsin General Testing
    Apparatus (WGTA), 262
Wolff-Chaikoff effect, 232
World Health Organization
    (WHO), and newborn
    screening programs, 63

Yersina enterocolitica, **230**
Yusho and yu-cheng
    (neurotoxicity from
    dioxin-like compounds), 251,
    252, **255,** 261, 262